PURE PRACTICE
FOR 12-LEAD ECGS

A Practice Workbook

Robin B. Purdie, RN, MS

Sam L. Earnest, MD

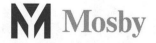 Mosby

St. Louis Baltimore Boston Carlsbad Chicago Naples New York Philadelphia Portland
London Madrid Mexico City Singapore Sydney Tokyo Toronto Wiesbaden

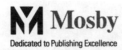
Mosby
Dedicated to Publishing Excellence

A Times Mirror
Company

Vice President and Publisher: Jacqueline Katz
Developmental Editor: Barbara Watts
Project Manager: Gayle Morris
Production Editor: Pamela G. Martin
Designer: David Zielinski
Manufacturing Manager: William A. Winneberger, Jr.

Printed in the United States of America
Composition by Accu-color
Printing/binding by Plus Communications

Mosby–Year Book, Inc.
11830 Westline Industrial Drive
St. Louis, Missouri 63146

International Standard Book Number 0-8151-4669-8
96 97 98 99 00 / 9 8 7 6 5 4 3 2 1

REVIEWERS

ABOUT THE AUTHORS

Robin B. Purdie, RN, MS

Ms. Purdie began her career in critical care nursing. Following a variety of experiences in intensive and coronary care, she became involved in cardiac rehabilitation at Oklahoma State University. While working with cardiac patients in the Department of Health and Exercise Physiology, she became interested in exercise physiology. Subsequently she gained a Master's Degree in Physiology of Exercise. In order to complement the degree she became certified by the American College of Sports Medicine as a Program Director. She has taught numerous classes and workshops in ECG interpretation. Her professional involvements include the American College of Sports Medicine, American Association of Cardiovascular Pulmonary Rehabilitation, Smoke Stoppers, and CPR instructor. Her research projects include grants with the American Heart Association and Oklahoma Center for the Advancement of Science and Technology. She has coauthored publications on blood lipid analysis and has been an invited speaker on the subjects of cardiopulmonary rehabilitation, ECG interpretation, and stress testing.

Sam L. Earnest, MD

Dr. Earnest graduated from the University of Oklahoma School of Medicine and specializes in Internal Medicine. He has had a successful private practice for over 20 years and recently joined the Warren Clinic as physician and medical representative. He has served as Chief of Staff and Director of Respiratory and Electrocardiography Services at Stillwater Medical Center. He has also been a medical representative for the Oklahoma State Peer Review Board. He is currently the Medical Director for the Oklahoma State University Wellness Center stress testing laboratory and for the cardiopulmonary rehabilitation program. Dr. Earnest is a member of the American Society of Internal Medicine, American College of Physicians and numerous other professional organizations. He is an entertaining speaker and has been invited to present seminars at many professional meetings.

ACKNOWLEDGMENTS

Our sincere appreciation is extended to Stillwater Medical Center, Oklahoma State University Wellness Center, and Cardiology of Stillwater for their support of this project.

RBP
SLE

To the three best nurses I know: Jean Green, Carolyn Williams, and Robin Purdie. Thanks.

SLE

To my daughter, for her patience and understanding like no other 9-year-old.
To my husband: my inspiration, my editor, and my best friend.

RBP

INTRODUCTION

Pure Practice for 12-Lead ECGs is designed to provide extensive practice and feedback in the interpretation of 12-lead electrocardiograms. A variety of experience may be gained from reading and analyzing ECG tracings that are within normal limits, as well as those with axis deviations, basic dysrhythmias, heart blocks, atrial enlargement, ventricular hypertrophy, myocardial infarctions, ischemia, pacemakers, and ECGs altered by medications. Patient tracings are provided with a detailed analysis that will assist you in becoming proficient in 12-lead ECG interpretation.

THE EIGHT PART WORKBOOK INCLUDES THE FOLLOWING:

Part I: Quick Review

Part IIa: 12-Lead ECGs Within Normal Limits

These are 12-lead ECG tracings in which rate, rhythm, waves, intervals, segments, and axes are within normal limits.

Part IIb: 12-Lead ECGs with Axis Deviations and/or Rate Disturbances

Prerequisite: A beginning level 12-lead ECG course and a sound understanding of basic electrophysiology and cardiac anatomy is recommended.

Part III: Basic Dysrhythmias and Blocks

These 12-lead ECG tracings depict basic cardiac dysrhythmias and atrial and ventricular heart blocks.

Prerequisite: A beginning level dysrhythmia course and/or an understanding of common cardiac dysrhythmias and heart blocks is recommended.

Part IV: Atrial and Ventricular Hypertrophy

These 12-lead ECG tracings indicate atrial and/or ventricular enlargement or hypertrophy.

Prerequisite: The same knowledge base as in Parts II and III is recommended with an emphasis on cardiac anatomy and physiology.

Part V: Myocardial Infarctions and Ischemia

These 12-lead ECG findings are consistent with ischemia and myocardial infarctions, ranging from acute to mature phase, subendocardial to transmural.

Prerequisite: An understanding of cardiac electrophysiology and the pathophysiology of ischemia and myocardial infarctions is recommended.

Part VI: Cardiac Pacemakers and Medication Effects

These 12-lead ECG tracings are altered by mechanical pacemakers and by commonly encountered medications.

Prerequisite: In addition to the above, an understanding of cardiac pacemakers is essential. In order to fully comprehend the variations that medications may cause on the electrocardiogram, a basic understanding of pharmacology is suggested.

Part VII: Analysis

Part VIII: Continuing Education

These 12-lead ECG tracings and corresponding multiple choice questions are designed to test your proficiency at basic and more complex interpretations. Instructions for completing this section and for meeting required continuing education criteria are provided.

OBJECTIVES

After completing this workbook, the student will be able to do the following:
1. Systematically assess and interpret a 12-lead ECG
2. Recognize basic dysrhythmias and heart blocks as they occur on the 12-lead ECG
3. Identify 12-lead ECG patterns that are consistent with atrial enlargement and ventricular hypertrophy
4. Recognize myocardial infarctions as they occur on the 12-lead ECG and delineate possible coronary artery involvement
5. Identify pacemaker rhythms and assess pacemaker function on the 12-lead ECG
6. Recognize abnormalities on the 12-lead ECG that could be caused by commonly used medications

PRODUCT ADAPTABILITY

Individuals: *Pure Practice for 12-Lead ECGs* is designed for health care professionals, including physicians, nurses, physician assistants, exercise physiologists, and ECG technicians who are required to interpret 12-lead ECGs. Students of medicine will also benefit from this text.

Instructors: *Pure Practice for 12-Lead ECGs Instructor's Kit* consists of the workbook and a complete set of slides that may be used to visually augment the learning process.

WORKBOOK FORMAT AND USE

The ECG tracings included in this text are designed to maximize the student's ability to quickly and accurately interpret the 12-lead ECG. To that end, each tracing is in a worksheet format that provides space for calculations and notations. When analyzing the tracings, you are encouraged to systematically analyze each portion of the 12-lead, draw conclusions from that analysis, and finally make an interpretation.

The 12-lead tracings included in the workbook are not in any particular order. Sections do not begin with less difficult and progress to more difficult tracings. If you find a tracing that is too difficult, finish all the tracings possible in that section. Then return to those 12-leads that you found more difficult.

The authors have provided a detailed analysis and interpretation that emphasizes key findings. As is often the case in medicine, there may be more than one correct answer to a complex tracing. However, in this workbook, the analysis provided will include accepted standards of ECG interpretation leaving the "art" of further interpretation up to you as you gain valuable experience. Always keep in mind that there is no substitute for an accurate patient history and assessment of signs and symptoms. Without such information an accurate interpretation is often impossible.

Many 12-lead ECGs are computer analyzed and it may, therefore, seem redundant to measure each interval and axis. However, it is difficult to truly learn ECG interpretation without a good deal of hands-on practice. This text is designed to provide that practice, and therefore it is recommended that each of the listed steps be followed.

FOR EACH 12-LEAD ECG THE STUDENT SHOULD RECORD THE FOLLOWING:*

1. Rate
Determine the atrial and ventricular rates and scan all leads in the assessment

2. Rhythm
Observe the rhythm for regularity—measure R to R

3. Intervals, Waves, and Segments

Intervals

P-R interval
Calculate the P-R interval

QRS complex
Measure the QRS complex and observe the morphology, especially in the precordial (chest) leads

* Ignore lead aVR in the interpretation as it is of little diagnostic value.

Q-T interval
Calculate the Q-T interval

Waves

P Waves
Inspect the ECG for presence, relation to QRS, and appearance

Q Waves
Inspect the ECG for significant or pathological Q waves

R Waves
Examine leads V_2 through V_4 for R wave progression

T Waves
Examine the T waves for their presence and morphology

U Waves
Observe for the presence of U waves

Segments

S-T Segment
Observe the S-T segment and J point for elevation or depression

4. Axis
Determine the frontal plane QRS axis of the ECG

5. Hypertrophy
Observe the ECG for signs of chamber enlargement

6. Myocardial Infarction and Ischemia
Examine the ECG for signs of acute, recent, or old infarction and/or ischemia

7. Pacemaker
Observe the ECG for the presence of a mechanical pacemaker

8. Medication Effects
Look for possible signs of a medication effect on the ECG

9. Data Analysis*
Analyze the above data to determine which values are outside normal limits
Analyze the above data to summarize these findings

10. Interpretation
Interpret the 12-lead ECG including the underlying rhythm and any abnormalities noted

After completing the 12-lead worksheet, turn to Part VII and compare your answers with those of the authors.

* Assume standard speed and voltage unless otherwise indicated

CONTENTS

Part I
Quick Review

ECG ANALYSIS GUIDE AND NORMAL VALUES

I. RATE

Atrial: To calculate the atrial rate, locate two consecutive P waves and measure the number of boxes between them. You may quickly apply the 300, 150, 100, 75, 60, 50, 40 rule if the rate is constant. You may also count the number of P waves in a 6-second strip and multiply by 10.

Ventricular: To calculate the ventricular rate, measure the distance between the R to R intervals and apply the same rules as above.

Normal range: The normal range is from 60 to 100 beats per minute (bpm); however, lower heart rates may be normal in highly trained individuals. Rate rulers may also be used to calculate rate quickly when the rhythm is regular.

2. RHYTHM

Observe the ECG for irregularities in the rhythm. Measure the R to R intervals and determine if the rhythm is essentially regular. Recall that slight variations in rhythm are considered within normal limits (e.g., off by one small box if the ventricular rate is greater than 100 bpm, or one to three boxes if the rate is less than 100 bpm).

3. INTERVALS, WAVES, AND SEGMENTS

Intervals:

P-R interval

Measure the P-R interval from the beginning of the P wave to the beginning of the QRS

Normal range: The normal range is from 0.12 to 0.20 seconds and is consistent.

QRS complex

The QRS is actually an interval, however more often it is referred to as a complex.

Measure the QRS complex from the beginning of the Q wave to the end of the S wave.

Normal range: The normal range is from 0.04 to 0.10 seconds. Note that some practitioners use the upper limit as 0.12 seconds with 0.10 being considered borderline for an intraventricular delay or bundle branch block.

Q-T interval

Measure the Q-T interval from the beginning of the Q wave to the end of the T wave.

Normal range: The normal range is no more than one half the duration of the preceding R to R interval with heart rates less than 100 bpm. The Q-T interval becomes shorter as the rate increases.

Some practitioners use the following guidelines as upper limits of the normal range:

$$\text{Rate } 100 \leq 0.34 \text{ seconds}$$
$$\text{Rate } 80 \leq 0.38 \text{ seconds}$$
$$\text{Rate } 60 \leq 0.42 \text{ seconds}$$

Waves:

P waves

Examine lead II for the P wave; it should be upright, and there should be a P wave for each QRS (i.e., 1:1 ratio).

Normal range: The normal range should not exceed 0.25 mV in amplitude, or 0.12 seconds in duration, in lead II. Lead V_1 lends supporting evidence for P wave abnormalities.

Q waves

Examine all leads for pathological Q waves
Exclude aVR from the analysis.

Normal range: Small, nonpathological Q waves can be normal in I, aVL, V_4, V_5, and V_6. Moderate to large-sized Q waves may be found in III, aVF, aVL, and V_1 and occasionally V_2 as isolated findings without associated pathology. Pathological Q waves are greater than 0.04 seconds in duration and/or at least one-third the amplitude of the R wave.

R waves

Examine leads V_2 through V_4 for R wave "progression"

Normal range: Each R wave should become progressively higher in amplitude from V_2 through V_4, then gradually become smaller again through V_6.

T waves

Examine all leads for T wave presence and morphology

Normal range: T waves should be slightly rounded and upright (may be inverted in III, aVF, aVL, and V_1 as a normal finding).

T waves should not be tall, peaked, biphasic, or notched.

U waves

Examine the ECG for the presence of U waves

Normal finding: The presence of U waves may be a normal finding, but the voltage should be low and deflection the same as the T wave.

Segments

S-T segment

Observe the S-T segment and J-point morphology. The "junction point" (J-point) is located at the end of the QRS where the T wave begins.

Normal Range: The S-T segment should be isoelectric (i.e., neither negative, positive, nor biphasic). To be clinically significant the S-T deviation should be greater than 1 mm. (Some practitioners use greater than or equal to 2 mm S-T depression as the point of significance.)

4. AXIS

Determine the net QRS axis of the ECG by either the simplified method or the two-step method given below.

Normal range:

Normal axis — the net QRS deflection lies between 0° and +90°

Normal left axis deviation (LAD) — 0° to -30° (normal horizontal)

Normal right axis — +90° to +110° (normal vertical)

Right axis deviation (RAD) — +110° to +180°

Indeterminate axis (extreme right axis deviation or "no man's land") — greater than +180°

Pathological left axis deviation (left anterior hemiblock [LAHB*]), or left anterior fascicular block — -30° to -180°

* This workbook will use the term left anterior hemiblock.

Simplified Method

Examine leads I and aVF for the net voltage of the QRS. Subtract the number of boxes that lay above the isoelectric or "equiphasic" line from the number of boxes below the isoelectric line. Thus, if the R wave amplitude (above the iso-

Quadrant/Axis Sketches

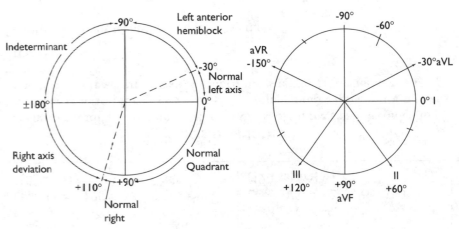

electric line) measured 7 mV, and the S amplitude (below the isoelectric line) measured 2 mV, the net voltage would be +5 mV and would be considered more *positive* than *negative*.

After determining the net voltage in leads I and aVF, simply apply the following guidelines:

Axis	Net QRS Deflection Lead I	Lead aVF
Normal Quadrant (0° to 90°)	+	+
Normal left axis deviation (LAD 0° to 30°)*	+	–
Pathological left axis deviation (LAHB ≥ -30°) and lead II is negative		
Right axis deviation (RAD > +110°)	–	+
Normal horizontal (0°)	+	Equiphasic
Normal vertical (+90°)	Equiphasic	+
Indeterminate (extreme right "no man's land" > +180°)	–	–

* If an LAD is found, look next at lead II. If lead II is positive, the axis lies between 0 and -30°. If lead II is equiphasic, the net QRS axis is -30°. If the net QRS deflection is *negative*, the axis lies beyond ≥30° and is considered *pathological* and often termed as a left anterior hemiblock or a left anterior fascicular block.

** This text will consider all left axis deviations of ≥ -30° as a left anterior hemiblock (LAHB).

Two-Step Method

The two-step method gives a more quantitative measure of the mean QRS axis of the heart and is expressed as a number of degrees rather than by simply the quadrant in which it falls. This is of particular importance when comparing old ECG tracings to more recent ones as an axis shift may be a diagnostic finding. Note that there is often a slight leftward shift of the axis with age and pregnancy, which is considered a normal variant. A normal left axis deviation may also be evident in obese patients.

The two-step method uses the Hexaxial Lead System below:

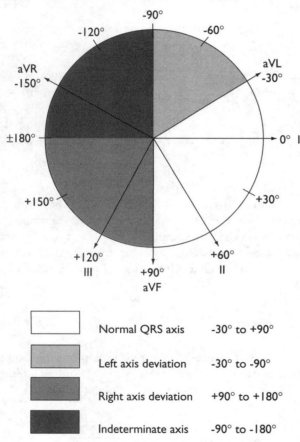

□	Normal QRS axis	-30° to +90°
▨	Left axis deviation	-30° to -90°
▨	Right axis deviation	+90° to +180°
▮	Indeterminate axis	-90° to -180°

Step I

Find the quadrant from the simplified method (normal, left, right, extreme right "no man's land").

Step II

Next observe all the limb leads, and find the most equiphasic lead (if two leads are equal, use the one with the lesser voltage). Then, using the hexaxial lead system either add or subtract 90° to that lead so that it lies within the quadrant found in Step I. If two leads have approximately the same NET voltage, the axis lies between those two leads.

Examples

Example 1
Step 1: The net QRS in leads I and aVF are positive, therefore it is known that the axis lies within the normal (0 to 90°) quadrant.
Step 2: After observing all the limb leads it is noted that lead aVL is the most isoelectric (or equiphasic). Lead aVL on the hexaxial lead system lies at -30°. From Step 1 it is known that the QRS axis is within the normal quadrant. Therefore 90° **is added** to aVL (-30°) making the axis +60°.

Example 2
Step 1: The net QRS deflection in lead I is positive, and lead aVF is negative, therefore the axis lies within the left quadrant.
Step 2: After observing all the limb leads it is noted that lead II is the most equiphasic. Knowing that the mean axis lies within the left quadrant, **subtract** +90° from +60° making the mean axis -30° (i.e., a nonpathological left axis deviation or LAD).

If the hexaxial lead system is not available, simply remember the following and then either add or subtract 90°:

Lead I = 0°	Lead aVL = -30°
Lead II = +60°	Lead aVF = +90°
Lead III = +120°	Lead aVR = +210° or -150°
(60° apart)	(120° apart)

Precision Method

When over-reading computer analyzed ECG's, often the axis is recorded in more precise terms, such as +57° or -29°. Although more difficult for humans to perform more accuracy may be gained by using the following method.

Step I

Find the quadrant from the simplified method.

Step II

Follow step II in the "two step method."

Step III

For greater accuracy in determining axis apply the following:
After finding the most isoelectric lead and either adding or subtracting 90°, observe that isoelectric lead to determine if it is slightly more negative or positive. If it is slightly more positive, the axis will be more toward the negative electrode.

If two limb leads are equally isoelectric, the QRS axis lies between those two leads.

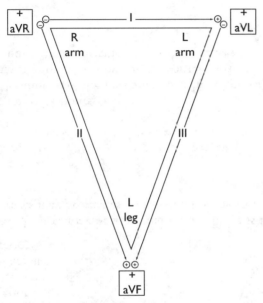

Einthoven's triangle shows the positive and negative lead placement of the limb leads.

Example 1

Step I

Lead I is positive and lead II is positive. Thus the QRS axis lies within the normal quadrant.

Step II

Following examination of all limb leads it is noted that lead III is the most isoelectric. Thus 90° is added to +120° for a net QRS axis of +30°.

Step III

To more accurately determine the axis note that lead III is the most isoelectric, however it is slightly more positive than negative. Because the positive electrode in lead III is located on the left foot, the positive deflection is lead III means that the axis is slightly more toward that positive electrode. Thus the more accurate QRS axis would be approximately +40°.

5. HYPERTROPHY/CHAMBER ENLARGEMENT

Patient history is quite valuable in the assessment of hypertrophy and chamber enlargement.

Ventricular Hypertrophy

Inspect the QRS in leads V_1 and V_5

Right Ventricular Hypertrophy (RVH)

Differentiation between RVH and pulmonary disease patterns is difficult without patient history.
ECG findings suggesting RVH include the following:
   a. R > S in lead V_1
      An R > S in V_1 that is also associated with posterior myocardial infarction
      Without patient history, the interpretation is RVH vs. true posterior MI
   b. Low overall voltage
   c. RAD (>110°) or indeterminate axis
   d. Incomplete right bundle branch block (rSr' in $V_1 \leq 0.10$ seconds)
   e. Poor R wave progression in precordial leads
   f. Often accompanied by "strain" pattern (slightly depressed S-T segment with flat T wave)

Left Ventricular Hypertrophy (LVH)

ECG findings suggestive of LVH include (for adult patients) the following:
   a. S wave amplitude in lead V_1 added to the R wave amplitude in $V_5 \geq$ 35 mV
   b. R wave amplitude in aVL ≥ 12 mV
   c. Often accompanied by strain pattern in V_5 and V_6
   d. May be accompanied by a left axis deviation

Atrial Enlargement

Look at the P waves in leads II and V_1 for evidence of atrial enlargement.

Right Atrial Enlargement (RAE)

P wave appears tall (≥ 2.5 mV) and peaked in lead II, often biphasic P in V_1 with more prominent *positive* portion.

Left Atrial Enlargement (LAE)

P wave appears wide (≥ 0.12 seconds) and notched in lead II, often biphasic P in V_1 with more prominent *negative* portion.

6. MYOCARDIAL INFARCTION AND ISCHEMIA

Examine all leads (with the exception of aVR) of the ECG for pathological Q waves, S-T segment displacement, and T wave inversion. The diagnosis of myocardial infarction (MI) is difficult without pertinent patient history.

Basic Lead Groups
(Indicating Area of Involvement)

Type of Infarct	Associated Leads
Inferior	II, III, aVF
Septal	$V_1 - V_2$
Anterior	$V_3 - V_4$
Low Lateral	$V_5 - V_6$
High Lateral	I, aVL
Posterior	V_1

Small, narrow Q waves may be a normal variant in leads I, aVL, and V_{4-6}. Larger Q waves may be seen as an isolated finding in III, aVR, aVF, and V_1.

Definitions

Acute MI
Immediate onset up to 24 hours
Marked by S-T elevation and often accompanied by reciprocal S-T depression (S-T) elevation may also be caused by coronary artery spasm and by coronary artery aneurysm, however the elevation from these causes is usually minimal [1 mm].

Recent MI
24 to 48 hours up to 1 week
S-T elevation is minimal, frequent T wave inversion, Q waves may begin to form, and reciprocal S-T depression is minimal or absent.

Old MI
Infarction is over 1 week old.
Pathological Q waves are formed.
There is infrequent T wave inversion.
Poor R wave progression in precordial leads is possible.

Subendocardial MI
There is involvement of the subendocardial layer of the myocardium. ECG findings include diffuse S-T depression with deep T wave inversion.

Transmural MI
Involvement includes the entire thickness of the myocardium. It is marked by S-T elevation at onset resolving to pathological Q waves.

Ischemia
A lack of oxygenated blood to an area of the heart
May be an isolated finding or precurser to more serious infarction
ECG findings for ischemia are similar to a subendocardial MI, however, ischemia is a reversible process.

7. MECHANICAL PACEMAKER

Examine the ECG for pacemaker spikes

Normal functioning:
a. Mechanical pacemaker "senses" that the ventricular rate falls below the preset value.
b. The pacemaker "captures" with a P wave or QRS following each spike.

8. MEDICATION EFFECTS AND ELECTROLYTE IMBALANCES

Examine the ECG for any abnormalities that may be caused by the effects of a medication or electrolyte imbalances.
• If an ECG tracing in this workbook has a possible medication effect, that medication will be listed.
• If an ECG tracing in this workbook is from a patient with an electrolyte imbalance, that will be noted.

Part II

12-Lead ECGs within Normal Limits, with Axis Deviations, and with Rate Disturbances

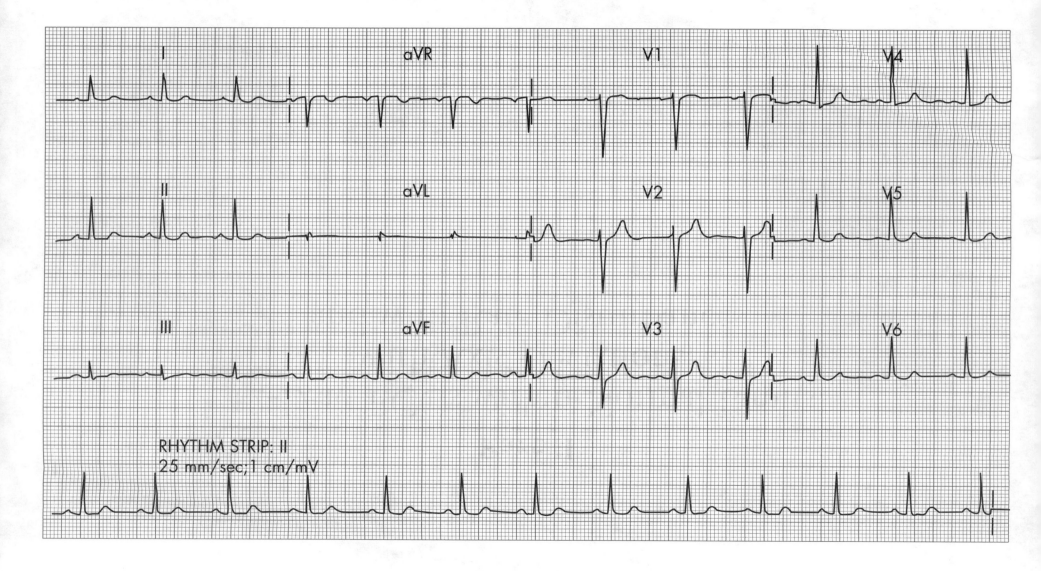

RHYTHM STRIP: II
25 mm/sec;1 cm/mV

Figure 2-1
Resting 12-Lead ECG

8

1. **RATE**

    Atrial:

    Ventricular:

2. **RHYTHM**

    Atrial:

    Ventricular:

3. **WAVES**

    P waves present:

    　　Appearance:

    　　Consistent:

    　　Relation to QRS:

    Q waves present:

    　　Leads:

    　　Pathological:

    T waves present:

    　　Morphology:

4. **INTERVALS**

    P-R interval:

    　　Consistent:

    QRS:

    　　Appearance:

    　　Consistent:

    Q-T interval:

5. **AXIS**

    Quadrant:

    Degrees:

6. **HYPERTROPHY**

    Atrial:

    Ventricular:

7. **MYOCARDIAL INFARCTION**

    Q waves:

    S-T displacement:

8. **ISCHEMIA**

    S-T displacement:

9. **POSSIBLE DRUG EFFECTS**

10. **ECG ANALYSIS**

11. **INTERPRETATION**

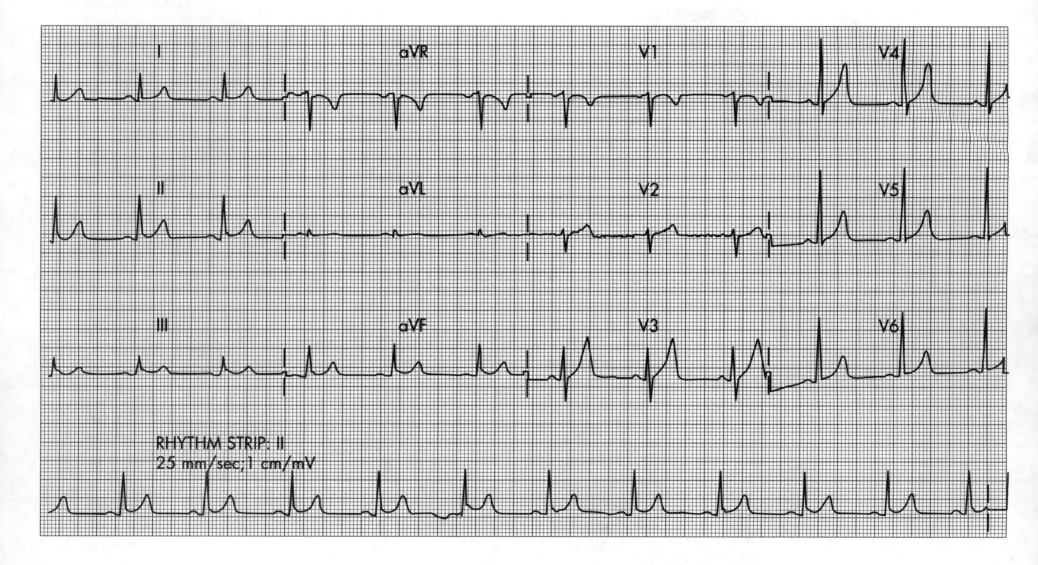

Figure 2-2
Resting 12-Lead ECG

I. RATE

    Atrial:

    Ventricular:

2. RHYTHM

    Atrial:

    Ventricular:

3. WAVES

    P waves present:

        Appearance:

        Consistent:

        Relation to QRS:

    Q waves present:

        Leads:

        Pathological:

    T waves present:

        Morphology:

4. INTERVALS

    P-R interval:

        Consistent:

    QRS:

        Appearance:

        Consistent:

    Q-T interval:

5. AXIS

    Quadrant:

    Degrees:

6. HYPERTROPHY

    Atrial:

    Ventricular:

7. MYOCARDIAL INFARCTION

    Q waves:

    S-T displacement:

8. ISCHEMIA

    S-T displacement:

9. POSSIBLE DRUG EFFECTS

10. ECG ANALYSIS

11. INTERPRETATION

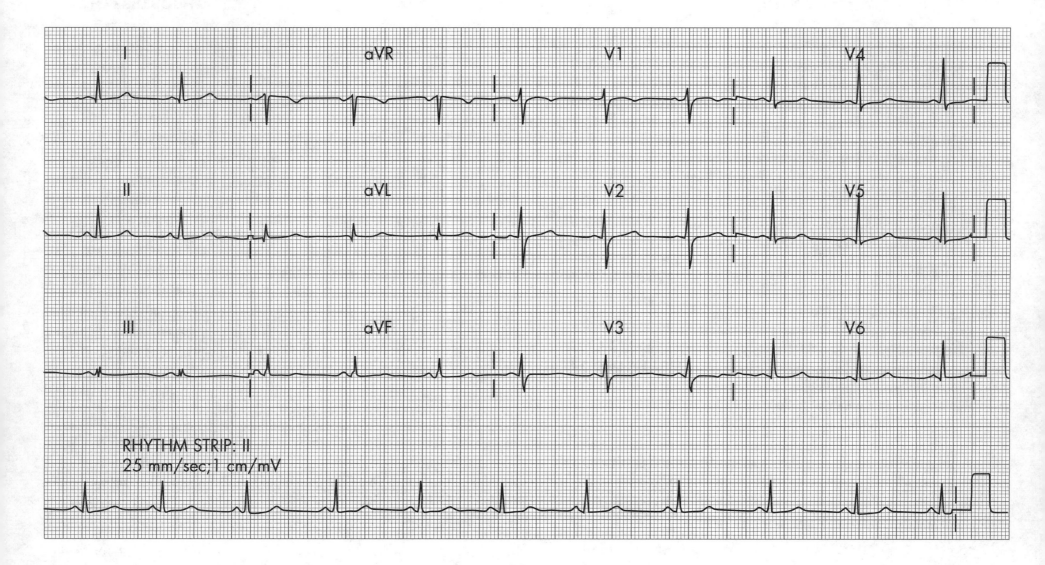

Figure 2-3
Resting 12-Lead ECG

1. **RATE**

   Atrial:

   Ventricular:

2. **RHYTHM**

   Atrial:

   Ventricular:

3. **WAVES**

   P waves present:

      Appearance:

      Consistent:

      Relation to QRS:

   Q waves present:

      Leads:

      Pathological:

   T waves present:

      Morphology:

4. **INTERVALS**

   P-R interval:

      Consistent:

   QRS:

      Appearance:

      Consistent:

   Q-T interval:

5. **AXIS**

   Quadrant:

   Degrees:

6. **HYPERTROPHY**

   Atrial:

   Ventricular:

7. **MYOCARDIAL INFARCTION**

   Q waves:

   S-T displacement:

8. **ISCHEMIA**

   S-T displacement:

9. **POSSIBLE DRUG EFFECTS**

10. **ECG ANALYSIS**

11. **INTERPRETATION**

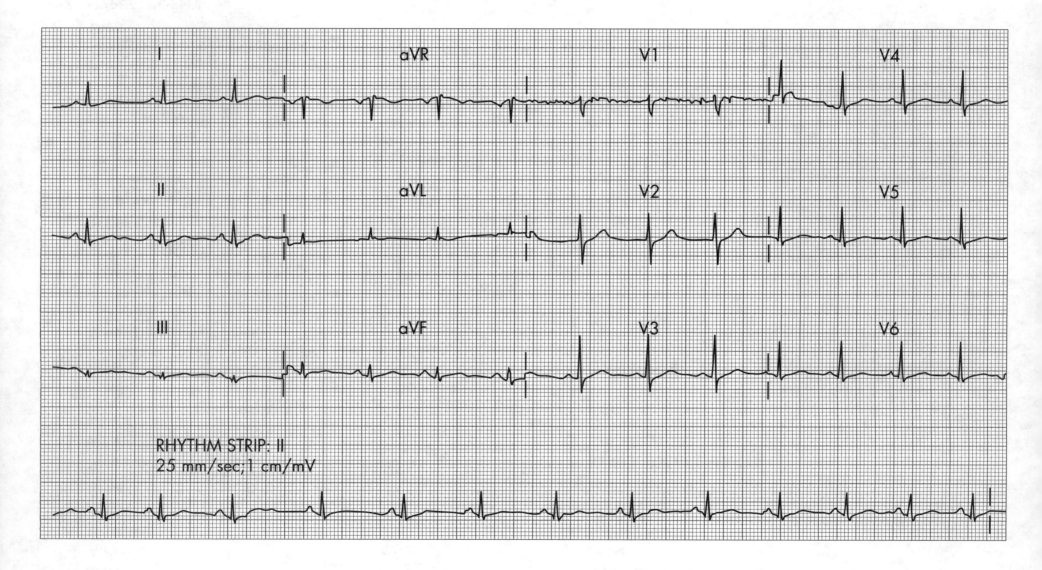

I   aVR   V1   V4

II   aVL   V2   V5

III   aVF   V3   V6

RHYTHM STRIP: II
25 mm/sec; 1 cm/mV

Figure 2-4
Resting 12-Lead ECG

14

1. RATE

Atrial:

Ventricular:

2. RHYTHM

Atrial:

Ventricular:

3. WAVES

P waves present:

Appearance:

Consistent:

Relation to QRS:

Q waves present:

Leads:

Pathological:

T waves present:

Morphology:

4. INTERVALS

P-R interval:

Consistent:

QRS:

Appearance:

Consistent:

Q-T interval:

5. AXIS

Quadrant:

Degrees:

6. HYPERTROPHY

Atrial:

Ventricular:

7. MYOCARDIAL INFARCTION

Q waves:

S-T displacement:

8. ISCHEMIA

S-T displacement:

9. POSSIBLE DRUG EFFECTS

10. ECG ANALYSIS

11. INTERPRETATION

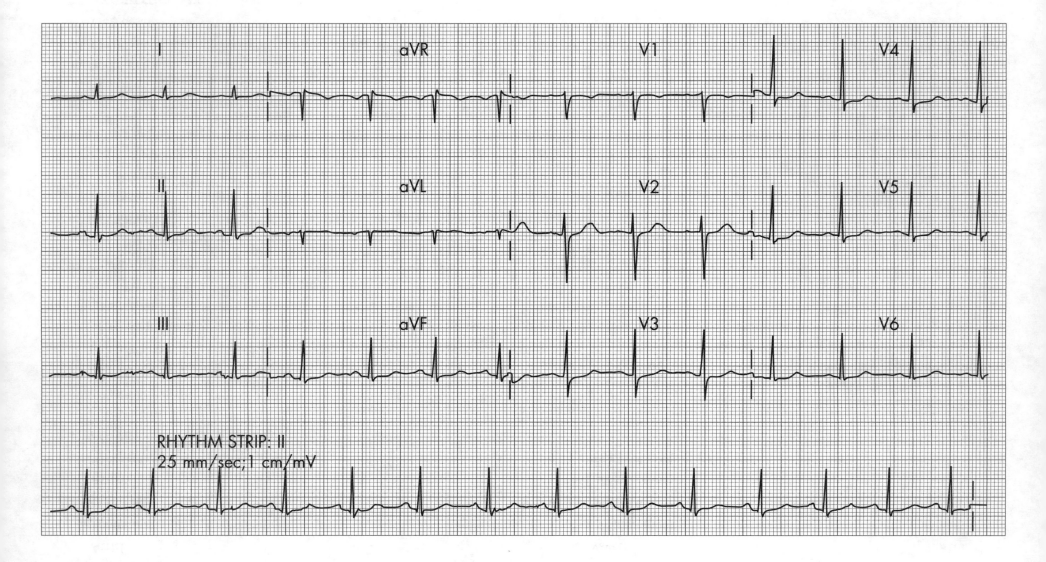

I	aVR	V1	V4
II	aVL	V2	V5
III	aVF	V3	V6

RHYTHM STRIP: II
25 mm/sec; 1 cm/mV

Figure 2-5
Resting 12-Lead ECG

1. RATE

    Atrial:

    Ventricular:

2. RHYTHM

    Atrial:

    Ventricular:

3. WAVES

    P waves present:

        Appearance:

        Consistent:

        Relation to QRS:

    Q waves present:

        Leads:

        Pathological:

    T waves present:

        Morphology:

4. INTERVALS

    P-R interval:

        Consistent:

    QRS:

        Appearance:

        Consistent:

    Q-T interval:

5. AXIS

    Quadrant:

    Degrees:

6. HYPERTROPHY

    Atrial:

    Ventricular:

7. MYOCARDIAL INFARCTION

    Q waves:

    S-T displacement:

8. ISCHEMIA

    S-T displacement:

9. POSSIBLE DRUG EFFECTS

10. ECG ANALYSIS

11. INTERPRETATION

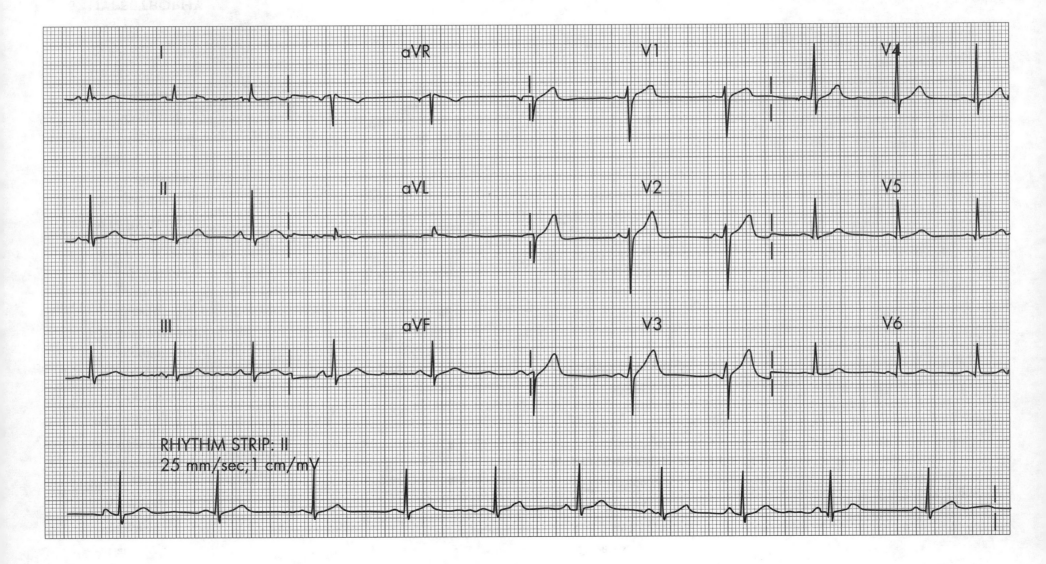

I

aVR

V1

V4

II

aVL

V2

V5

III

aVF

V3

V6

RHYTHM STRIP: II
25 mm/sec;1 cm/mV

Figure 2-6
Resting 12-Lead ECG

18

1. **RATE**

   Atrial:

   Ventricular:

2. **RHYTHM**

   Atrial:

   Ventricular:

3. **WAVES**

   P waves present:

      Appearance:

      Consistent:

      Relation to QRS:

   Q waves present:

      Leads:

      Pathological:

   T waves present:

      Morphology:

4. **INTERVALS**

   P-R interval:

      Consistent:

   QRS:

      Appearance:

      Consistent:

   Q-T interval:

5. **AXIS**

   Quadrant:

   Degrees:

6. **HYPERTROPHY**

   Atrial:

   Ventricular:

7. **MYOCARDIAL INFARCTION**

   Q waves:

   S-T displacement:

8. **ISCHEMIA**

   S-T displacement:

9. **POSSIBLE DRUG EFFECTS**

10. **ECG ANALYSIS**

11. **INTERPRETATION**

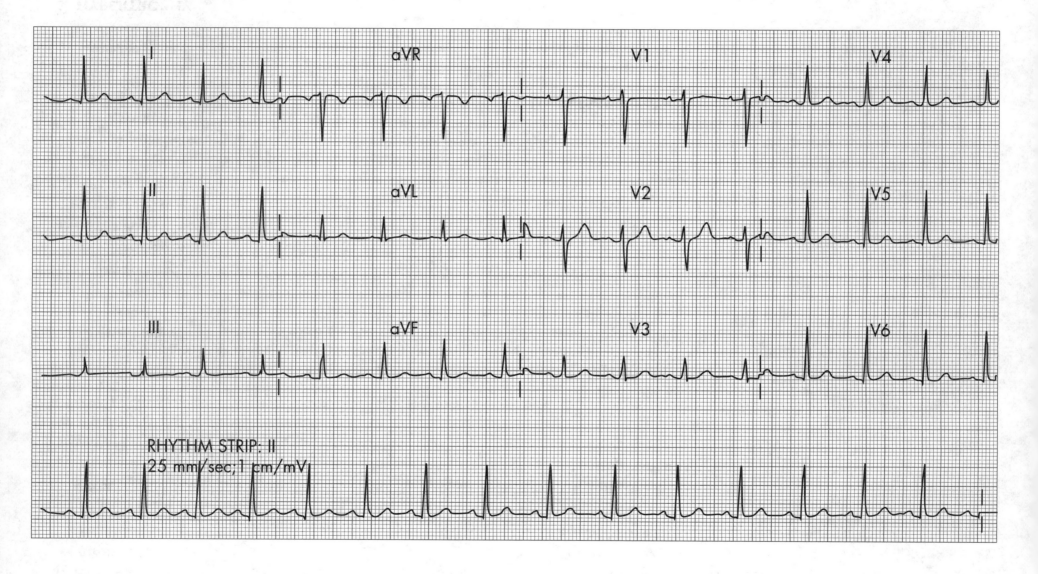

I aVR V1 V4

II aVL V2 V5

III aVF V3 V6

RHYTHM STRIP: II
25 mm/sec; 1 cm/mV

Figure 2-7
Resting 12-Lead ECG

20

1. RATE

Atrial:

Ventricular:

2. RHYTHM

Atrial:

Ventricular:

3. WAVES

P waves present:

Appearance:

Consistent:

Relation to QRS:

Q waves present:

Leads:

Pathological:

T waves present:

Morphology:

4. INTERVALS

P-R interval:

Consistent:

QRS:

Appearance:

Consistent:

Q-T interval:

5. AXIS

Quadrant:

Degrees:

6. HYPERTROPHY

Atrial:

Ventricular:

7. MYOCARDIAL INFARCTION

Q waves:

S-T displacement:

8. ISCHEMIA

S-T displacement:

9. POSSIBLE DRUG EFFECTS

10. ECG ANALYSIS

11. INTERPRETATION

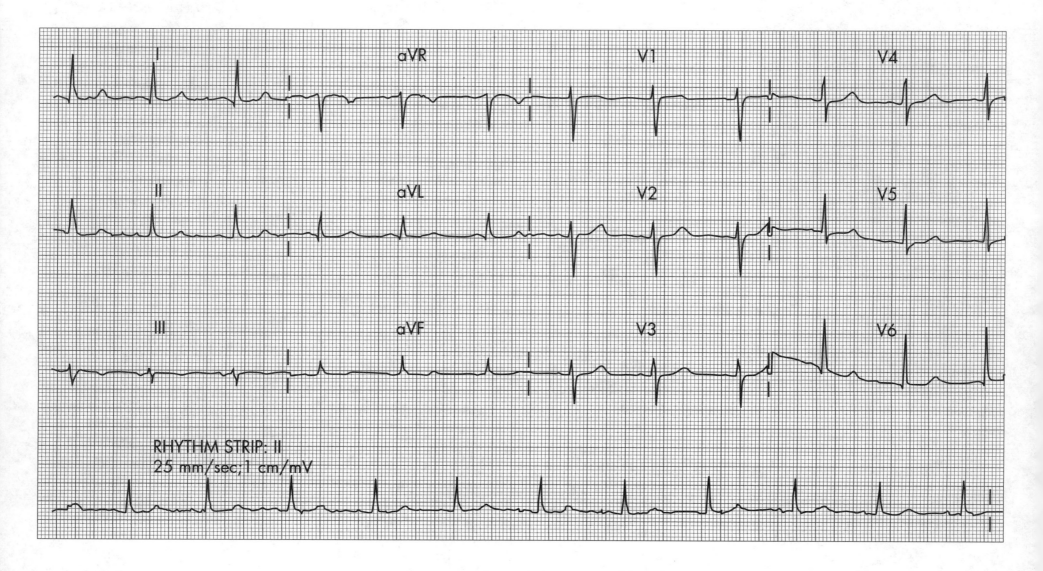

I aVR V1 V4

II aVL V2 V5

III aVF V3 V6

RHYTHM STRIP: II
25 mm/sec; 1 cm/mV

Figure 2-8
Resting 12-Lead ECG

22

1. RATE

Atrial:

Ventricular:

2. RHYTHM

Atrial:

Ventricular:

3. WAVES

P waves present:

Appearance:

Consistent:

Relation to QRS:

Q waves present:

Leads:

Pathological:

T waves present:

Morphology:

4. INTERVALS

P-R interval:

Consistent:

QRS:

Appearance:

Consistent:

Q-T interval:

5. AXIS

Quadrant:

Degrees:

6. HYPERTROPHY

Atrial:

Ventricular:

7. MYOCARDIAL INFARCTION

Q waves:

S-T displacement:

8. ISCHEMIA

S-T displacement:

9. POSSIBLE DRUG EFFECTS

10. ECG ANALYSIS

11. INTERPRETATION

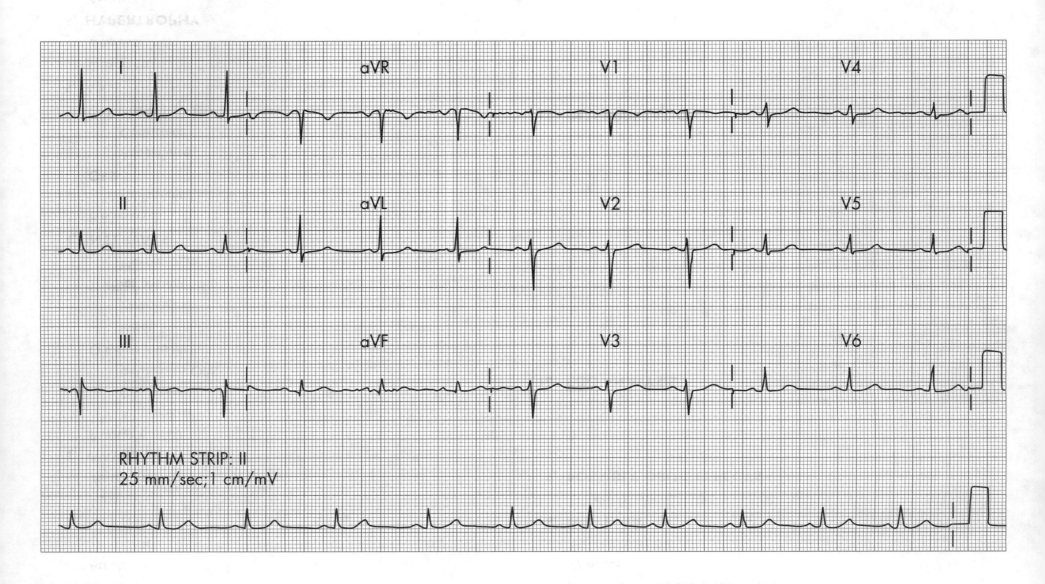

I aVR V1 V4

II aVL V2 V5

III aVF V3 V6

RHYTHM STRIP: II
25 mm/sec; 1 cm/mV

Figure 2-9
Resting 12-Lead ECG

1. **RATE**

   Atrial:

   Ventricular:

2. **RHYTHM**

   Atrial:

   Ventricular:

3. **WAVES**

   P waves present:

       Appearance:

       Consistent:

       Relation to QRS:

   Q waves present:

       Leads:

       Pathological:

   T waves present:

       Morphology:

4. **INTERVALS**

   P-R interval:

       Consistent:

   QRS:

       Appearance:

       Consistent:

   Q-T interval:

5. **AXIS**

   Quadrant:

   Degrees:

6. **HYPERTROPHY**

   Atrial:

   Ventricular:

7. **MYOCARDIAL INFARCTION**

   Q waves:

   S-T displacement:

8. **ISCHEMIA**

   S-T displacement:

9. **POSSIBLE DRUG EFFECTS**

10. **ECG ANALYSIS**

11. **INTERPRETATION**

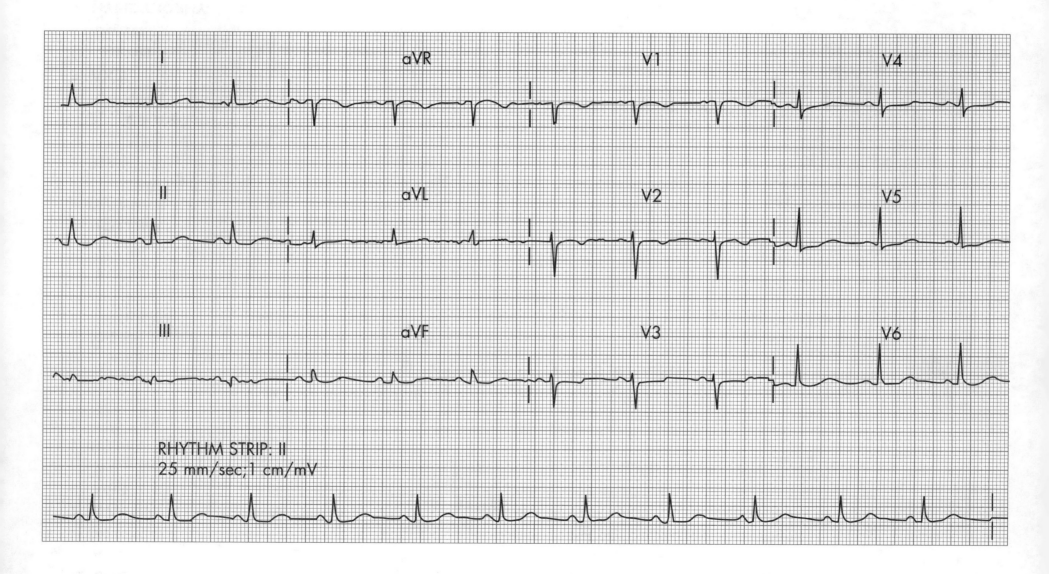

I aVR V1 V4

II aVL V2 V5

III aVF V3 V6

RHYTHM STRIP: II
25 mm/sec; 1 cm/mV

Figure 2-10
Resting 12-Lead ECG

26

1. RATE

    Atrial:

    Ventricular:

2. RHYTHM

    Atrial:

    Ventricular:

3. WAVES

    P waves present:

        Appearance:

        Consistent:

        Relation to QRS:

    Q waves present:

        Leads:

        Pathological:

    T waves present:

        Morphology:

4. INTERVALS

    P-R interval:

        Consistent:

    QRS:

        Appearance:

        Consistent:

    Q-T interval:

5. AXIS

    Quadrant:

    Degrees:

6. HYPERTROPHY

    Atrial:

    Ventricular:

7. MYOCARDIAL INFARCTION

    Q waves:

    S-T displacement:

8. ISCHEMIA

    S-T displacement:

9. POSSIBLE DRUG EFFECTS

10. ECG ANALYSIS

11. INTERPRETATION

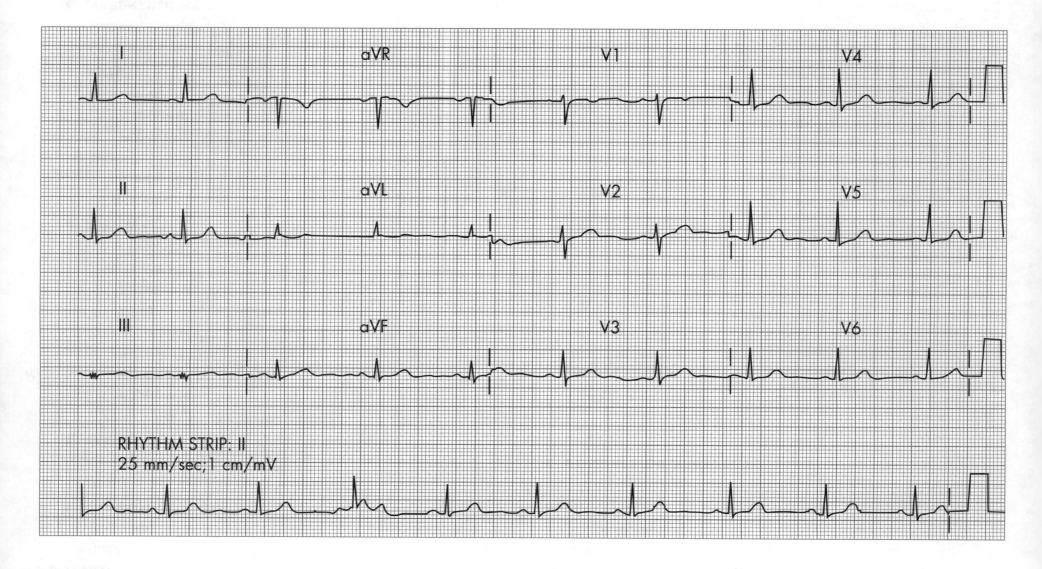

I   aVR   V1   V4

II   aVL   V2   V5

III   aVF   V3   V6

RHYTHM STRIP: II
25 mm/sec; 1 cm/mV

Figure 2-11
Resting 12-Lead ECG

28

1. **RATE**

   Atrial:

   Ventricular:

2. **RHYTHM**

   Atrial:

   Ventricular:

3. **WAVES**

   P waves present:

   Appearance:

   Consistent:

   Relation to QRS:

   Q waves present:

   Leads:

   Pathological:

   T waves present:

   Morphology:

4. **INTERVALS**

   P-R interval:

   Consistent:

   QRS:

   Appearance:

   Consistent:

   Q-T interval:

5. **AXIS**

   Quadrant:

   Degrees:

6. **HYPERTROPHY**

   Atrial:

   Ventricular:

7. **MYOCARDIAL INFARCTION**

   Q waves:

   S-T displacement:

8. **ISCHEMIA**

   S-T displacement:

9. **POSSIBLE DRUG EFFECTS**

10. **ECG ANALYSIS**

11. **INTERPRETATION**

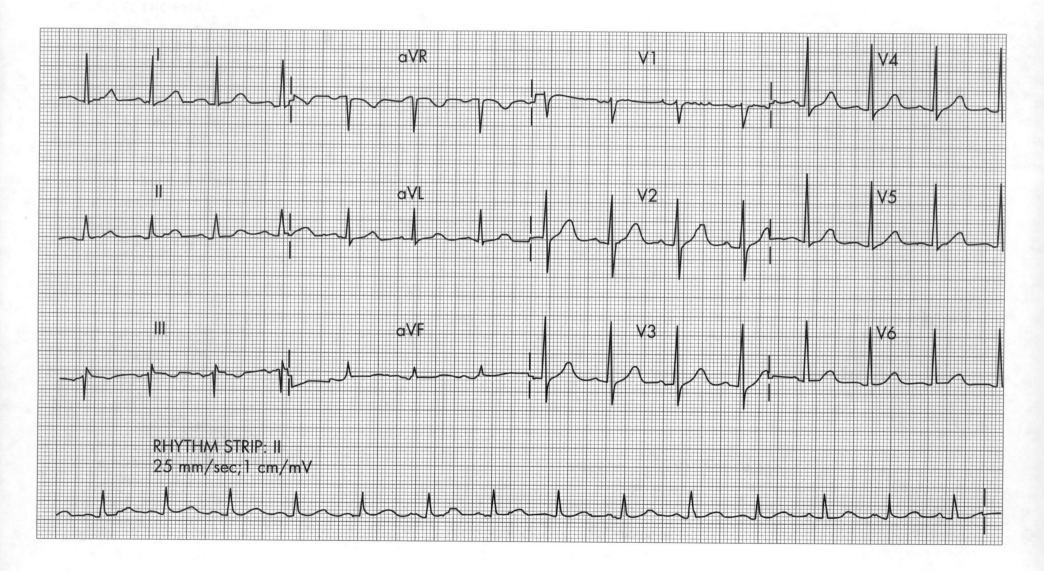

aVR   V1   V4

II   aVL   V2   V5

III   aVF   V3   V6

RHYTHM STRIP: II
25 mm/sec;1 cm/mV

Figure 2-12
Resting 12-Lead ECG

30

1. RATE

Atrial:

Ventricular:

2. RHYTHM

Atrial:

Ventricular:

3. WAVES

P waves present:

Appearance:

Consistent:

Relation to QRS:

Q waves present:

Leads:

Pathological:

T waves present:

Morphology:

4. INTERVALS

P-R interval:

Consistent:

QRS:

Appearance:

Consistent:

Q-T interval:

5. AXIS

Quadrant:

Degrees:

6. HYPERTROPHY

Atrial:

Ventricular:

7. MYOCARDIAL INFARCTION

Q waves:

S-T displacement:

8. ISCHEMIA

S-T displacement:

9. POSSIBLE DRUG EFFECTS

10. ECG ANALYSIS

11. INTERPRETATION

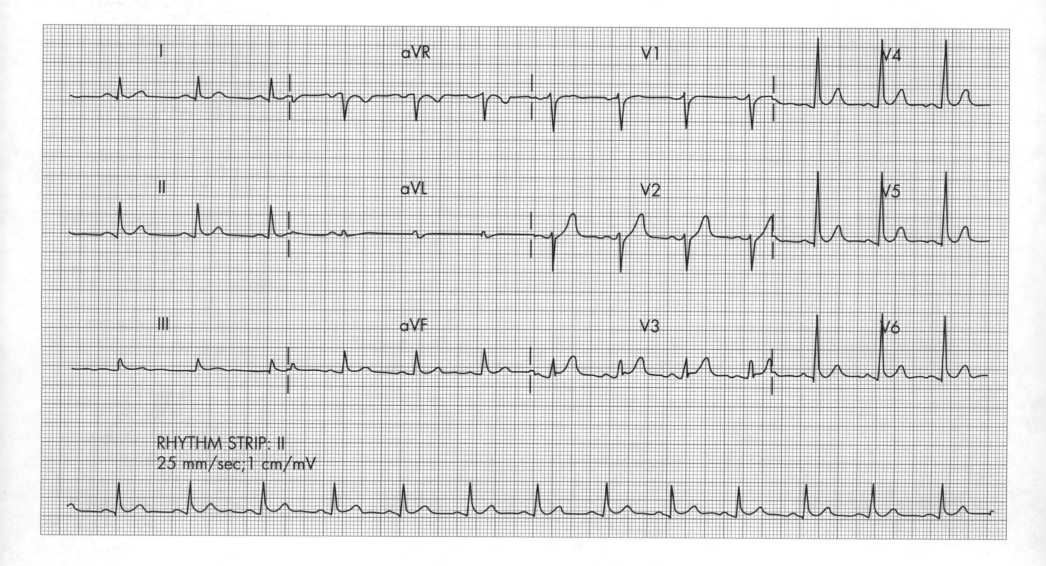

Figure 2-13
Resting 12-Lead ECG

1. RATE

Atrial:

Ventricular:

2. RHYTHM

Atrial:

Ventricular:

3. WAVES

P waves present:

Appearance:

Consistent:

Relation to QRS:

Q waves present:

Leads:

Pathological:

T waves present:

Morphology:

4. INTERVALS

P-R interval:

Consistent:

QRS:

Appearance:

Consistent:

Q-T interval:

5. AXIS

Quadrant:

Degrees:

6. HYPERTROPHY

Atrial:

Ventricular:

7. MYOCARDIAL INFARCTION

Q waves:

S-T displacement:

8. ISCHEMIA

S-T displacement:

9. POSSIBLE DRUG EFFECTS

10. ECG ANALYSIS

11. INTERPRETATION

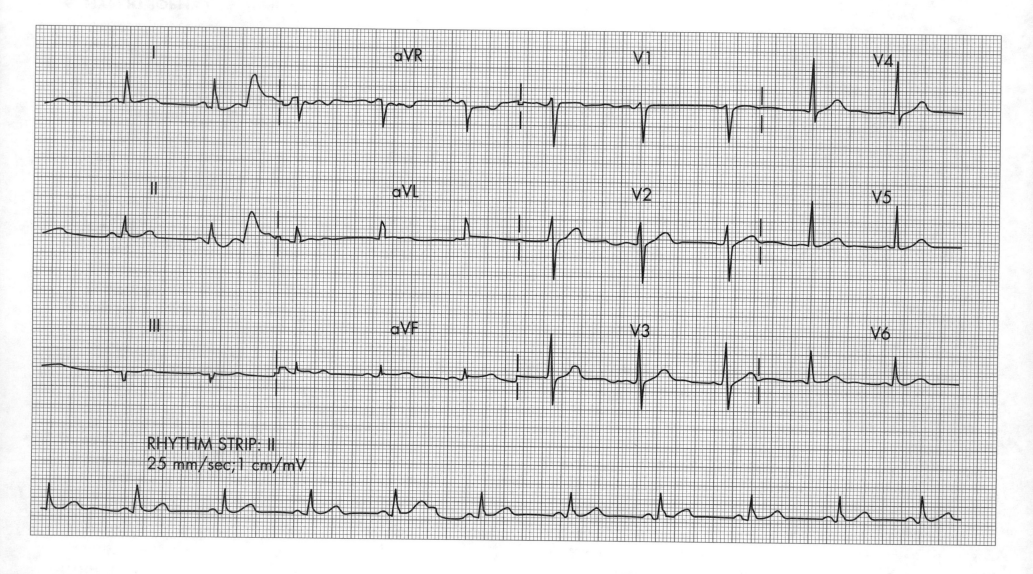

Figure 2-14
Resting 12-Lead ECG

34

1. RATE

Atrial:

Ventricular:

2. RHYTHM

Atrial:

Ventricular:

3. WAVES

P waves present:

Appearance:

Consistent:

Relation to QRS:

Q waves present:

Leads:

Pathological:

T waves present:

Morphology:

4. INTERVALS

P-R interval:

Consistent:

QRS:

Appearance:

Consistent:

Q-T interval:

5. AXIS

Quadrant:

Degrees:

6. HYPERTROPHY

Atrial:

Ventricular:

7. MYOCARDIAL INFARCTION

Q waves:

S-T displacement:

8. ISCHEMIA

S-T displacement:

9. POSSIBLE DRUG EFFECTS

10. ECG ANALYSIS

11. INTERPRETATION

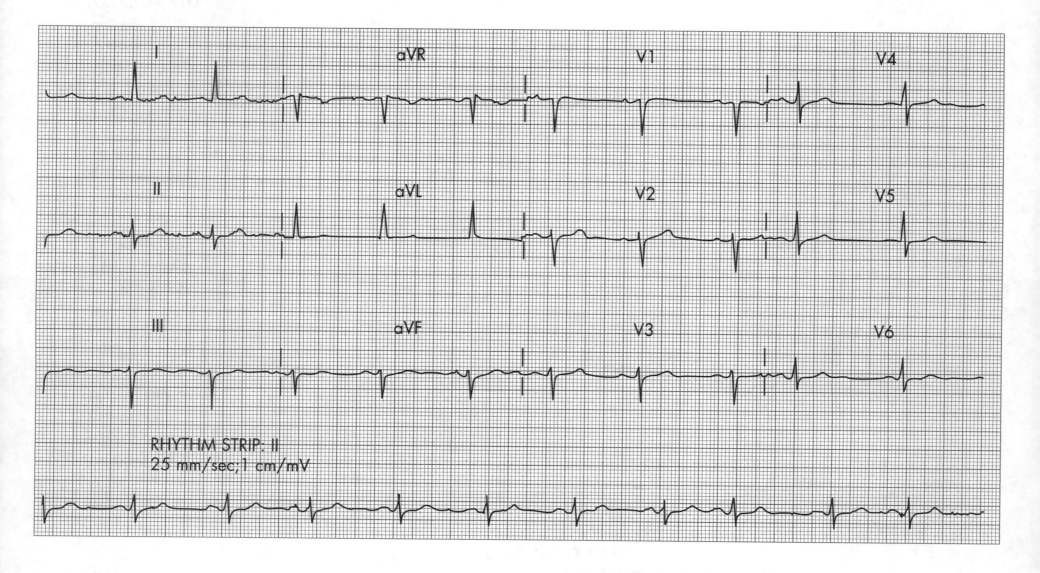

Figure 2-15
Resting 12-Lead ECG

1. RATE

Atrial:

Ventricular:

2. RHYTHM

Atrial:

Ventricular:

3. WAVES

P waves present:

    Appearance:

    Consistent:

    Relation to QRS:

Q waves present:

    Leads:

    Pathological:

T waves present:

    Morphology:

4. INTERVALS

P-R interval:

    Consistent:

QRS:

    Appearance:

    Consistent:

Q-T interval:

5. AXIS

Quadrant:

Degrees:

6. HYPERTROPHY

Atrial:

Ventricular:

7. MYOCARDIAL INFARCTION

Q waves:

S-T displacement:

8. ISCHEMIA

S-T displacement:

9. POSSIBLE DRUG EFFECTS

10. ECG ANALYSIS

11. INTERPRETATION

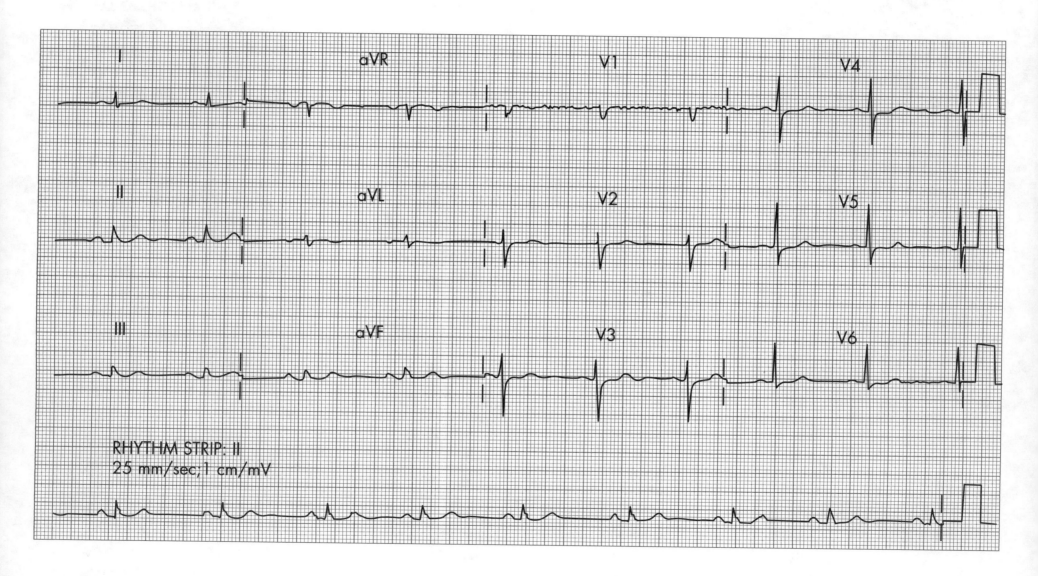

Figure 2-16
Resting 12-Lead ECG

38

1. **RATE**

  Atrial:

  Ventricular:

2. **RHYTHM**

  Atrial:

  Ventricular:

3. **WAVES**

  P waves present:

  Appearance:

  Consistent:

  Relation to QRS:

  Q waves present:

  Leads:

  Pathological:

  T waves present:

  Morphology:

4. **INTERVALS**

  P-R interval:

  Consistent:

  QRS:

  Appearance:

  Consistent:

  Q-T interval:

5. **AXIS**

  Quadrant:

  Degrees:

6. **HYPERTROPHY**

  Atrial:

  Ventricular:

7. **MYOCARDIAL INFARCTION**

  Q waves:

  S-T displacement:

8. **ISCHEMIA**

  S-T displacement:

9. **POSSIBLE DRUG EFFECTS**

10. **ECG ANALYSIS**

11. **INTERPRETATION**

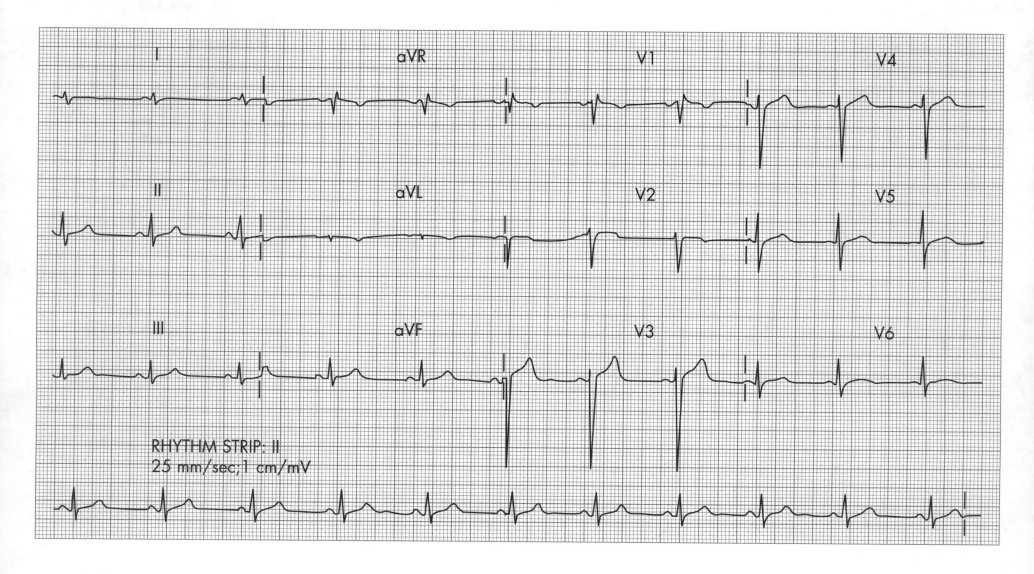

Figure 2-17
Resting 12-Lead ECG

40

1. RATE

Atrial:

Ventricular:

2. RHYTHM

Atrial:

Ventricular:

3. WAVES

P waves present:

Appearance:

Consistent:

Relation to QRS:

Q waves present:

Leads:

Pathological:

T waves present:

Morphology:

4. INTERVALS

P-R interval:

Consistent:

QRS:

Appearance:

Consistent:

Q-T interval:

5. AXIS

Quadrant:

Degrees:

6. HYPERTROPHY

Atrial:

Ventricular:

7. MYOCARDIAL INFARCTION

Q waves:

S-T displacement:

8. ISCHEMIA

S-T displacement:

9. POSSIBLE DRUG EFFECTS

10. ECG ANALYSIS

11. INTERPRETATION

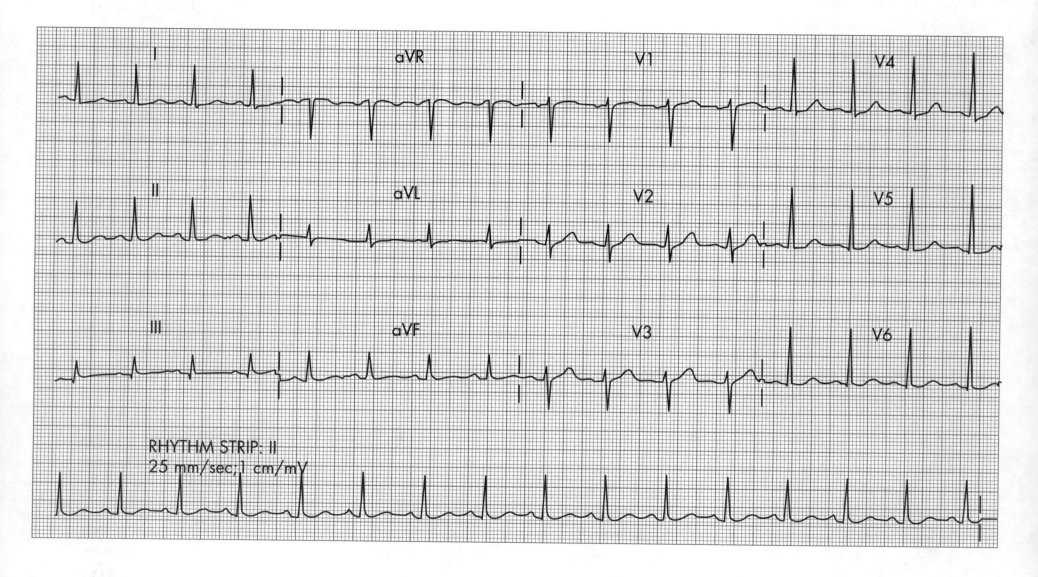

Figure 2-18
Resting 12-Lead ECG

1. RATE

    Atrial:

    Ventricular:

2. RHYTHM

    Atrial:

    Ventricular:

3. WAVES

    P waves present:

        Appearance:

        Consistent:

        Relation to QRS:

    Q waves present:

        Leads:

        Pathological:

    T waves present:

        Morphology:

4. INTERVALS

    P-R interval:

        Consistent:

    QRS:

        Appearance:

        Consistent:

    Q-T interval:

5. AXIS

    Quadrant:

    Degrees:

6. HYPERTROPHY

    Atrial:

    Ventricular:

7. MYOCARDIAL INFARCTION

    Q waves:

    S-T displacement:

8. ISCHEMIA

    S-T displacement:

9. POSSIBLE DRUG EFFECTS

10. ECG ANALYSIS

11. INTERPRETATION

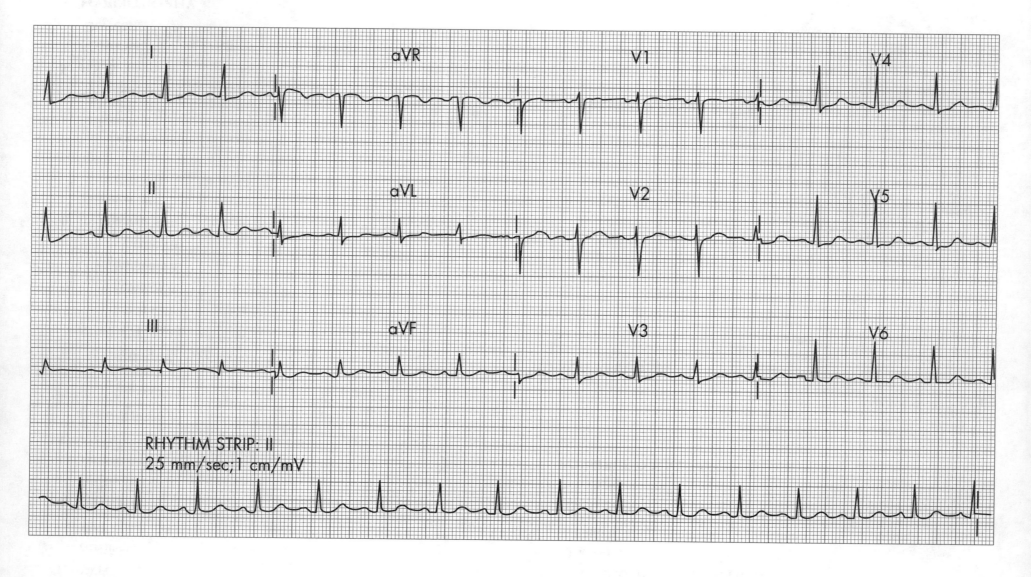

I aVR V1 V4

II aVL V2 V5

III aVF V3 V6

RHYTHM STRIP: II
25 mm/sec; 1 cm/mV

Figure 2-19
Resting 12-Lead ECG

44

1. RATE

Atrial:

Ventricular:

2. RHYTHM

Atrial:

Ventricular:

3. WAVES

P waves present:

Appearance:

Consistent:

Relation to QRS:

Q waves present:

Leads:

Pathological:

T waves present:

Morphology:

4. INTERVALS

P-R interval:

Consistent:

QRS:

Appearance:

Consistent:

Q-T interval:

5. AXIS

Quadrant:

Degrees:

6. HYPERTROPHY

Atrial:

Ventricular:

7. MYOCARDIAL INFARCTION

Q waves:

S-T displacement:

8. ISCHEMIA

S-T displacement:

9. POSSIBLE DRUG EFFECTS

10. ECG ANALYSIS

11. INTERPRETATION

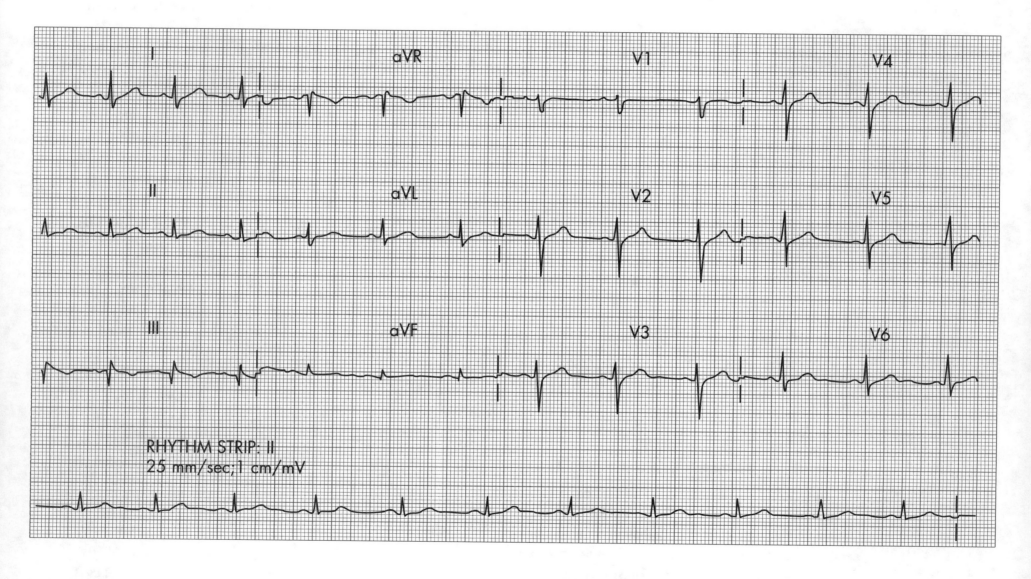

Figure 2-20
Resting 12-Lead ECG

46

1. **RATE**

    Atrial:

    Ventricular:

2. **RHYTHM**

    Atrial:

    Ventricular:

3. **WAVES**

    P waves present:

        Appearance:

        Consistent:

        Relation to QRS:

    Q waves present:

        Leads:

        Pathological:

    T waves present:

        Morphology:

4. **INTERVALS**

    P-R interval:

        Consistent:

    QRS:

        Appearance:

        Consistent:

    Q-T interval:

5. **AXIS**

    Quadrant:

    Degrees:

6. **HYPERTROPHY**

    Atrial:

    Ventricular:

7. **MYOCARDIAL INFARCTION**

    Q waves:

    S-T displacement:

8. **ISCHEMIA**

    S-T displacement:

9. **POSSIBLE DRUG EFFECTS**

10. **ECG ANALYSIS**

11. **INTERPRETATION**

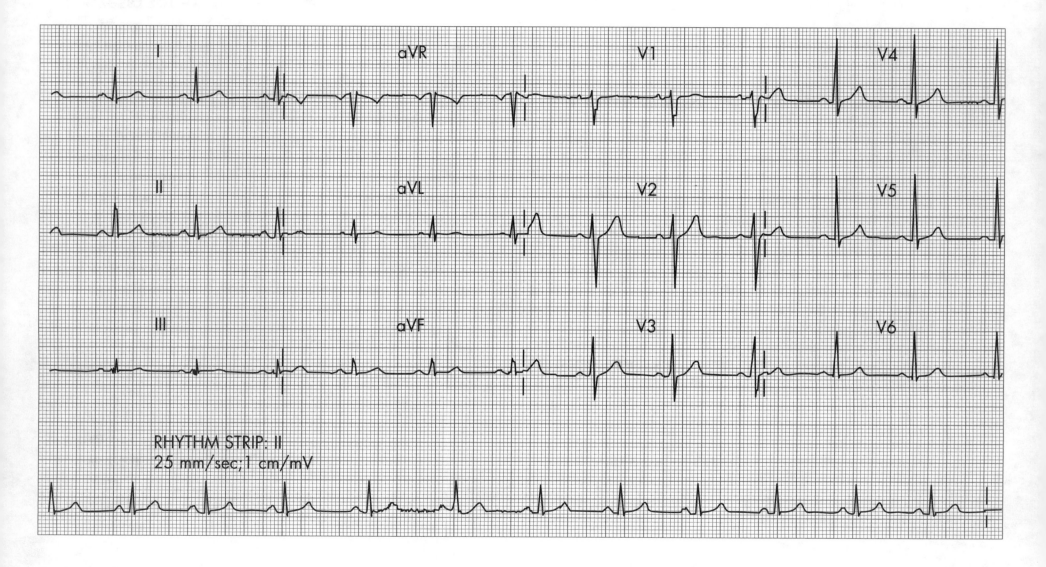

RHYTHM STRIP: II
25 mm/sec; 1 cm/mV

Figure 2-21
Resting 12-Lead ECG

48

1. **RATE**

   Atrial:

   Ventricular:

2. **RHYTHM**

   Atrial:

   Ventricular:

3. **WAVES**

   P waves present:

   　　Appearance:

   　　Consistent:

   　　Relation to QRS:

   Q waves present:

   　　Leads:

   　　Pathological:

   T waves present:

   　　Morphology:

4. **INTERVALS**

   P-R interval:

   　　Consistent:

   QRS:

   　　Appearance:

   　　Consistent:

   Q-T interval:

5. **AXIS**

   Quadrant:

   Degrees:

6. **HYPERTROPHY**

   Atrial:

   Ventricular:

7. **MYOCARDIAL INFARCTION**

   Q waves:

   S-T displacement:

8. **ISCHEMIA**

   S-T displacement:

9. **POSSIBLE DRUG EFFECTS**

10. **ECG ANALYSIS**

11. **INTERPRETATION**

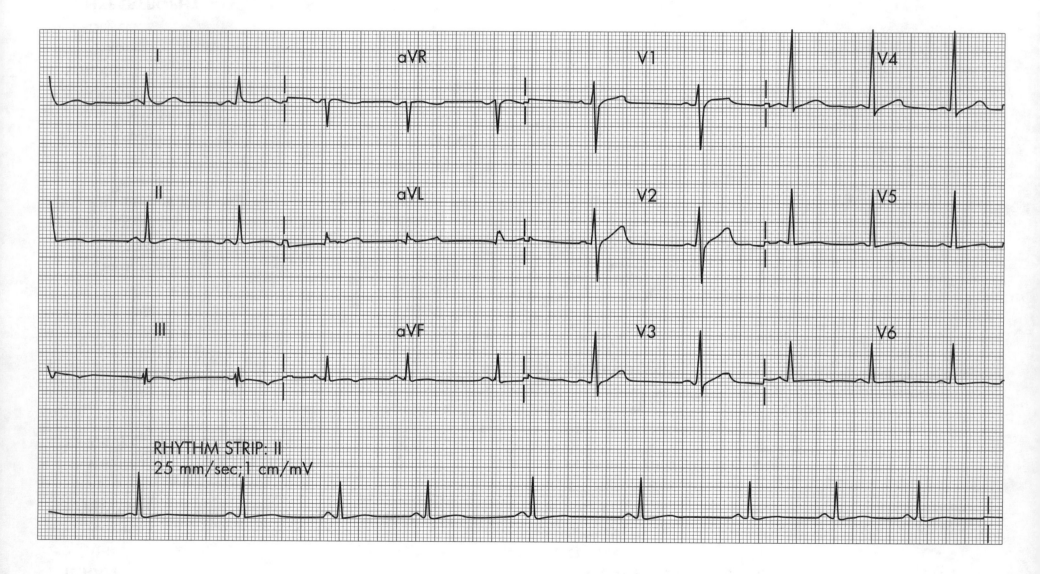

I aVR V1 V4

II aVL V2 V5

III aVF V3 V6

RHYTHM STRIP: II
25 mm/sec; 1 cm/mV

Figure 2-22
Resting 12-Lead ECG

1. **RATE**

   Atrial:

   Ventricular:

2. **RHYTHM**

   Atrial:

   Ventricular:

3. **WAVES**

   P waves present:

      Appearance:

      Consistent:

      Relation to QRS:

   Q waves present:

      Leads:

      Pathological:

   T waves present:

      Morphology:

4. **INTERVALS**

   P-R interval:

      Consistent:

   QRS:

      Appearance:

      Consistent:

   Q-T interval:

5. **AXIS**

   Quadrant:

   Degrees:

6. **HYPERTROPHY**

   Atrial:

   Ventricular:

7. **MYOCARDIAL INFARCTION**

   Q waves:

   S-T displacement:

8. **ISCHEMIA**

   S-T displacement:

9. **POSSIBLE DRUG EFFECTS**

10. **ECG ANALYSIS**

11. **INTERPRETATION**

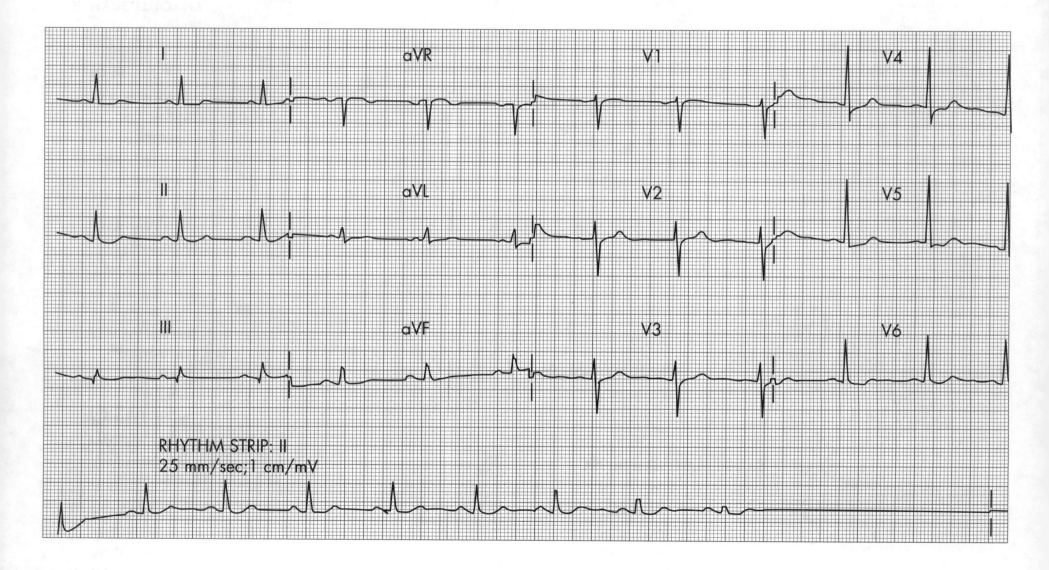

Figure 2-23
Resting 12-Lead ECG

52

1. RATE

Atrial:

Ventricular:

2. RHYTHM

Atrial:

Ventricular:

3. WAVES

P waves present:

    Appearance:

    Consistent:

    Relation to QRS:

Q waves present:

    Leads:

    Pathological:

T waves present:

    Morphology:

4. INTERVALS

P-R interval:

    Consistent:

QRS:

    Appearance:

    Consistent:

Q-T interval:

5. AXIS

Quadrant:

Degrees:

6. HYPERTROPHY

Atrial:

Ventricular:

7. MYOCARDIAL INFARCTION

Q waves:

S-T displacement:

8. ISCHEMIA

S-T displacement:

9. POSSIBLE DRUG EFFECTS

10. ECG ANALYSIS

11. INTERPRETATION

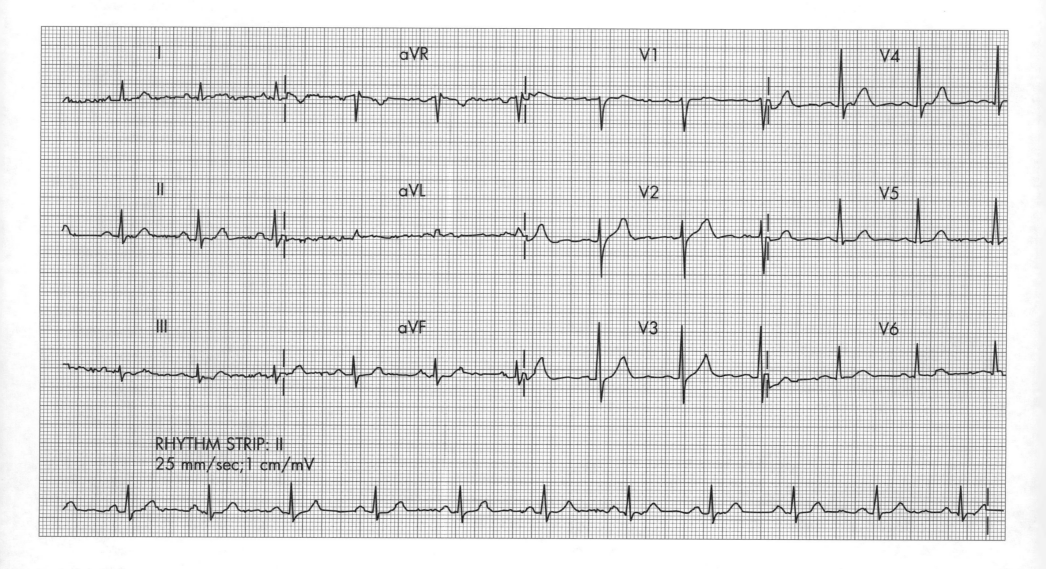

I

aVR

V1

V4

II

aVL

V2

V5

III

aVF

V3

V6

RHYTHM STRIP: II
25 mm/sec;1 cm/mV

Figure 2-24
Resting 12-Lead ECG

1. RATE

Atrial:

Ventricular:

2. RHYTHM

Atrial:

Ventricular:

3. WAVES

P waves present:

Appearance:

Consistent:

Relation to QRS:

Q waves present:

Leads:

Pathological:

T waves present:

Morphology:

4. INTERVALS

P-R interval:

Consistent:

QRS:

Appearance:

Consistent:

Q-T interval:

5. AXIS

Quadrant:

Degrees:

6. HYPERTROPHY

Atrial:

Ventricular:

7. MYOCARDIAL INFARCTION

Q waves:

S-T displacement:

8. ISCHEMIA

S-T displacement:

9. POSSIBLE DRUG EFFECTS

10. ECG ANALYSIS

11. INTERPRETATION

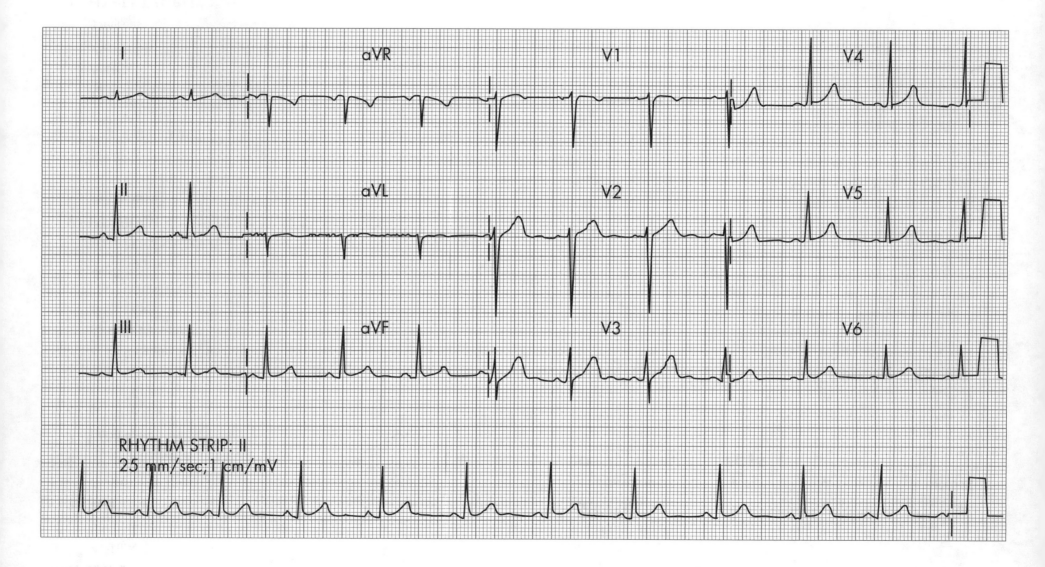

I   aVR   V1   V4

II   aVL   V2   V5

III   aVF   V3   V6

RHYTHM STRIP: II
25 mm/sec; 1 cm/mV

Figure 2-25
Resting 12-Lead ECG

I. RATE

    Atrial:

    Ventricular:

2. RHYTHM

    Atrial:

    Ventricular:

3. WAVES

    P waves present:

        Appearance:

        Consistent:

        Relation to QRS:

    Q waves present:

        Leads:

        Pathological:

    T waves present:

        Morphology:

4. INTERVALS

    P-R interval:

        Consistent:

    QRS:

        Appearance:

        Consistent:

    Q-T interval:

5. AXIS

    Quadrant:

    Degrees:

6. HYPERTROPHY

    Atrial:

    Ventricular:

7. MYOCARDIAL INFARCTION

    Q waves:

    S-T displacement:

8. ISCHEMIA

    S-T displacement:

9. POSSIBLE DRUG EFFECTS

10. ECG ANALYSIS

11. INTERPRETATION

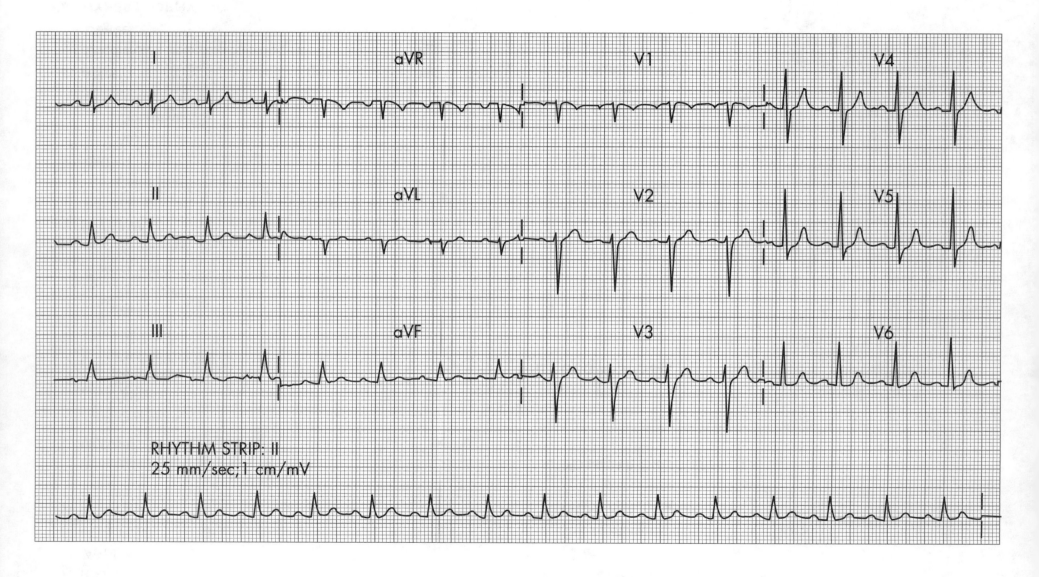

RHYTHM STRIP: II
25 mm/sec; 1 cm/mV

Figure 2-26
Resting 12-Lead ECG
58

1. RATE

   Atrial:

   Ventricular:

2. RHYTHM

   Atrial:

   Ventricular:

3. WAVES

   P waves present:

       Appearance:

       Consistent:

       Relation to QRS:

   Q waves present:

       Leads:

       Pathological:

   T waves present:

       Morphology:

4. INTERVALS

   P-R interval:

       Consistent:

   QRS:

       Appearance:

       Consistent:

   Q-T interval:

5. AXIS

   Quadrant:

   Degrees:

6. HYPERTROPHY

   Atrial:

   Ventricular:

7. MYOCARDIAL INFARCTION

   Q waves:

   S-T displacement:

8. ISCHEMIA

   S-T displacement:

9. POSSIBLE DRUG EFFECTS

10. ECG ANALYSIS

11. INTERPRETATION

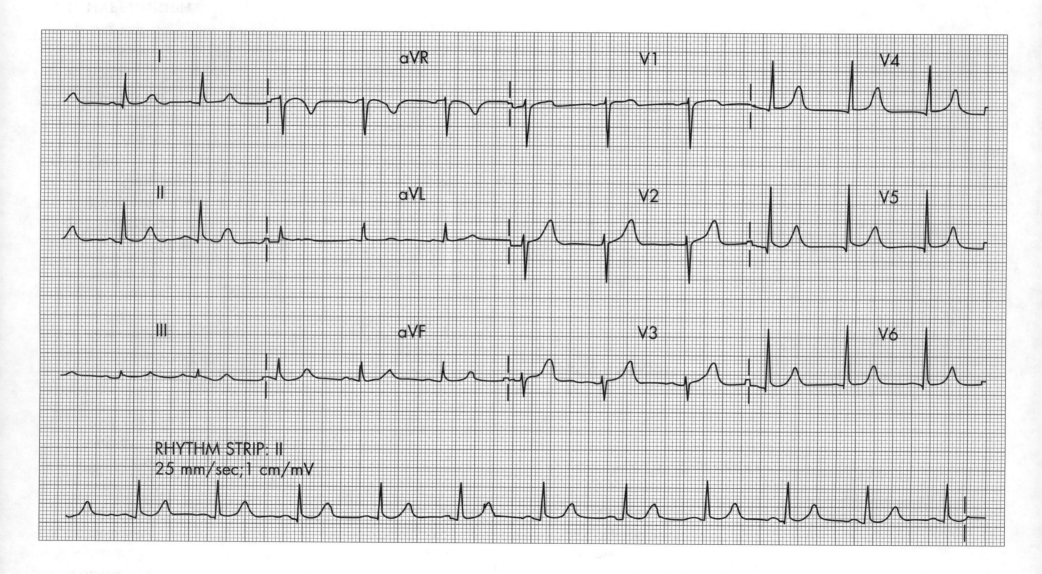

I aVR V1 V4

II aVL V2 V5

III aVF V3 V6

RHYTHM STRIP: II
25 mm/sec; 1 cm/mV

Figure 2-27
Resting 12-Lead ECG

60

I. RATE

    Atrial:

    Ventricular:

2. RHYTHM

    Atrial:

    Ventricular:

3. WAVES

    P waves present:

        Appearance:

        Consistent:

        Relation to QRS:

    Q waves present:

        Leads:

        Pathological:

    T waves present:

        Morphology:

4. INTERVALS

    P-R interval:

        Consistent:

    QRS:

        Appearance:

        Consistent:

    Q-T interval:

5. AXIS

    Quadrant:

    Degrees:

6. HYPERTROPHY

    Atrial:

    Ventricular:

7. MYOCARDIAL INFARCTION

    Q waves:

    S-T displacement:

8. ISCHEMIA

    S-T displacement:

9. POSSIBLE DRUG EFFECTS

10. ECG ANALYSIS

11. INTERPRETATION

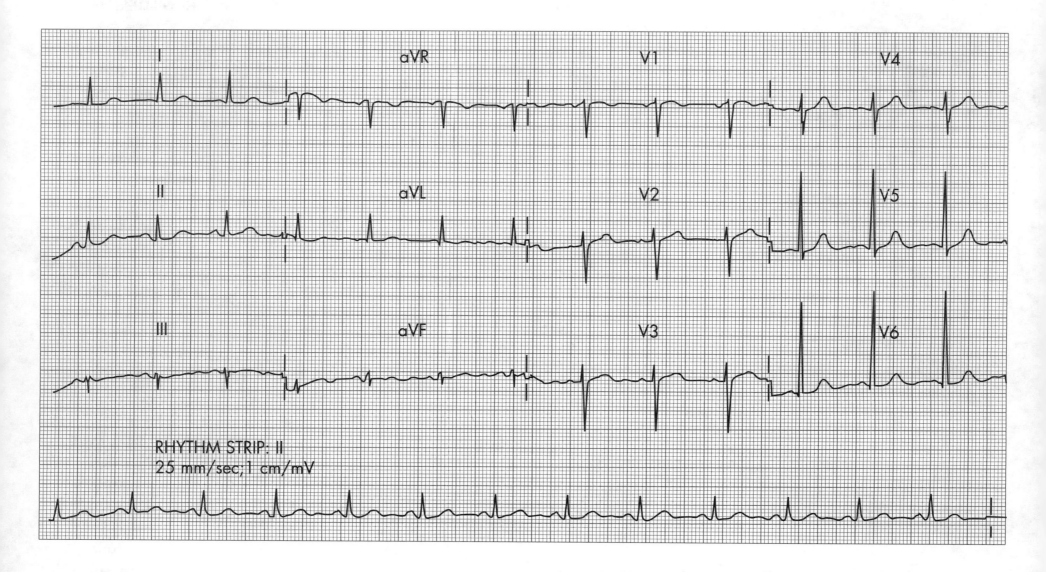

Figure 2-28
Resting 12-Lead ECG

62

1. RATE

Atrial:

Ventricular:

2. RHYTHM

Atrial:

Ventricular:

3. WAVES

P waves present:

Appearance:

Consistent:

Relation to QRS:

Q waves present:

Leads:

Pathological:

T waves present:

Morphology:

4. INTERVALS

P-R interval:

Consistent:

QRS:

Appearance:

Consistent:

Q-T interval:

5. AXIS

Quadrant:

Degrees:

6. HYPERTROPHY

Atrial:

Ventricular:

7. MYOCARDIAL INFARCTION

Q waves:

S-T displacement:

8. ISCHEMIA

S-T displacement:

9. POSSIBLE DRUG EFFECTS

10. ECG ANALYSIS

11. INTERPRETATION

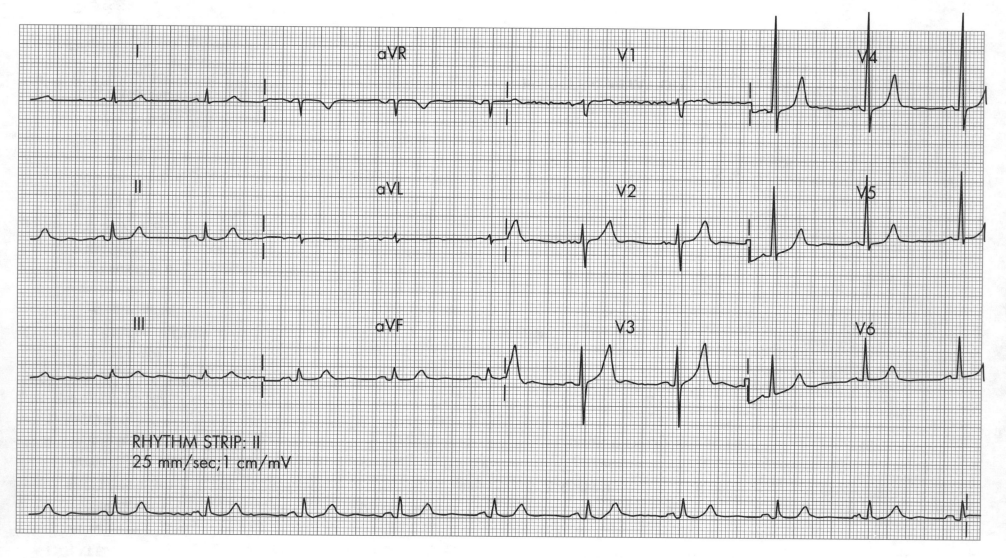

I aVR V1 V4

II aVL V2 V5

III aVF V3 V6

RHYTHM STRIP: II
25 mm/sec;1 cm/mV

Figure 2-29
Resting 12-Lead ECG

1. **RATE**

   Atrial:

   Ventricular:

2. **RHYTHM**

   Atrial:

   Ventricular:

3. **WAVES**

   P waves present:

      Appearance:

      Consistent:

      Relation to QRS:

   Q waves present:

      Leads:

      Pathological:

   T waves present:

      Morphology:

4. **INTERVALS**

   P-R interval:

      Consistent:

   QRS:

      Appearance:

      Consistent:

   Q-T interval:

5. **AXIS**

   Quadrant:

   Degrees:

6. **HYPERTROPHY**

   Atrial:

   Ventricular:

7. **MYOCARDIAL INFARCTION**

   Q waves:

   S-T displacement:

8. **ISCHEMIA**

   S-T displacement:

9. **POSSIBLE DRUG EFFECTS**

10. **ECG ANALYSIS**

11. **INTERPRETATION**

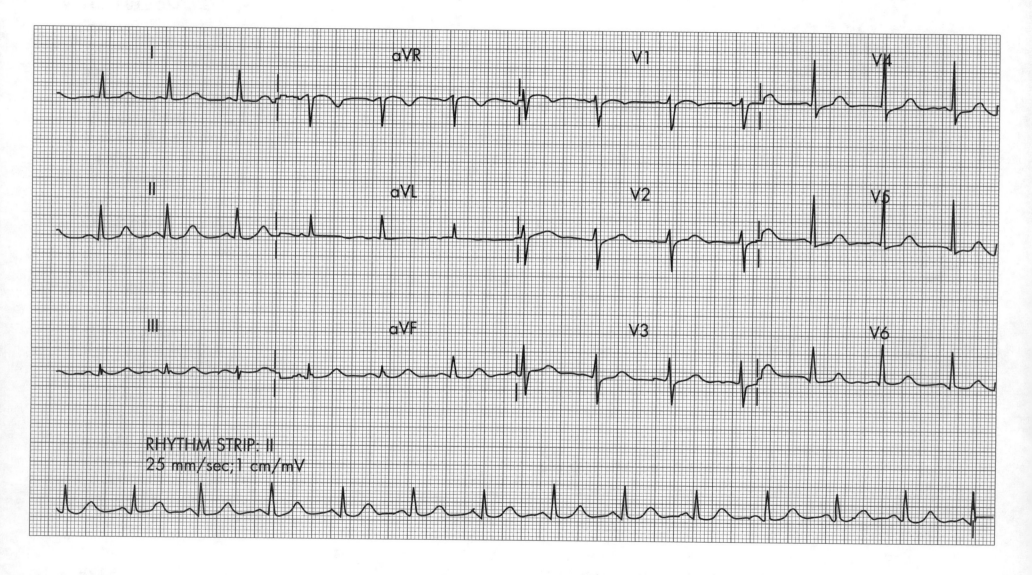

Figure 2-30
Resting 12-Lead ECG

1. RATE

Atrial:

Ventricular:

2. RHYTHM

Atrial:

Ventricular:

3. WAVES

P waves present:

Appearance:

Consistent:

Relation to QRS:

Q waves present:

Leads:

Pathological:

T waves present:

Morphology:

4. INTERVALS

P-R interval:

Consistent:

QRS:

Appearance:

Consistent:

Q-T interval:

5. AXIS

Quadrant:

Degrees:

6. HYPERTROPHY

Atrial:

Ventricular:

7. MYOCARDIAL INFARCTION

Q waves:

S-T displacement:

8. ISCHEMIA

S-T displacement:

9. POSSIBLE DRUG EFFECTS

10. ECG ANALYSIS

11. INTERPRETATION

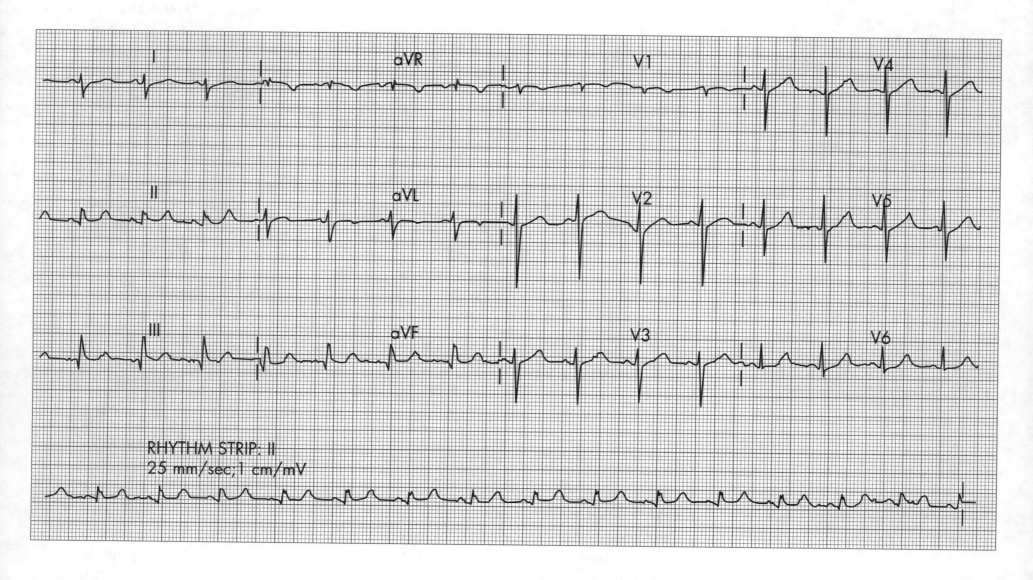

Figure 2-31
Resting 12-Lead ECG

1. **RATE**

   Atrial:

   Ventricular:

2. **RHYTHM**

   Atrial:

   Ventricular:

3. **WAVES**

   P waves present:

       Appearance:

       Consistent:

       Relation to QRS:

   Q waves present:

       Leads:

       Pathological:

   T waves present:

       Morphology:

4. **INTERVALS**

   P-R interval:

       Consistent:

   QRS:

       Appearance:

       Consistent:

   Q-T interval:

5. **AXIS**

   Quadrant:

   Degrees:

6. **HYPERTROPHY**

   Atrial:

   Ventricular:

7. **MYOCARDIAL INFARCTION**

   Q waves:

   S-T displacement:

8. **ISCHEMIA**

   S-T displacement:

9. **POSSIBLE DRUG EFFECTS**

10. **ECG ANALYSIS**

11. **INTERPRETATION**

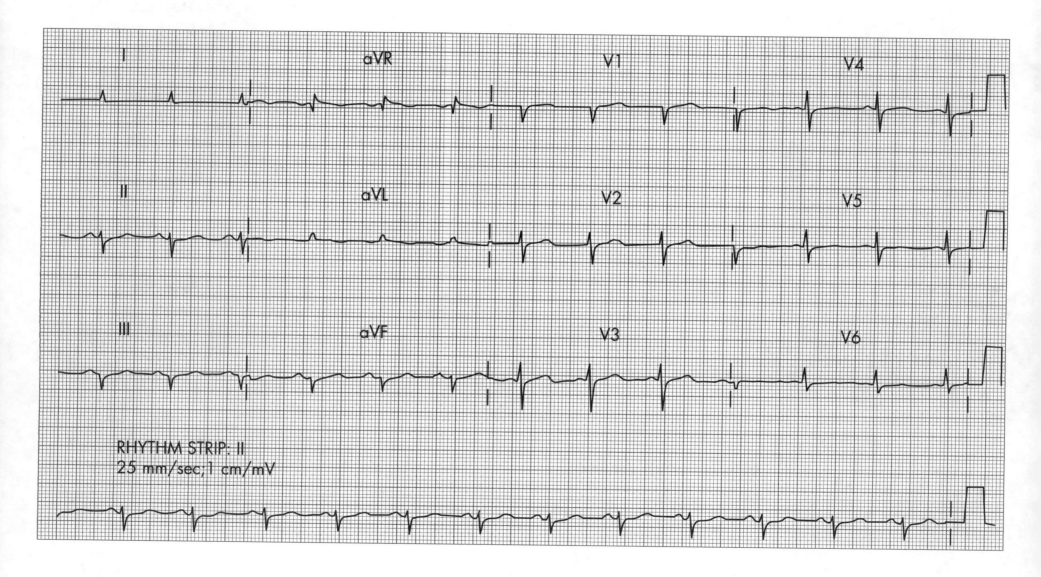

I aVR V1 V4

II aVL V2 V5

III aVF V3 V6

RHYTHM STRIP: II
25 mm/sec; 1 cm/mV

Figure 2-32
Resting 12-Lead ECG

I. RATE

Atrial:

Ventricular:

2. RHYTHM

Atrial:

Ventricular:

3. WAVES

P waves present:

Appearance:

Consistent:

Relation to QRS:

Q waves present:

Leads:

Pathological:

T waves present:

Morphology:

4. INTERVALS

P-R interval:

Consistent:

QRS:

Appearance:

Consistent:

Q-T interval:

5. AXIS

Quadrant:

Degrees:

6. HYPERTROPHY

Atrial:

Ventricular:

7. MYOCARDIAL INFARCTION

Q waves:

S-T displacement:

8. ISCHEMIA

S-T displacement:

9. POSSIBLE DRUG EFFECTS

10. ECG ANALYSIS

11. INTERPRETATION

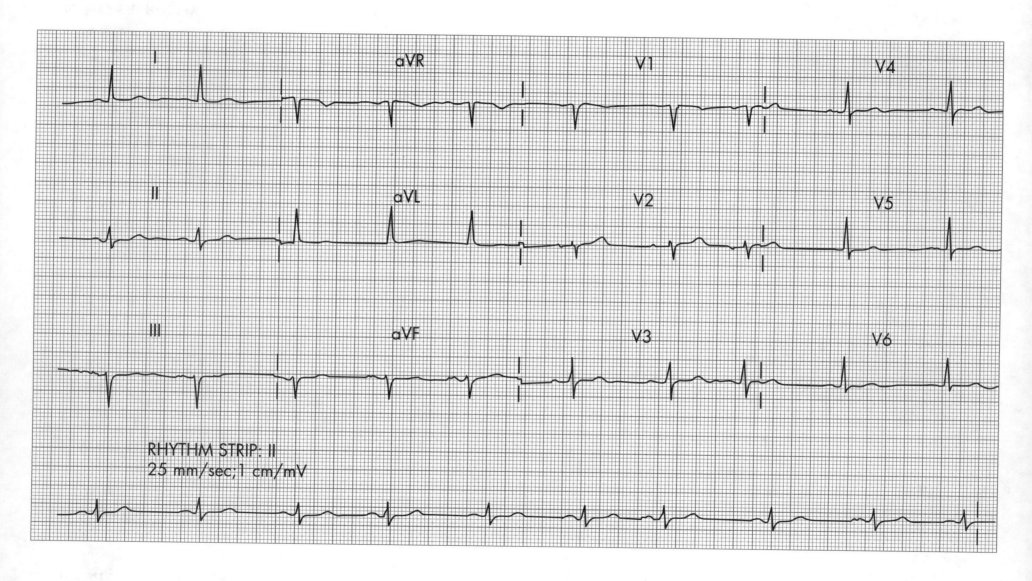

Figure 2-33
Resting 12-Lead ECG

1. RATE

Atrial:

Ventricular:

2. RHYTHM

Atrial:

Ventricular:

3. WAVES

P waves present:

Appearance:

Consistent:

Relation to QRS:

Q waves present:

Leads:

Pathological:

T waves present:

Morphology:

4. INTERVALS

P-R interval:

Consistent:

QRS:

Appearance:

Consistent:

Q-T interval:

5. AXIS

Quadrant:

Degrees:

6. HYPERTROPHY

Atrial:

Ventricular:

7. MYOCARDIAL INFARCTION

Q waves:

S-T displacement:

8. ISCHEMIA

S-T displacement:

9. POSSIBLE DRUG EFFECTS

10. ECG ANALYSIS

11. INTERPRETATION

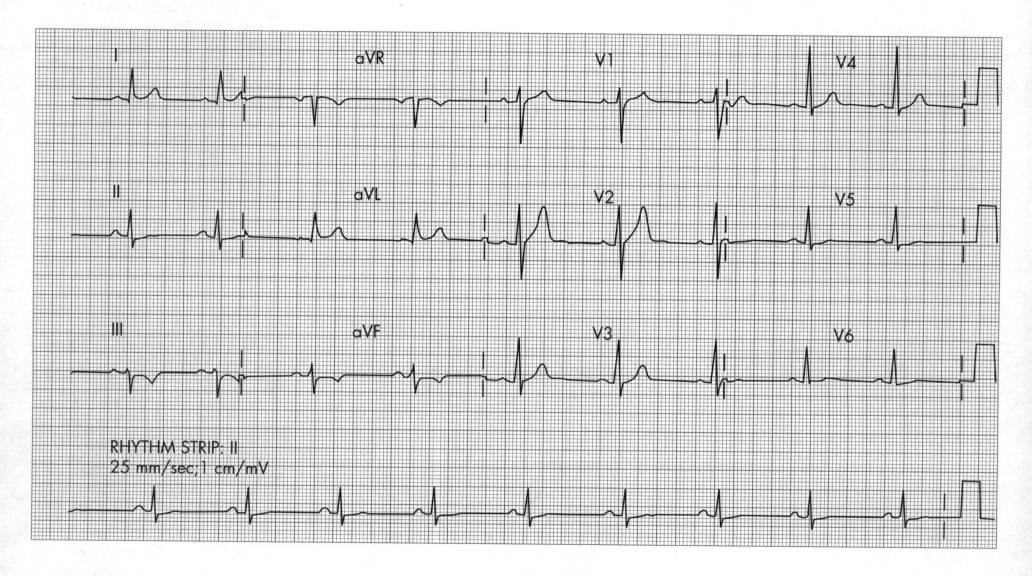

Figure 2-34
Resting 12-Lead ECG

74

1. RATE

Atrial:

Ventricular:

2. RHYTHM

Atrial:

Ventricular:

3. WAVES

P waves present:

Appearance:

Consistent:

Relation to QRS:

Q waves present:

Leads:

Pathological:

T waves present:

Morphology:

4. INTERVALS

P-R interval:

Consistent:

QRS:

Appearance:

Consistent:

Q-T interval:

5. AXIS

Quadrant:

Degrees:

6. HYPERTROPHY

Atrial:

Ventricular:

7. MYOCARDIAL INFARCTION

Q waves:

S-T displacement:

8. ISCHEMIA

S-T displacement:

9. POSSIBLE DRUG EFFECTS

10. ECG ANALYSIS

11. INTERPRETATION

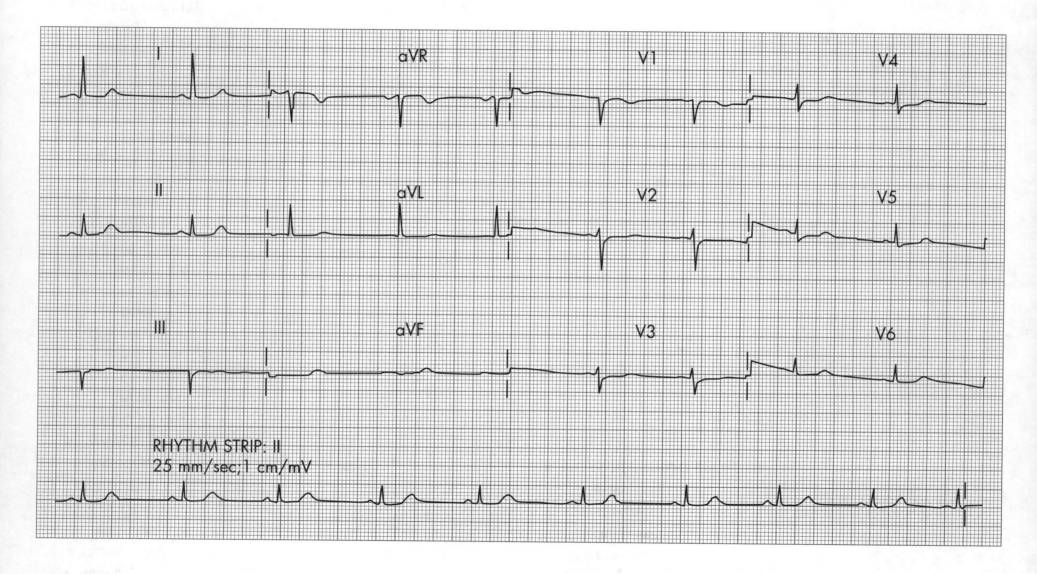

Figure 2-35
Resting 12-Lead ECG
76

1. RATE

Atrial:

Ventricular:

2. RHYTHM

Atrial:

Ventricular:

3. WAVES

P waves present:

Appearance:

Consistent:

Relation to QRS:

Q waves present:

Leads:

Pathological:

T waves present:

Morphology:

4. INTERVALS

P-R interval:

Consistent:

QRS:

Appearance:

Consistent:

Q-T interval:

5. AXIS

Quadrant:

Degrees:

6. HYPERTROPHY

Atrial:

Ventricular:

7. MYOCARDIAL INFARCTION

Q waves:

S-T displacement:

8. ISCHEMIA

S-T d splacement:

9. POSSIBLE DRUG EFFECTS

10. ECG ANALYSIS

11. INTERPRETATION

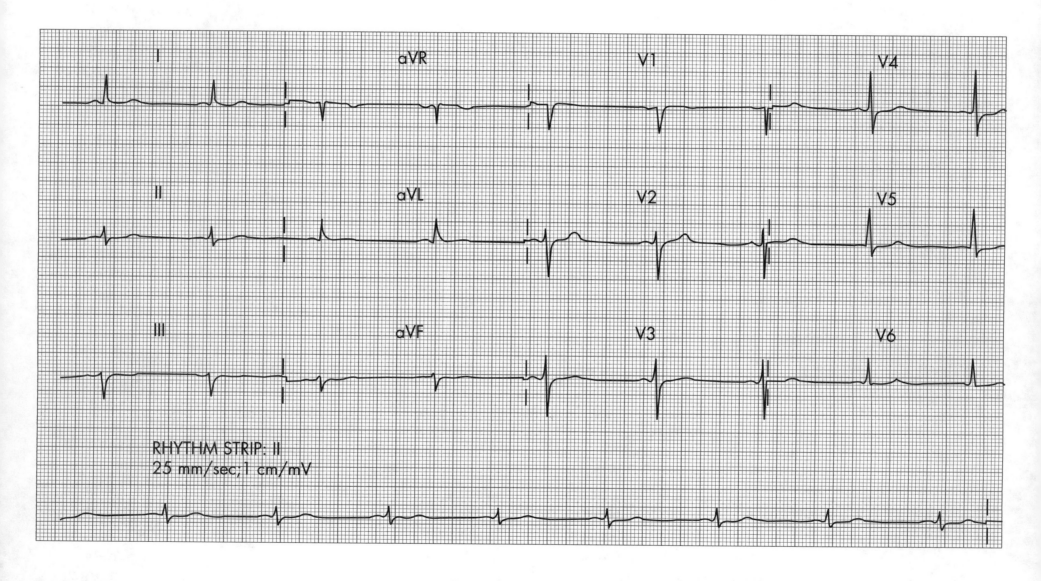

Figure 2-36
Resting 12-Lead ECG

1. **RATE**

   Atrial:

   Ventricular:

2. **RHYTHM**

   Atrial:

   Ventricular:

3. **WAVES**

   P waves present:

   Appearance:

   Consistent:

   Relation to QRS:

   Q waves present:

   Leads:

   Pathological:

   T waves present:

   Morphology:

4. **INTERVALS**

   P-R interval:

   Consistent:

   QRS:

   Appearance:

   Consistent:

   Q-T interval:

5. **AXIS**

   Quadrant:

   Degrees:

6. **HYPERTROPHY**

   Atrial:

   Ventricular:

7. **MYOCARDIAL INFARCTION**

   Q waves:

   S-T displacement:

8. **ISCHEMIA**

   S-T displacement:

9. **POSSIBLE DRUG EFFECTS**

10. **ECG ANALYSIS**

11. **INTERPRETATION**

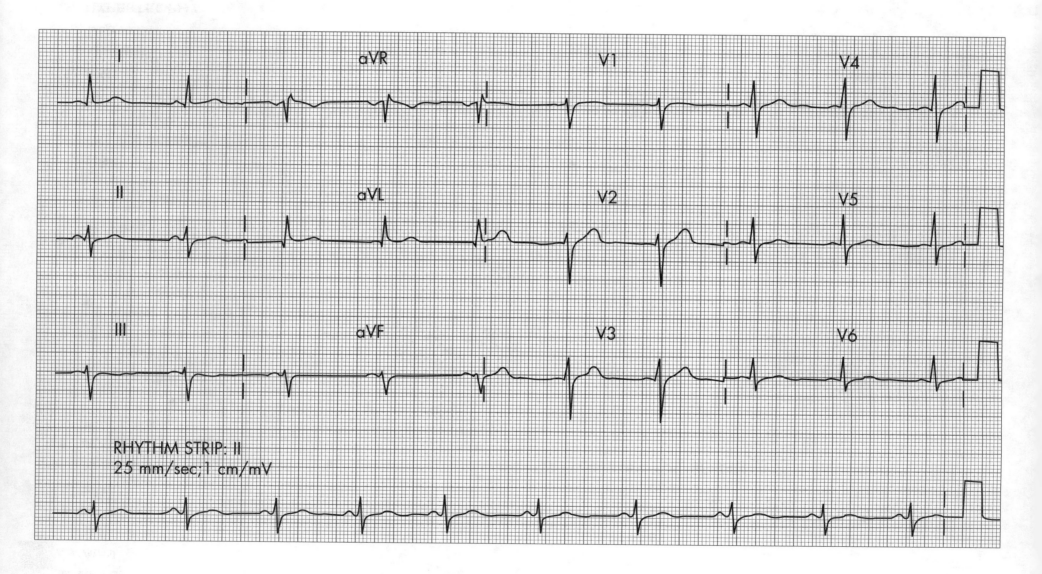

I   aVR   V1   V4

II   aVL   V2   V5

III   aVF   V3   V6

RHYTHM STRIP: II
25 mm/sec;1 cm/mV

Figure 2-37
Resting 12-Lead ECG

1. **RATE**

   Atrial:

   Ventricular:

2. **RHYTHM**

   Atrial:

   Ventricular:

3. **WAVES**

   P waves present:

   Appearance:

   Consistent:

   Relation to QRS:

   Q waves present:

   Leads:

   Pathological:

   T waves present:

   Morphology:

4. **INTERVALS**

   P-R interval:

   Consistent:

   QRS:

   Appearance:

   Consistent:

   Q-T interval:

5. **AXIS**

   Quadrant:

   Degrees:

6. **HYPERTROPHY**

   Atrial:

   Ventricular:

7. **MYOCARDIAL INFARCTION**

   Q waves:

   S-T displacement:

8. **ISCHEMIA**

   S-T displacement:

9. **POSSIBLE DRUG EFFECTS**

10. **ECG ANALYSIS**

11. **INTERPRETATION**

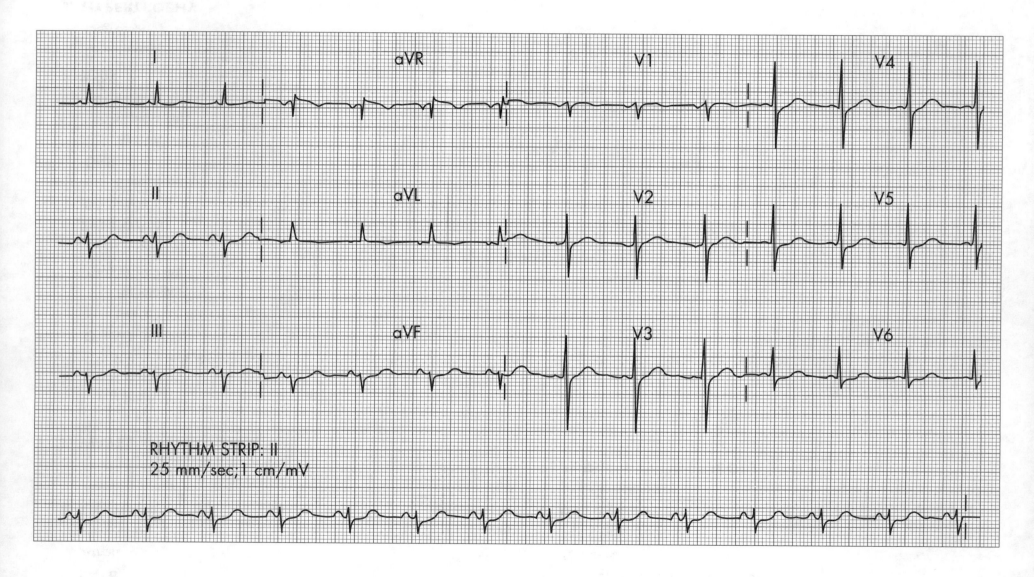

I aVR V1 V4

II aVL V2 V5

III aVF V3 V6

RHYTHM STRIP: II
25 mm/sec; 1 cm/mV

Figure 2-38
Resting 12-Lead ECG

82

1. RATE

Atrial:

Ventricular:

2. RHYTHM

Atrial:

Ventricular:

3. WAVES

P waves present:

Appearance:

Consistent:

Relation to QRS:

Q waves present:

Leads:

Pathological:

T waves present:

Morphology:

4. INTERVALS

P-R interval:

Consistent:

QRS:

Appearance:

Consistent:

Q-T interval:

5. AXIS

Quadrant:

Degrees:

6. HYPERTROPHY

Atrial:

Ventricular:

7. MYOCARDIAL INFARCTION

Q waves:

S-T displacement:

8. ISCHEMIA

S-T displacement:

9. POSSIBLE DRUG EFFECTS

10. ECG ANALYSIS

11. INTERPRETATION

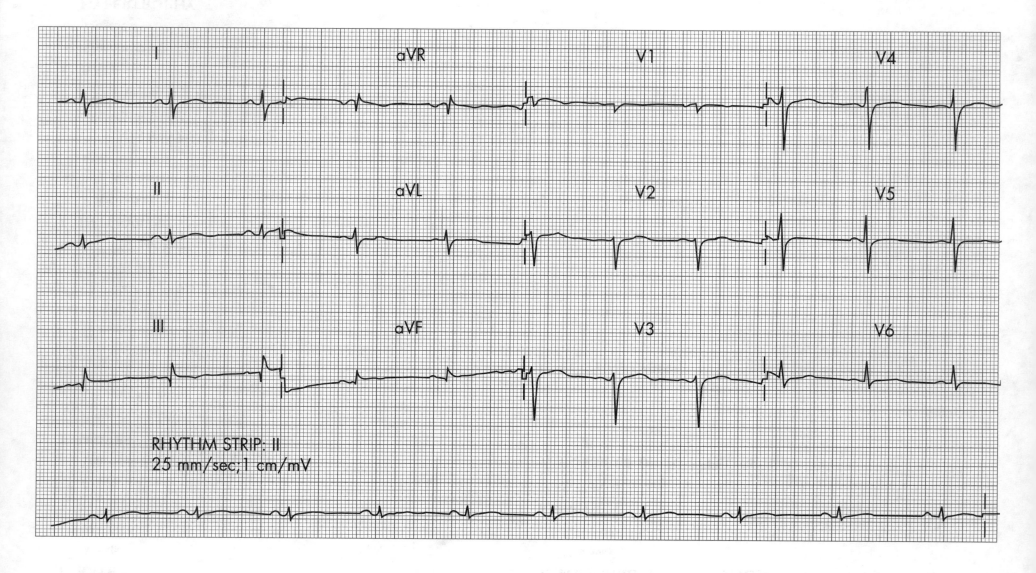

Figure 2-39
Resting 12-Lead ECG

1. RATE

Atrial:

Ventricular:

2. RHYTHM

Atrial:

Ventricular:

3. WAVES

P waves present:

    Appearance:

    Consistent:

    Relation to QRS:

Q waves present:

    Leads:

    Pathological:

T waves present:

    Morphology:

4. INTERVALS

P-R interval:

    Consistent:

QRS:

    Appearance:

    Consistent:

Q-T interval:

5. AXIS

Quadrant:

Degrees:

6. HYPERTROPHY

Atrial:

Ventricular:

7. MYOCARDIAL INFARCTION

Q waves:

S-T displacement:

8. ISCHEMIA

S-T displacement:

9. POSSIBLE DRUG EFFECTS

10. ECG ANALYSIS

11. INTERPRETATION

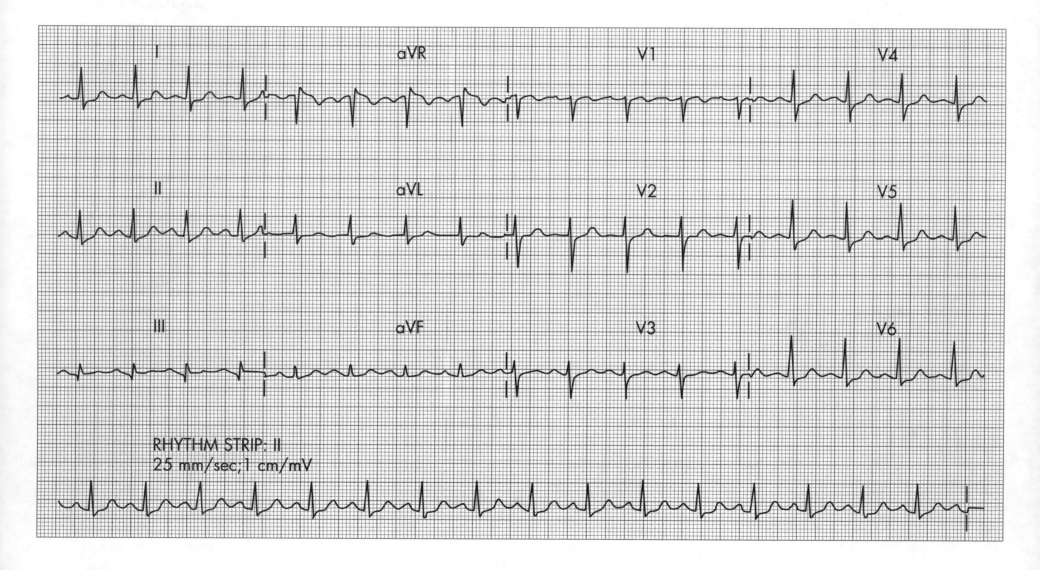

Figure 2-40
Resting 12-Lead ECG

1. **RATE**

   Atrial:

   Ventricular:

2. **RHYTHM**

   Atrial:

   Ventricular:

3. **WAVES**

   P waves present:

       Appearance:

       Consistent:

       Relation to QRS:

   Q waves present:

       Leads:

       Pathological:

   T waves present:

       Morphology:

4. **INTERVALS**

   P-R interval:

       Consistent:

   QRS:

       Appearance:

       Consistent:

   Q-T interval:

5. **AXIS**

   Quadrant:

   Degrees:

6. **HYPERTROPHY**

   Atrial:

   Ventricular:

7. **MYOCARDIAL INFARCTION**

   Q waves:

   S-T displacement:

8. **ISCHEMIA**

   S-T displacement:

9. **POSSIBLE DRUG EFFECTS**

10. **ECG ANALYSIS**

11. **INTERPRETATION**

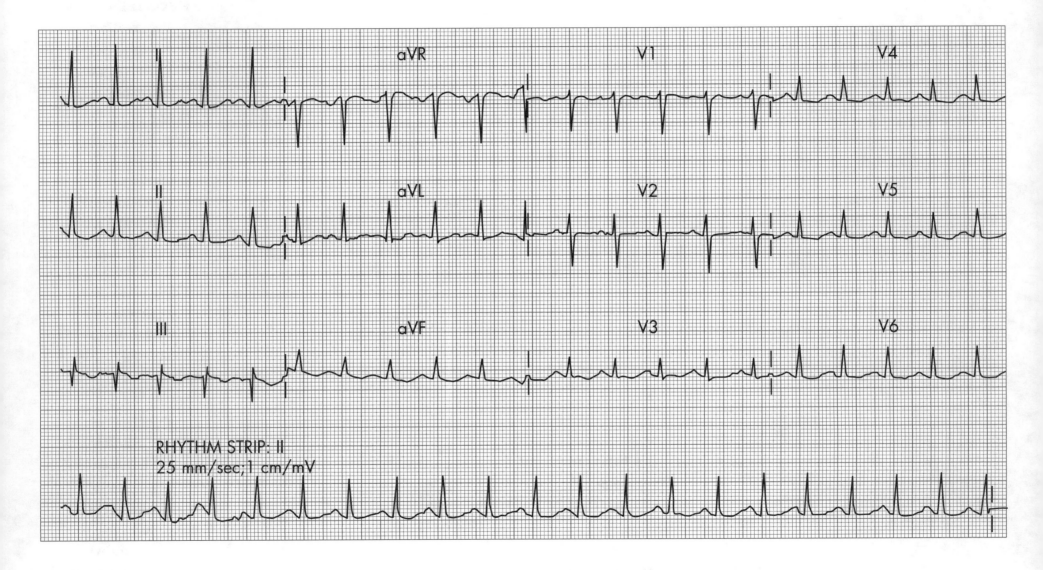

aVR V1 V4

II aVL V2 V5

III aVF V3 V6

RHYTHM STRIP: II
25 mm/sec;1 cm/mV

Figure 2-41
Resting 12-Lead ECG

88

1. RATE

    Atrial:

    Ventricular:

2. RHYTHM

    Atrial:

    Ventricular:

3. WAVES

    P waves present:

        Appearance:

        Consistent:

        Relation to QRS:

    Q waves present:

        Leads:

        Pathological:

    T waves present:

        Morphology:

4. INTERVALS

    P-R interval:

        Consistent:

    QRS:

        Appearance:

        Consistent:

    Q-T interval:

5. AXIS

    Quadrant:

    Degrees:

6. HYPERTROPHY

    Atrial:

    Ventricular:

7. MYOCARDIAL INFARCTION

    Q waves:

    S-T displacement:

8. ISCHEMIA

    S-T displacement:

9. POSSIBLE DRUG EFFECTS

10. ECG ANALYSIS

11. INTERPRETATION

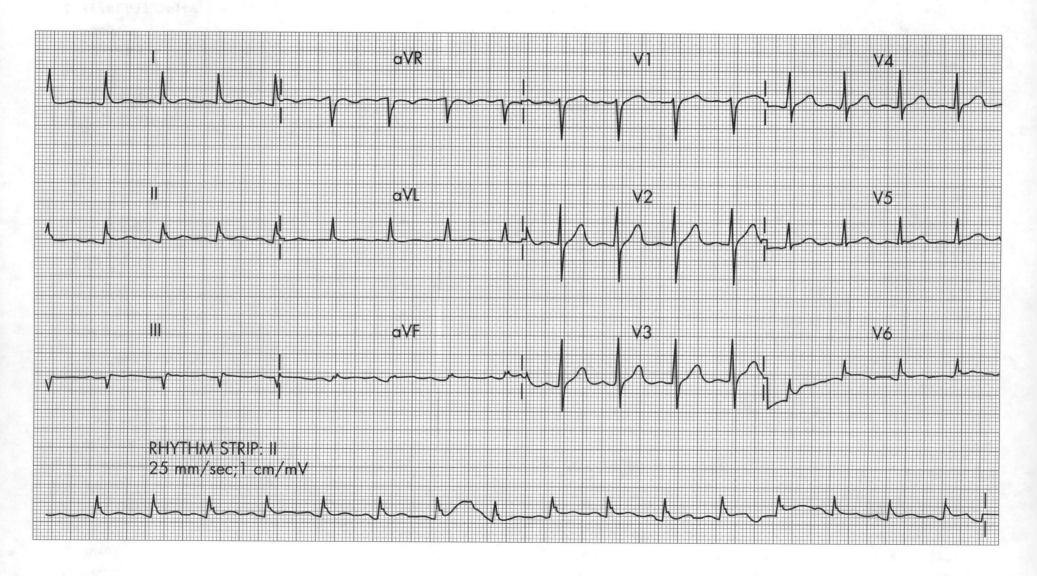

Figure 2-42
Resting 12-Lead ECG

I. RATE

Atrial:

Ventricular:

2. RHYTHM

Atrial:

Ventricular:

3. WAVES

P waves present:

    Appearance:

    Consistent:

    Relation to QRS:

Q waves present:

    Leads:

    Pathological:

T waves present:

    Morphology:

4. INTERVALS

P-R interval:

    Consistent:

QRS:

    Appearance:

    Consistent:

Q-T interval:

5. AXIS

Quadrant:

Degrees:

6. HYPERTROPHY

Atrial:

Ventricular:

7. MYOCARDIAL INFARCTION

Q waves:

S-T displacement:

8. ISCHEMIA

S-T displacement:

9. POSSIBLE DRUG EFFECTS

10. ECG ANALYSIS

11. INTERPRETATION

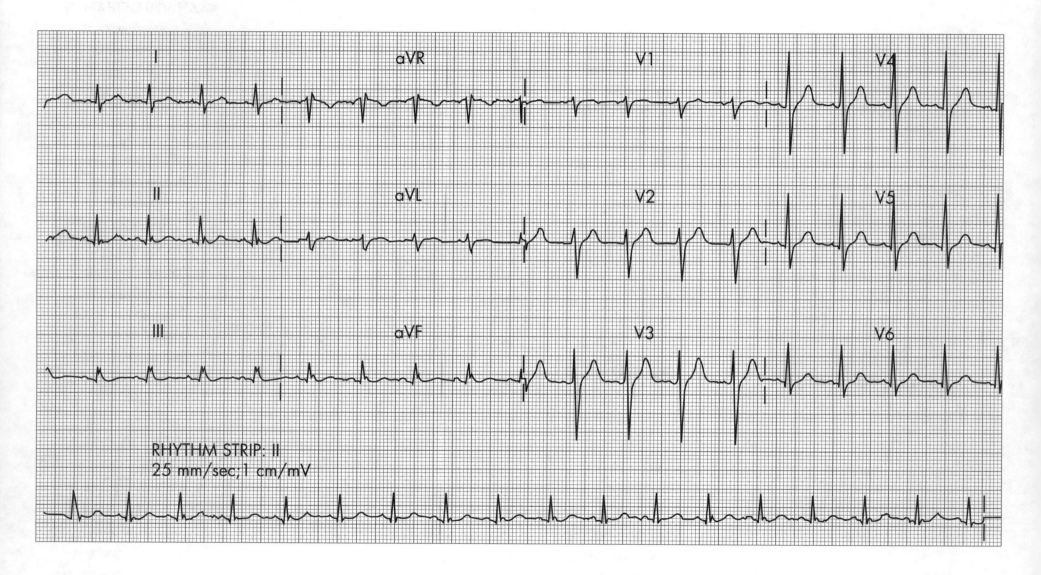

I aVR V1 V4

II aVL V2 V5

III aVF V3 V6

RHYTHM STRIP: II
25 mm/sec; 1 cm/mV

Figure 2-43
Resting 12-Lead ECG

92

1. **RATE**

    Atrial:

    Ventricular:

2. **RHYTHM**

    Atrial:

    Ventricular:

3. **WAVES**

    P waves present:

        Appearance:

        Consistent:

        Relation to QRS:

    Q waves present:

        Leads:

        Pathological:

    T waves present:

        Morphology:

4. **INTERVALS**

    P-R interval:

        Consistent:

    QRS:

        Appearance:

        Consistent:

    Q-T interval:

5. **AXIS**

    Quadrant:

    Degrees:

6. **HYPERTROPHY**

    Atrial:

    Ventricular:

7. **MYOCARDIAL INFARCTION**

    Q waves:

    S-T displacement:

8. **ISCHEMIA**

    S-T displacement:

9. **POSSIBLE DRUG EFFECTS**

10. **ECG ANALYSIS**

11. **INTERPRETATION**

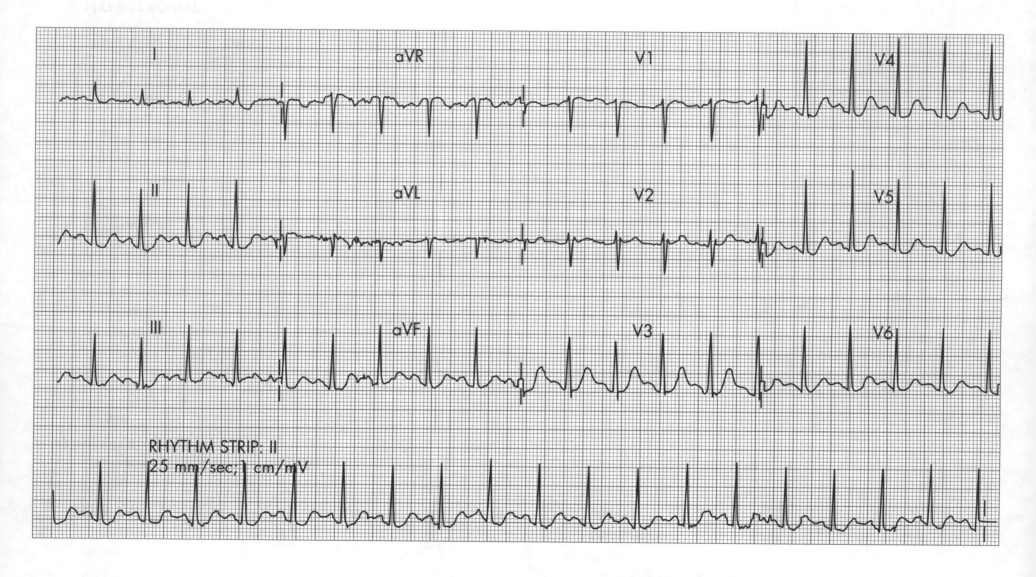

Figure 2-44
Resting 12-Lead ECG

I. RATE

Atrial:

Ventricular:

2. RHYTHM

Atrial:

Ventricular:

3. WAVES

P waves present:

Appearance:

Consistent:

Relation to QRS:

Q waves present:

Leads:

Pathological:

T waves present:

Morphology:

4. INTERVALS

P-R interval:

Consistent:

QRS:

Appearance:

Consistent:

Q-T interval:

5. AXIS

Quadrant:

Degrees:

6. HYPERTROPHY

Atrial:

Ventricular:

7. MYOCARDIAL INFARCTION

Q waves:

S-T displacement:

8. ISCHEMIA

S-T displacement:

9. POSSIBLE DRUG EFFECTS

10. ECG ANALYSIS

11. INTERPRETATION

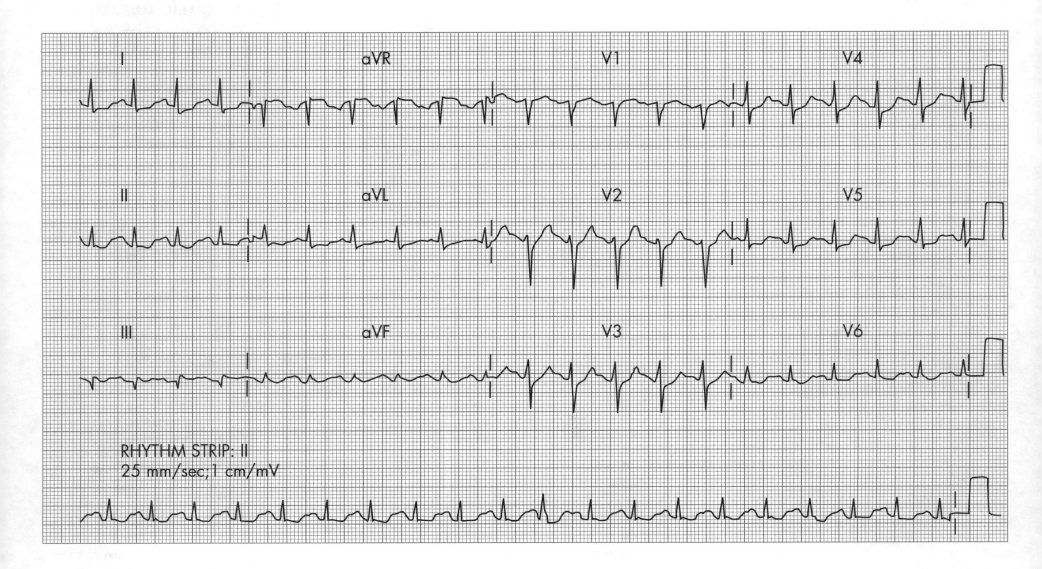

Figure 2-45
Resting 12-Lead ECG

1. **RATE**

   Atrial:

   Ventricular:

2. **RHYTHM**

   Atrial:

   Ventricular:

3. **WAVES**

   P waves present:

   Appearance:

   Consistent:

   Relation to QRS:

   Q waves present:

   Leads:

   Pathological:

   T waves present:

   Morphology:

4. **INTERVALS**

   P-R interval:

   Consistent:

   QRS:

   Appearance:

   Consistent:

   Q-T interval:

5. **AXIS**

   Quadrant:

   Degrees:

6. **HYPERTROPHY**

   Atrial:

   Ventricular:

7. **MYOCARDIAL INFARCTION**

   Q waves:

   S-T displacement:

8. **ISCHEMIA**

   S-T displacement:

9. **POSSIBLE DRUG EFFECTS**

10. **ECG ANALYSIS**

11. **INTERPRETATION**

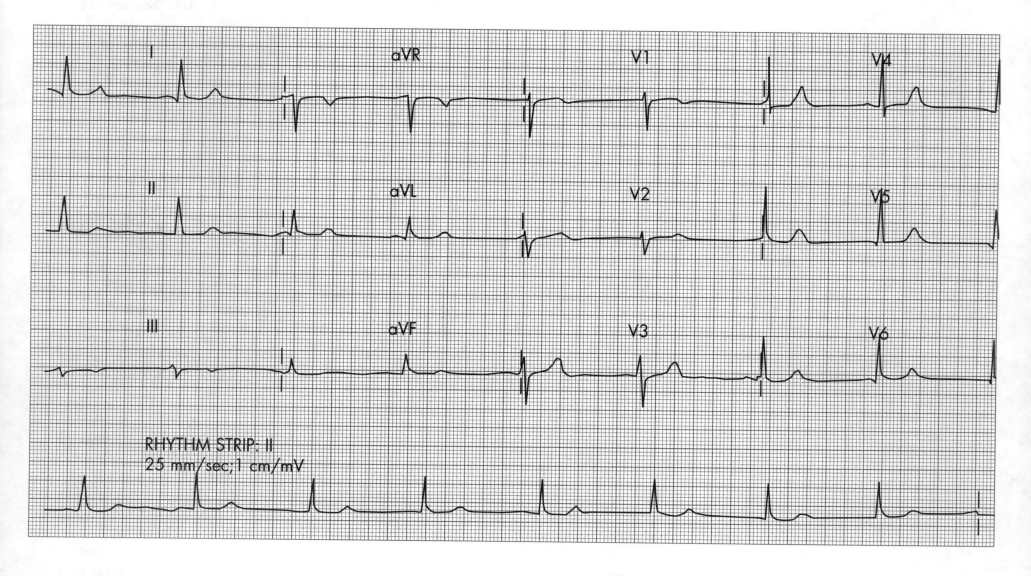

I   aVR   V1   V4

II   aVL   V2   V5

III   aVF   V3   V6

RHYTHM STRIP: II
25 mm/sec; 1 cm/mV

Figure 2-46
Resting 12-Lead ECG

1. **RATE**

   Atrial:

   Ventricular:

2. **RHYTHM**

   Atrial:

   Ventricular:

3. **WAVES**

   P waves present:

       Appearance:

       Consistent:

       Relation to QRS:

   Q waves present:

       Leads:

       Pathological:

   T waves present:

       Morphology:

4. **INTERVALS**

   P-R interval:

       Consistent:

   QRS:

       Appearance:

       Consistent:

   Q-T interval:

5. **AXIS**

   Quadrant:

   Degrees:

6. **HYPERTROPHY**

   Atrial:

   Ventricular:

7. **MYOCARDIAL INFARCTION**

   Q waves:

   S-T displacement:

8. **ISCHEMIA**

   S-T displacement:

9. **POSSIBLE DRUG EFFECTS**

10. **ECG ANALYSIS**

11. **INTERPRETATION**

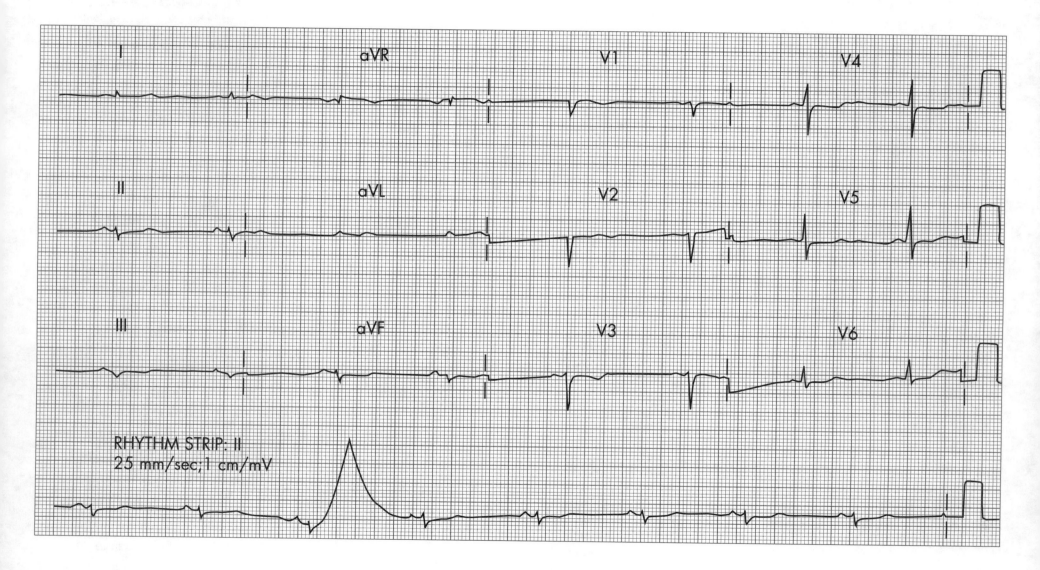

Figure 2-47
Resting 12-Lead ECG
100

1. RATE

Atrial:

Ventricular:

2. RHYTHM

Atrial:

Ventricular:

3. WAVES

P waves present:

Appearance:

Consistent:

Relation to QRS:

Q waves present:

Leads:

Pathological:

T waves present:

Morphology:

4. INTERVALS

P-R interval:

Consistent:

QRS:

Appearance:

Consistent:

Q-T interval:

5. AXIS

Quadrant:

Degrees:

6. HYPERTROPHY

Atrial:

Ventricular:

7. MYOCARDIAL INFARCTION

Q waves:

S-T displacement:

8. ISCHEMIA

S-T displacement:

9. POSSIBLE DRUG EFFECTS

10. ECG ANALYSIS

11. INTERPRETATION

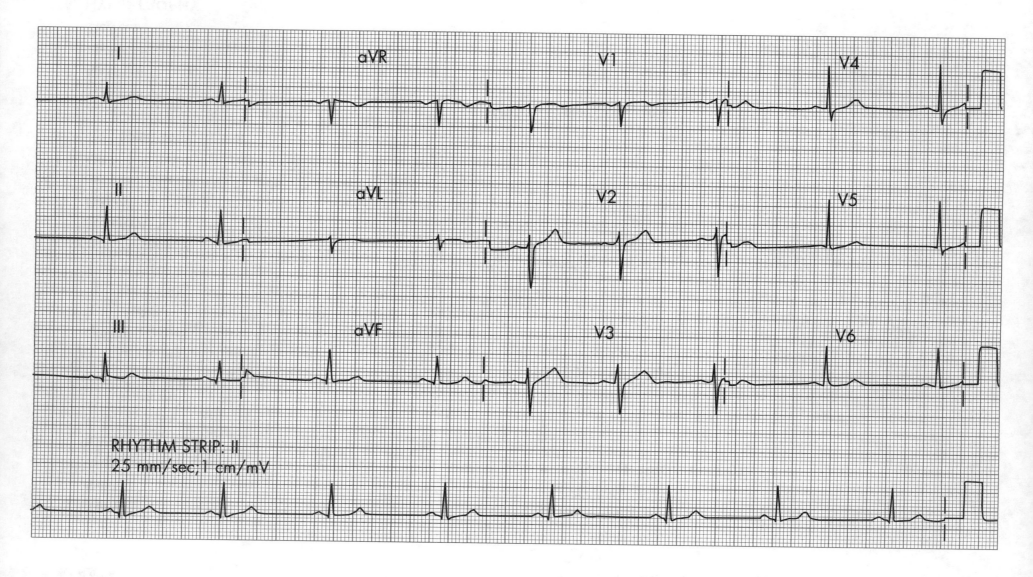

I

aVR

V1

V4

II

aVL

V2

V5

III

aVF

V3

V6

RHYTHM STRIP: II
25 mm/sec; 1 cm/mV

Figure 2-48
Resting 12-Lead ECG

102

1. RATE

Atrial:

Ventricular:

2. RHYTHM

Atrial:

Ventricular:

3. WAVES

P waves present:

Appearance:

Consistent:

Relation to QRS:

Q waves present:

Leads:

Pathological:

T waves present:

Morphology:

4. INTERVALS

P-R interval:

Consistent:

QRS:

Appearance:

Consistent:

Q-T interval:

5. AXIS

Quadrant:

Degrees:

6. HYPERTROPHY

Atrial:

Ventricular:

7. MYOCARDIAL INFARCTION

Q waves:

S-T displacement:

8. ISCHEMIA

S-T displacement:

9. POSSIBLE DRUG EFFECTS

10. ECG ANALYSIS

11. INTERPRETATION

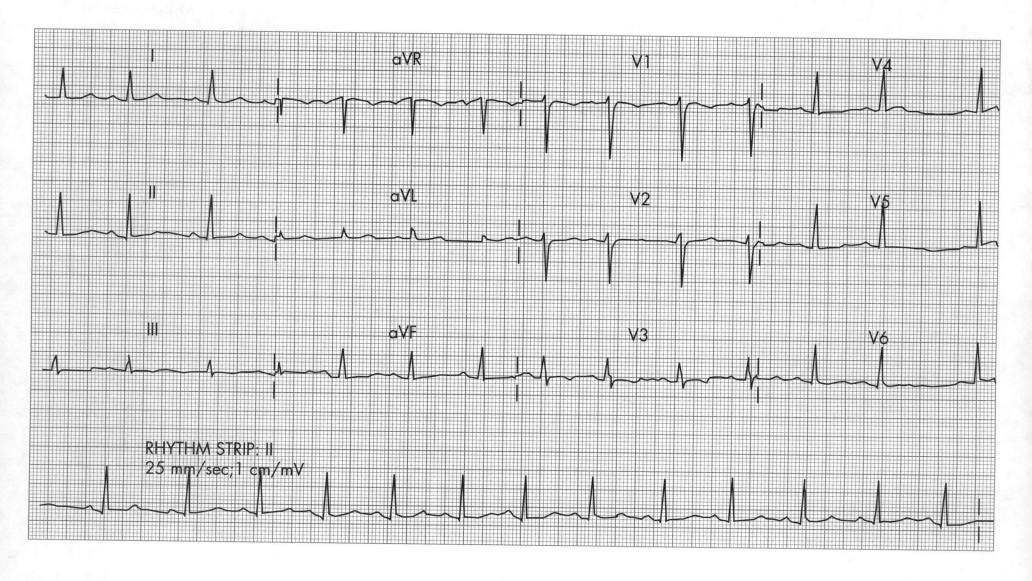

I aVR V1 V4

II aVL V2 V5

III aVF V3 V6

RHYTHM STRIP: II
25 mm/sec; 1 cm/mV

Figure 2-49
Resting 12-Lead ECG
104

1. RATE

Atrial:

Ventricular:

2. RHYTHM

Atrial:

Ventricular:

3. WAVES

P waves present:

    Appearance:

    Consistent:

    Relation to QRS:

Q waves present:

    Leads:

    Pathological:

T waves present:

    Morphology:

4. INTERVALS

P-R interval:

    Consistent:

QRS:

    Appearance:

    Consistent:

Q-T interval:

5. AXIS

Quadrant:

Degrees:

6. HYPERTROPHY

Atrial:

Ventricular:

7. MYOCARDIAL INFARCTION

Q waves:

S-T displacement:

8. ISCHEMIA

S-T displacement:

9. POSSIBLE DRUG EFFECTS

10. ECG ANALYSIS

11. INTERPRETATION

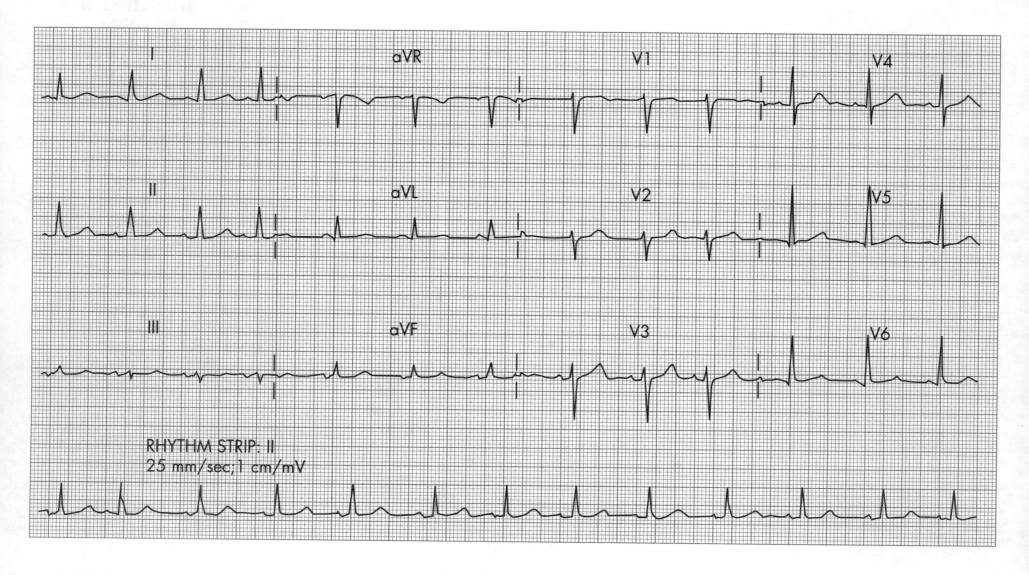

I aVR V1 V4

II aVL V2 V5

III aVF V3 V6

RHYTHM STRIP: II
25 mm/sec;1 cm/mV

Figure 2-50
Resting 12-Lead ECG

1. RATE

Atrial:

Ventricular:

2. RHYTHM

Atrial:

Ventricular:

3. WAVES

P waves present:

Appearance:

Consistent:

Relation to QRS:

Q waves present:

Leads:

Pathological:

T waves present:

Morphology:

4. INTERVALS

P-R interval:

Consistent:

QRS:

Appearance:

Consistent:

Q-T interval:

5. AXIS

Quadrant:

Degrees:

6. HYPERTROPHY

Atrial:

Ventricular:

7. MYOCARDIAL INFARCTION

Q waves:

S-T displacement:

8. ISCHEMIA

S-T displacement:

9. POSSIBLE DRUG EFFECTS

10. ECG ANALYSIS

11. INTERPRETATION

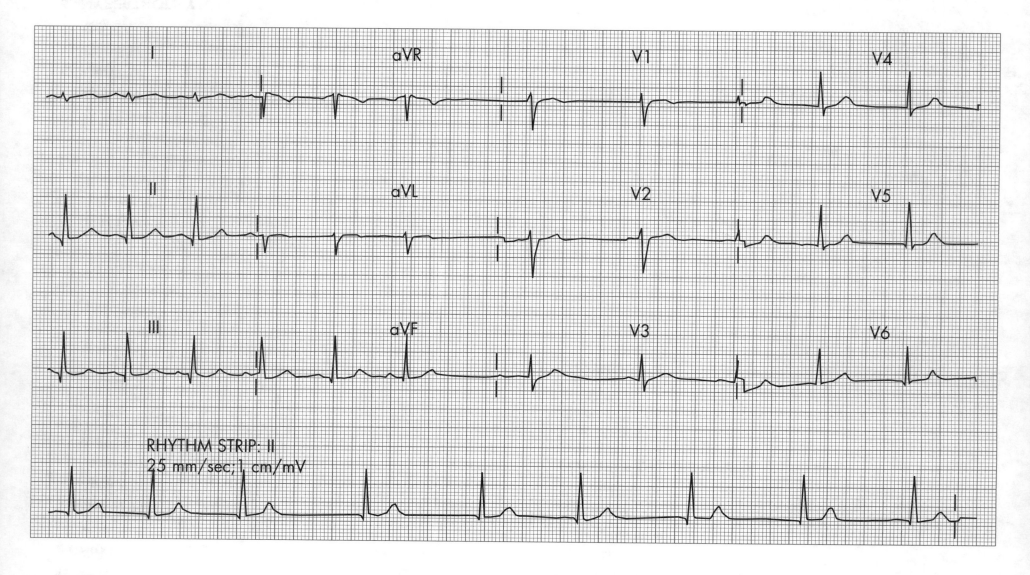

Figure 2-51
Resting 12-Lead ECG

108

1. **RATE**

   Atrial:

   Ventricular:

2. **RHYTHM**

   Atrial:

   Ventricular:

3. **WAVES**

   P waves present:

   Appearance:

   Consistent:

   Relation to QRS:

   Q waves present:

   Leads:

   Pathological:

   T waves present:

   Morphology:

4. **INTERVALS**

   P-R interval:

   Consistent:

   QRS:

   Appearance:

   Consistent:

   Q-T interval:

5. **AXIS**

   Quadrant:

   Degrees:

6. **HYPERTROPHY**

   Atrial:

   Ventricular:

7. **MYOCARDIAL INFARCTION**

   Q waves:

   S-T displacement:

8. **ISCHEMIA**

   S-T displacement:

9. **POSSIBLE DRUG EFFECTS**

10. **ECG ANALYSIS**

11. **INTERPRETATION**

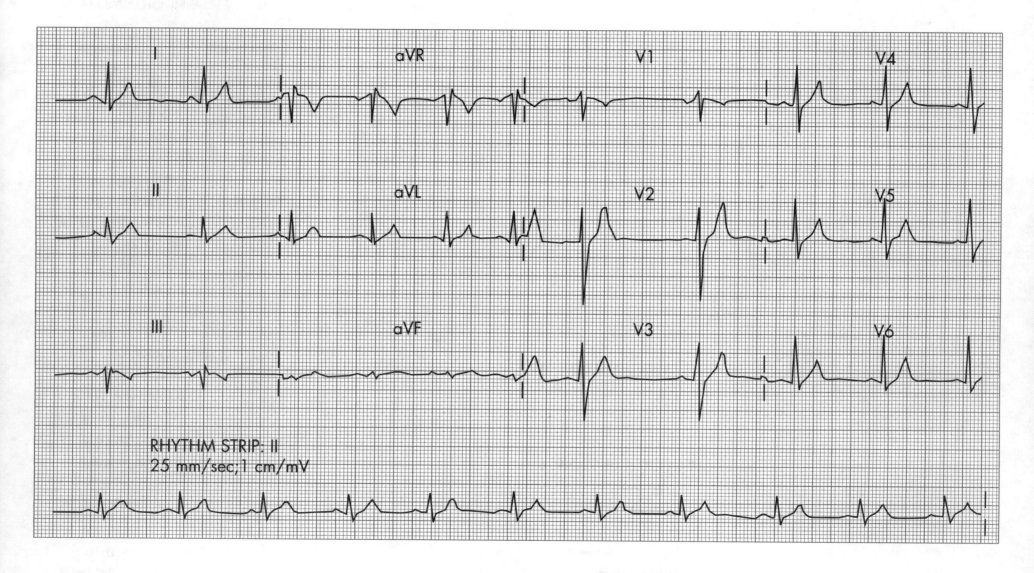

RHYTHM STRIP: II
25 mm/sec;1 cm/mV

Figure 2-52
Resting 12-Lead ECG

1. RATE

Atrial:

Ventricular:

2. RHYTHM

Atrial:

Ventricular:

3. WAVES

P waves present:

    Appearance:

    Consistent:

    Relation to QRS:

Q waves present:

    Leads:

    Pathological:

T waves present:

    Morphology:

4. INTERVALS

P-R interval:

    Consistent:

QRS:

    Appearance:

    Consistent:

Q-T interval:

5. AXIS

Quadrant:

Degrees:

6. HYPERTROPHY

Atrial:

Ventricular:

7. MYOCARDIAL INFARCTION

Q waves:

S-T displacement:

8. ISCHEMIA

S-T displacement:

9. POSSIBLE DRUG EFFECTS

10. ECG ANALYSIS

11. INTERPRETATION

Part III
Basic Dysrhythmias and Blocks

BASIC DYSRHYTHMIAS AND BLOCKS

Common Dysrhythmias

Dysrhythmias of the sinus node

Sinus tachycardia
Sinus bradycardia
Sinus arrhythmia
Sinus pause/arrest
Sinus exit block

Atrial dysrhythmias

Premature atrial contraction (PAC, APC)
Wandering atrial pacemaker (WAP)
Atrial tachycardia
Paroxysmal atrial tachycardia
Paroxysmal supraventricular tachycardia
Atrial flutter
Atrial fibrillation

Junctional dysrhythmias

Premature junctional contraction (PJC, PNC)
Junctional rhythm (slow or accelerated)
Junctional escape beats

Ventricular dysrhythmias

Premature ventricular contraction
Ventricular tachycardia
Ventricular fibrillation/flutter
Idioventricular rhythm (slow or accelerated)

Common Blocks

Atrioventricular blocks

First degree AV block (1° AVB)
Second degree AV block (2° AVB)
Type I (Wenchebach)
Type II
Third-degree AV block (3° AVB, complete heart block [CHB])

Bundle branch blocks and fascicular blocks

Right bundle branch block (RBBB)
Left bundle branch block (LBBB)
Left anterior fascicular block (left anterior hemiblock [LAHB])
Left posterior fascicular block (left posterior hemiblock [LPHB])
Bifascicular block (RBBB + LAHB or LPHB)

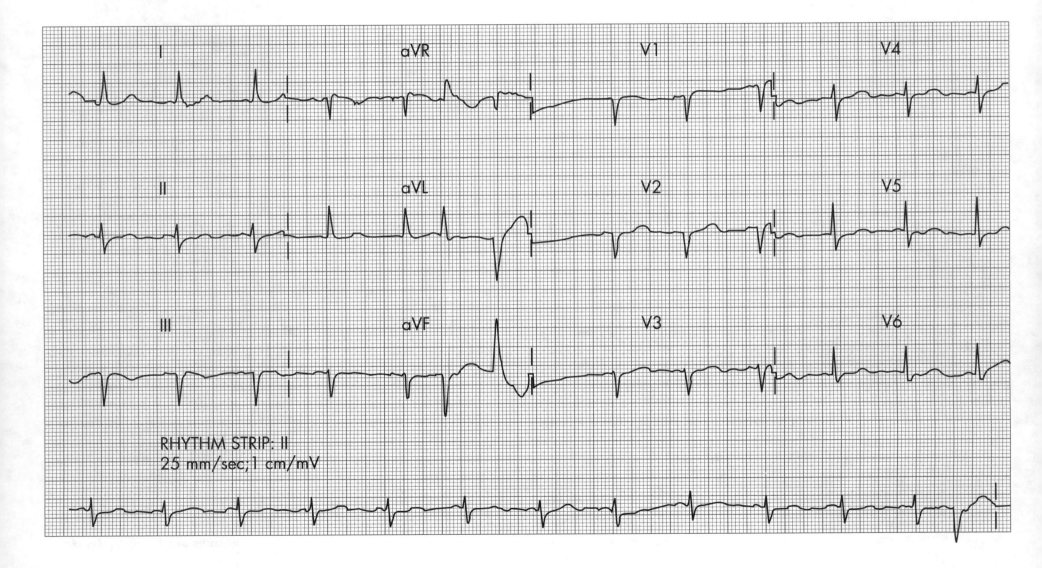

RHYTHM STRIP: II
25 mm/sec; 1 cm/mV

Figure 3-1
Resting 12-Lead ECG

1. RATE

    Atrial:

    Ventricular:

2. RHYTHM

    Atrial:

    Ventricular:

3. WAVES

    P waves present:

        Appearance:

        Consistent:

        Relation to QRS:

    Q waves present:

        Leads:

        Pathological:

    T waves present:

        Morphology:

4. INTERVALS

    P-R interval:

        Consistent:

    QRS:

        Appearance:

        Consistent:

    Q-T interval:

5. AXIS

    Quadrant:

    Degrees:

6. HYPERTROPHY

    Atrial:

    Ventricular:

7. MYOCARDIAL INFARCTION

    Q waves:

    S-T displacement:

8. ISCHEMIA

    S-T displacement:

9. POSSIBLE DRUG EFFECTS

10. ECG ANALYSIS

11. INTERPRETATION

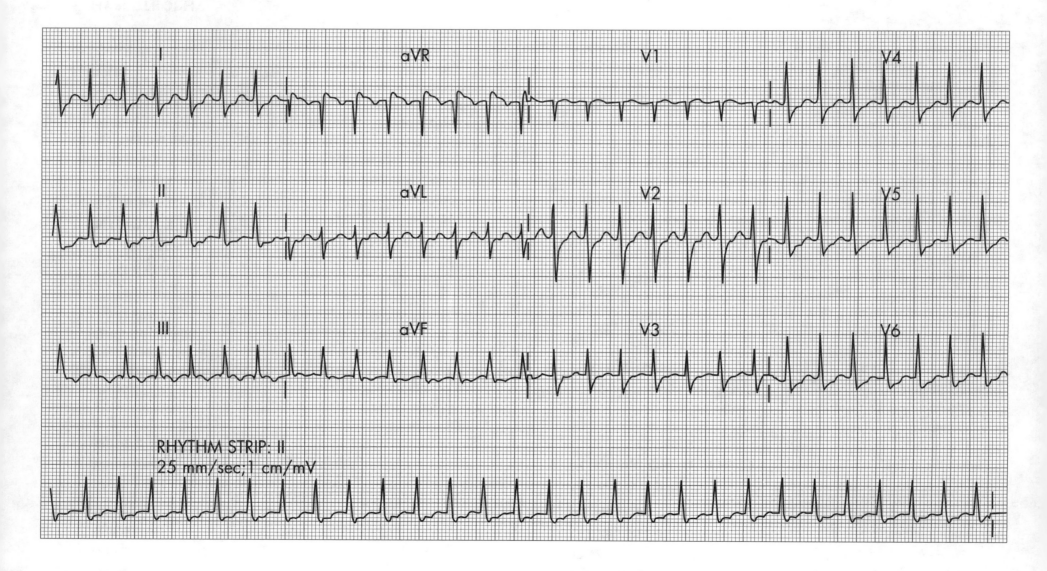

I aVR V1 V4

II aVL V2 V5

III aVF V3 V6

RHYTHM STRIP: II
25 mm/sec; 1 cm/mV

Figure 3-2
Resting 12-Lead ECG

118

1. **RATE**

   Atrial:

   Ventricular:

2. **RHYTHM**

   Atrial:

   Ventricular:

3. **WAVES**

   P waves present:

       Appearance:

       Consistent:

       Relation to QRS:

   Q waves present:

       Leads:

       Pathological:

   T waves present:

       Morphology:

4. **INTERVALS**

   P-R interval:

       Consistent:

   QRS:

       Appearance:

       Consistent:

   Q-T interval:

5. **AXIS**

   Quadrant:

   Degrees:

6. **HYPERTROPHY**

   Atrial:

   Ventricular:

7. **MYOCARDIAL INFARCTION**

   Q waves:

   S-T displacement:

8. **ISCHEMIA**

   S-T displacement:

9. **POSSIBLE DRUG EFFECTS**

10. **ECG ANALYSIS**

11. **INTERPRETATION**

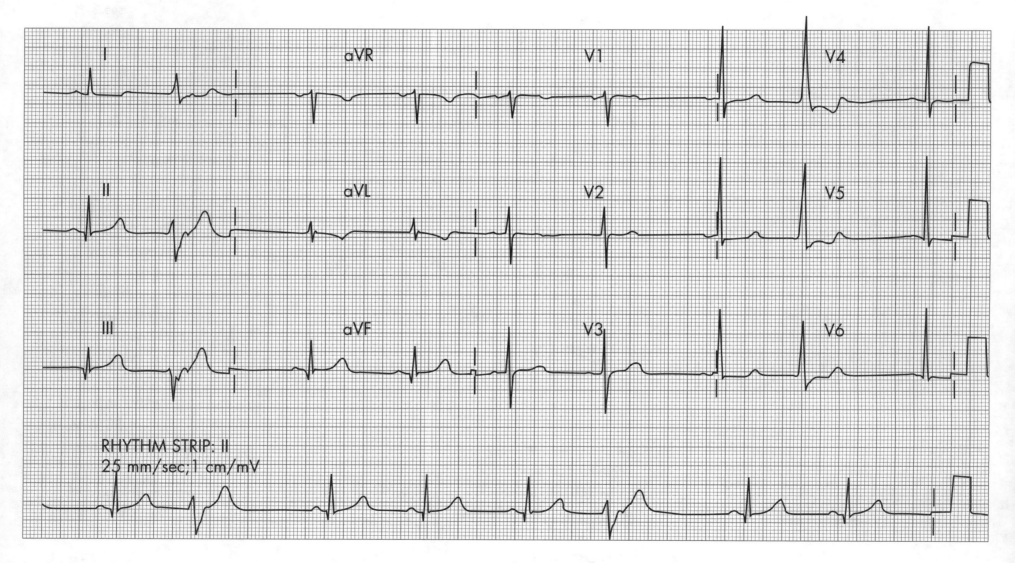

I aVR V1 V4

II aVL V2 V5

III aVF V3 V6

RHYTHM STRIP: II
25 mm/sec; 1 cm/mV

Figure 3-3
Resting 12-Lead ECG

1. **RATE**

   Atrial:

   Ventricular:

2. **RHYTHM**

   Atrial:

   Ventricular:

3. **WAVES**

   P waves present:

   Appearance:

   Consistent:

   Relation to QRS:

   Q waves present:

   Leads:

   Pathological:

   T waves present:

   Morphology:

4. **INTERVALS**

   P-R interval:

   Consistent:

   QRS:

   Appearance:

   Consistent:

   Q-T interval:

5. **AXIS**

   Quadrant:

   Degrees:

6. **HYPERTROPHY**

   Atrial:

   Ventricular:

7. **MYOCARDIAL INFARCTION**

   Q waves:

   S-T displacement:

8. **ISCHEMIA**

   S-T displacement:

9. **POSSIBLE DRUG EFFECTS**

10. **ECG ANALYSIS**

11. **INTERPRETATION**

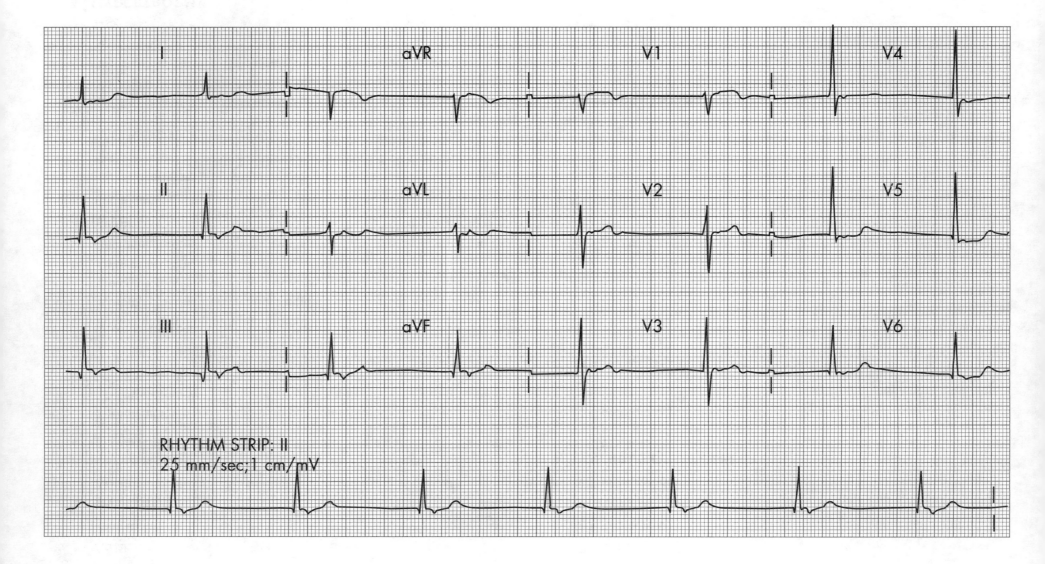

I aVR V1 V4

II aVL V2 V5

III aVF V3 V6

RHYTHM STRIP: II
25 mm/sec; 1 cm/mV

Figure 3-4
Resting 12-Lead ECG
122

1. RATE

Atrial:

Ventricular:

2. RHYTHM

Atrial:

Ventricular:

3. WAVES

P waves present:

Appearance:

Consistent:

Relation to QRS:

Q waves present:

Leads:

Pathological:

T waves present:

Morphology:

4. INTERVALS

P-R interval:

Consistent:

QRS:

Appearance:

Consistent:

Q-T interval:

5. AXIS

Quadrant:

Degrees:

6. HYPERTROPHY

Atrial:

Ventricular:

7. MYOCARDIAL INFARCTION

Q waves:

S-T displacement:

8. ISCHEMIA

S-T displacement:

9. POSSIBLE DRUG EFFECTS

10. ECG ANALYSIS

11. INTERPRETATION

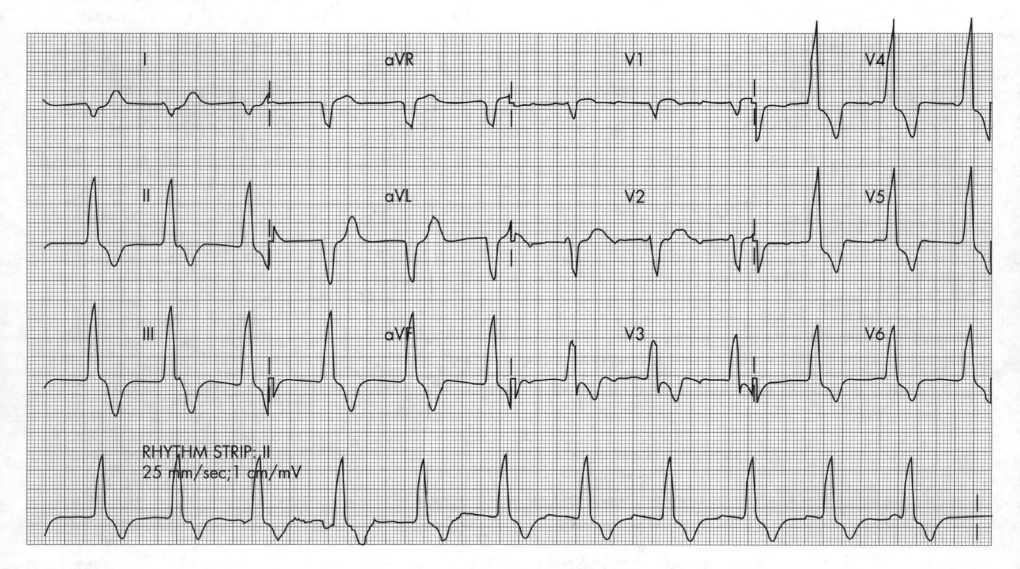

I aVR V1 V4

II aVL V2 V5

III aVF V3 V6

RHYTHM STRIP: II
25 mm/sec; 1 cm/mV

Figure 3-5
Resting 12-Lead ECG

124

1. RATE

Atrial:

Ventricular:

2. RHYTHM

Atrial:

Ventricular:

3. WAVES

P waves present:

Appearance:

Consistent:

Relation to QRS:

Q waves present:

Leads:

Pathological:

T waves present:

Morphology:

4. INTERVALS

P-R interval:

Consistent:

QRS:

Appearance:

Consistent:

Q-T interval:

5. AXIS

Quadrant:

Degrees:

6. HYPERTROPHY

Atrial:

Ventricular:

7. MYOCARDIAL INFARCTION

Q waves:

S-T displacement:

8. ISCHEMIA

S-T displacement:

9. POSSIBLE DRUG EFFECTS

10. ECG ANALYSIS

11. INTERPRETATION

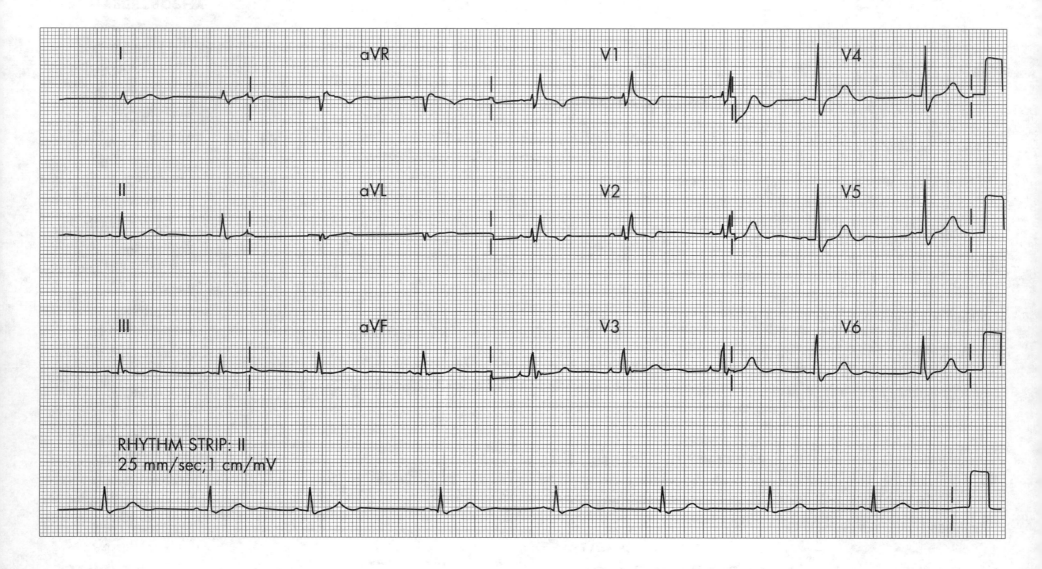

I   aVR   V1   V4

II   aVL   V2   V5

III   aVF   V3   V6

RHYTHM STRIP: II
25 mm/sec; 1 cm/mV

Figure 3-6
Resting 12-Lead ECG

1. RATE
Atrial:

Ventricular:

2. RHYTHM
Atrial:

Ventricular:

3. WAVES
P waves present:

    Appearance:

    Consistent:

    Relation to QRS:

Q waves present:

    Leads:

    Pathological:

T waves present:

    Morphology:

4. INTERVALS
P-R interval:

    Consistent:

QRS:

    Appearance:

    Consistent:

Q-T interval:

5. AXIS
Quadrant:

Degrees:

6. HYPERTROPHY
Atrial:

Ventricular:

7. MYOCARDIAL INFARCTION
Q waves:

S-T displacement:

8. ISCHEMIA
S-T displacement:

9. POSSIBLE DRUG EFFECTS

10. ECG ANALYSIS

11. INTERPRETATION

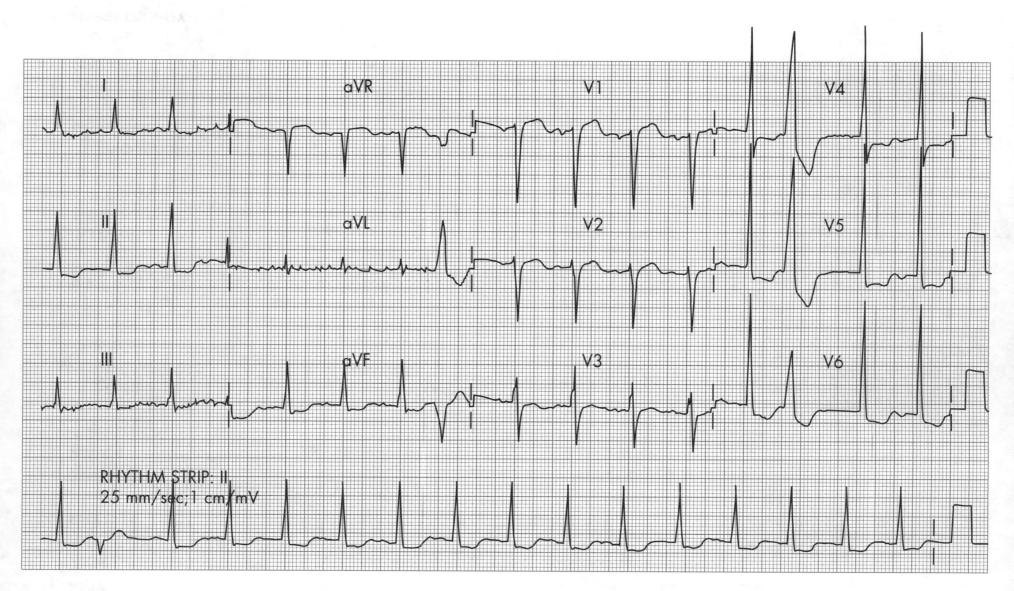

I aVR V1 V4

II aVL V2 V5

III aVF V3 V6

RHYTHM STRIP: II
25 mm/sec; 1 cm/mV

Figure 3-7
Resting 12-Lead ECG

128

1. **RATE**

   Atrial:

   Ventricular:

2. **RHYTHM**

   Atrial:

   Ventricular:

3. **WAVES**

   P waves present:

   Appearance:

   Consistent:

   Relation to QRS:

   Q waves present:

   Leads:

   Pathological:

   T waves present:

   Morphology:

4. **INTERVALS**

   P-R interval:

   Consistent:

   QRS:

   Appearance:

   Consistent:

   Q-T interval:

5. **AXIS**

   Quadrant:

   Degrees:

6. **HYPERTROPHY**

   Atrial:

   Ventricular:

7. **MYOCARDIAL INFARCTION**

   Q waves:

   S-T displacement:

8. **ISCHEMIA**

   S-T displacement:

9. **POSSIBLE DRUG EFFECTS**

10. **ECG ANALYSIS**

11. **INTERPRETATION**

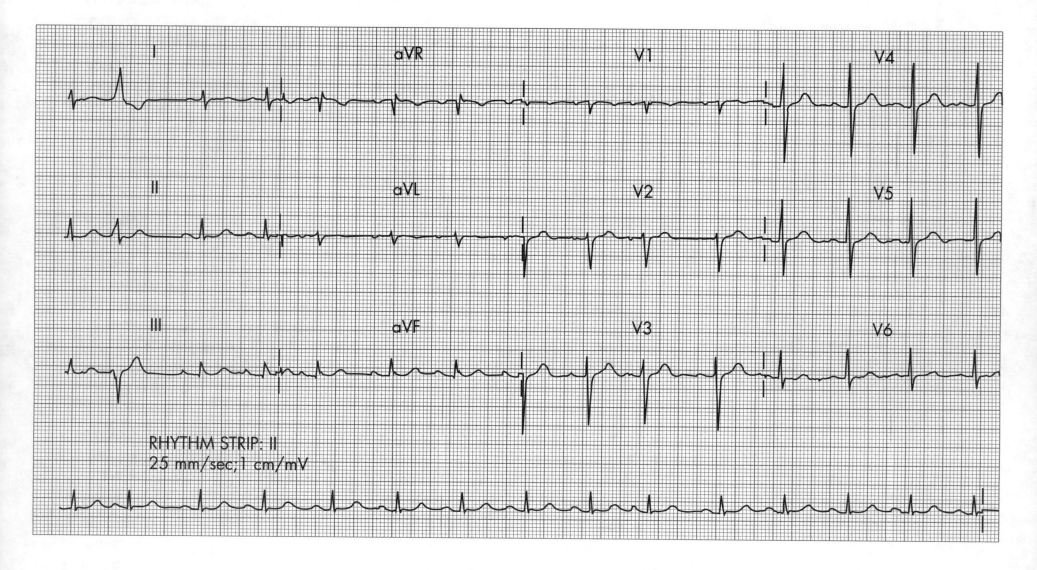

I aVR V1 V4

II aVL V2 V5

III aVF V3 V6

RHYTHM STRIP: II
25 mm/sec; 1 cm/mV

Figure 3-8
Resting 12-Lead ECG
130

1. **RATE**

   Atrial:

   Ventricular:

2. **RHYTHM**

   Atrial:

   Ventricular:

3. **WAVES**

   P waves present:

      Appearance:

      Consistent:

      Relation to QRS:

   Q waves present:

      Leads:

      Pathological:

   T waves present:

      Morphology:

4. **INTERVALS**

   P-R interval:

      Consistent:

   QRS:

      Appearance:

      Consistent:

   Q-T interval:

5. **AXIS**

   Quadrant:

   Degrees:

6. **HYPERTROPHY**

   Atrial:

   Ventricular:

7. **MYOCARDIAL INFARCTION**

   Q waves:

   S-T displacement:

8. **ISCHEMIA**

   S-T displacement:

9. **POSSIBLE DRUG EFFECTS**

10. **ECG ANALYSIS**

11. **INTERPRETATION**

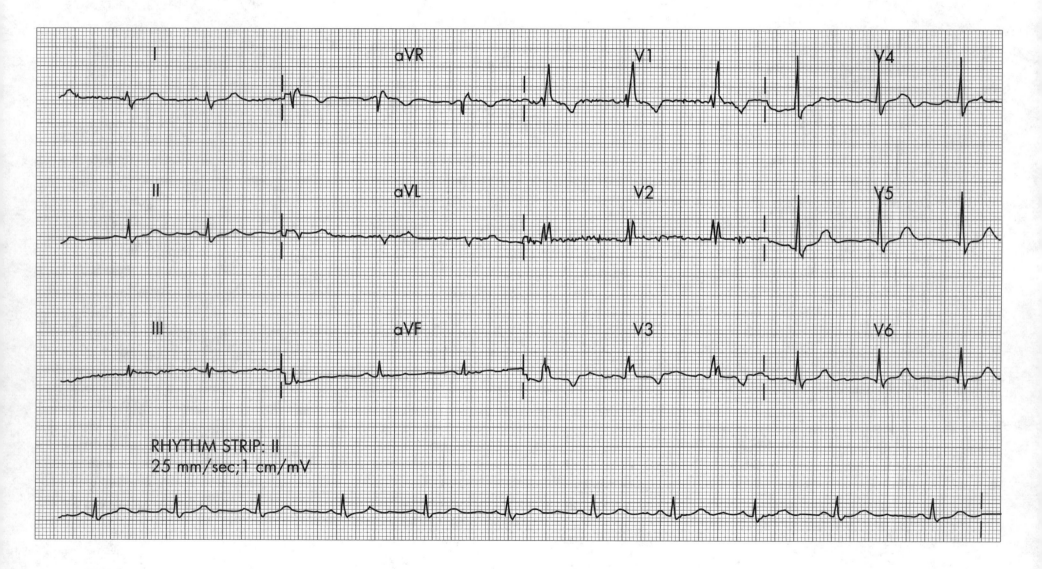

I   aVR   V1   V4

II   aVL   V2   V5

III   aVF   V3   V6

RHYTHM STRIP: II
25 mm/sec; 1 cm/mV

Figure 3-9
Resting 12-Lead ECG

132

I. RATE

   Atrial:

   Ventricular:

2. RHYTHM

   Atrial:

   Ventricular:

3. WAVES

   P waves present:

      Appearance:

      Consistent:

      Relation to QRS:

   Q waves present:

      Leads:

      Pathological:

   T waves present:

      Morphology:

4. INTERVALS

   P-R interval:

      Consistent:

   QRS:

      Appearance:

      Consistent:

   Q-T interval:

5. AXIS

   Quadrant:

   Degrees:

6. HYPERTROPHY

   Atrial:

   Ventricular:

7. MYOCARDIAL INFARCTION

   Q waves:

   S-T displacement:

8. ISCHEMIA

   S-T displacement:

9. POSSIBLE DRUG EFFECTS

10. ECG ANALYSIS

11. INTERPRETATION

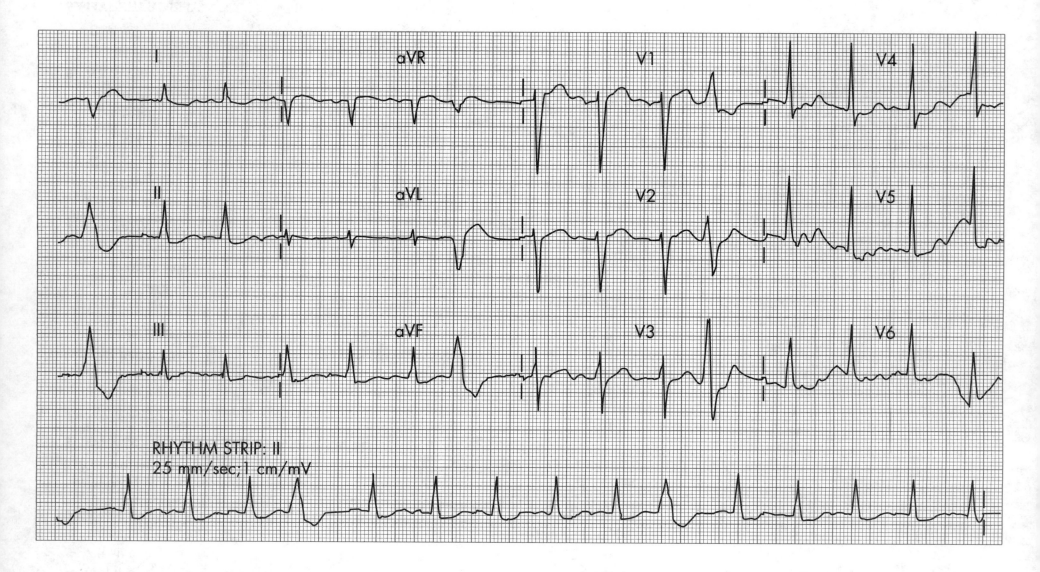

Figure 3-10
Resting 12-Lead ECG

1. RATE

Atrial:

Ventricular:

2. RHYTHM

Atrial:

Ventricular:

3. WAVES

P waves present:

Appearance:

Consistent:

Relation to QRS:

Q waves present:

Leads:

Pathological:

T waves present:

Morphology:

4. INTERVALS

P-R interval:

Consistent:

QRS:

Appearance:

Consistent:

Q-T interval:

5. AXIS

Quadrant:

Degrees:

6. HYPERTROPHY

Atrial:

Ventricular:

7. MYOCARDIAL INFARCTION

Q waves:

S-T displacement:

8. ISCHEMIA

S-T displacement:

9. POSSIBLE DRUG EFFECTS

10. ECG ANALYSIS

11. INTERPRETATION

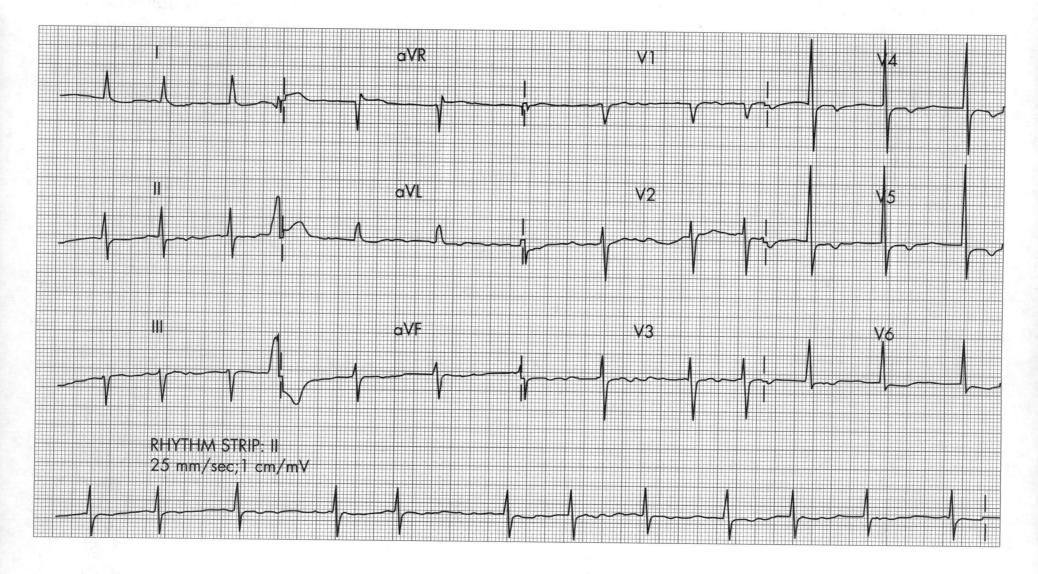

RHYTHM STRIP: II
25 mm/sec; 1 cm/mV

Figure 3-11
Resting 12-Lead ECG

136

1. RATE

    Atrial:

    Ventricular:

2. RHYTHM

    Atrial:

    Ventricular:

3. WAVES

    P waves present:

        Appearance:

        Consistent:

        Relation to QRS:

    Q waves present:

        Leads:

        Pathological:

    T waves present:

        Morphology:

4. INTERVALS

    P-R interval:

        Consistent:

    QRS:

        Appearance:

        Consistent:

    Q-T interval:

5. AXIS

    Quadrant:

    Degrees:

6. HYPERTROPHY

    Atrial:

    Ventricular:

7. MYOCARDIAL INFARCTION

    Q waves:

    S-T displacement:

8. ISCHEMIA

    S-T displacement:

9. POSSIBLE DRUG EFFECTS

10. ECG ANALYSIS

11. INTERPRETATION

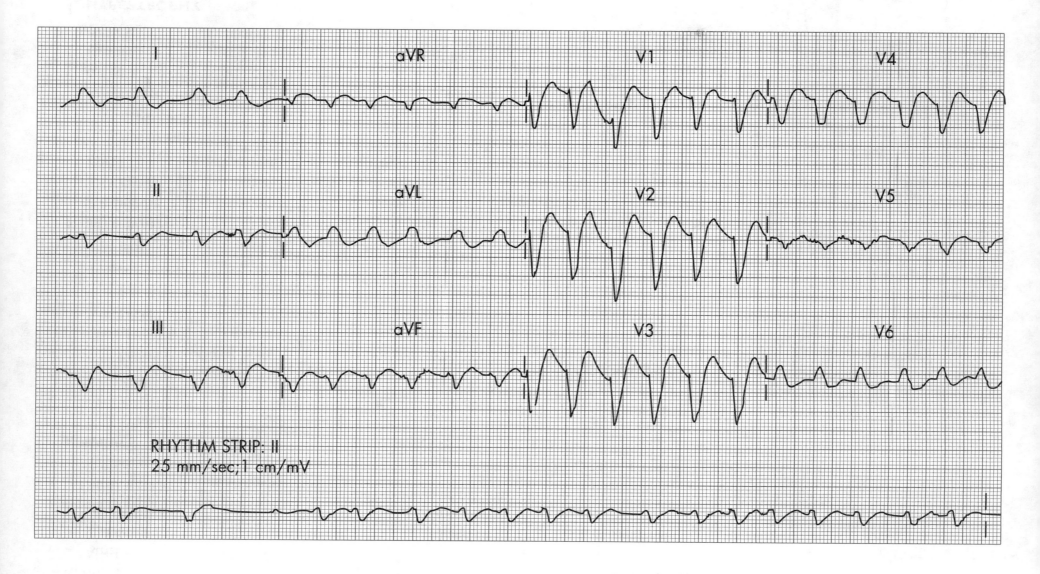

Figure 3-12
Resting 12-Lead ECG
138

1. RATE

Atrial:

Ventricular:

2. RHYTHM

Atrial:

Ventricular:

3. WAVES

P waves present:

Appearance:

Consistent:

Relation to QRS:

Q waves present:

Leads:

Pathological:

T waves present:

Morphology:

4. INTERVALS

P-R interval:

Consistent:

QRS:

Appearance:

Consistent:

Q-T interval:

5. AXIS

Quadrant:

Degrees:

6. HYPERTROPHY

Atrial:

Ventricular:

7. MYOCARDIAL INFARCTION

Q waves:

S-T displacement:

8. ISCHEMIA

S-T displacement:

9. POSSIBLE DRUG EFFECTS

10. ECG ANALYSIS

11. INTERPRETATION

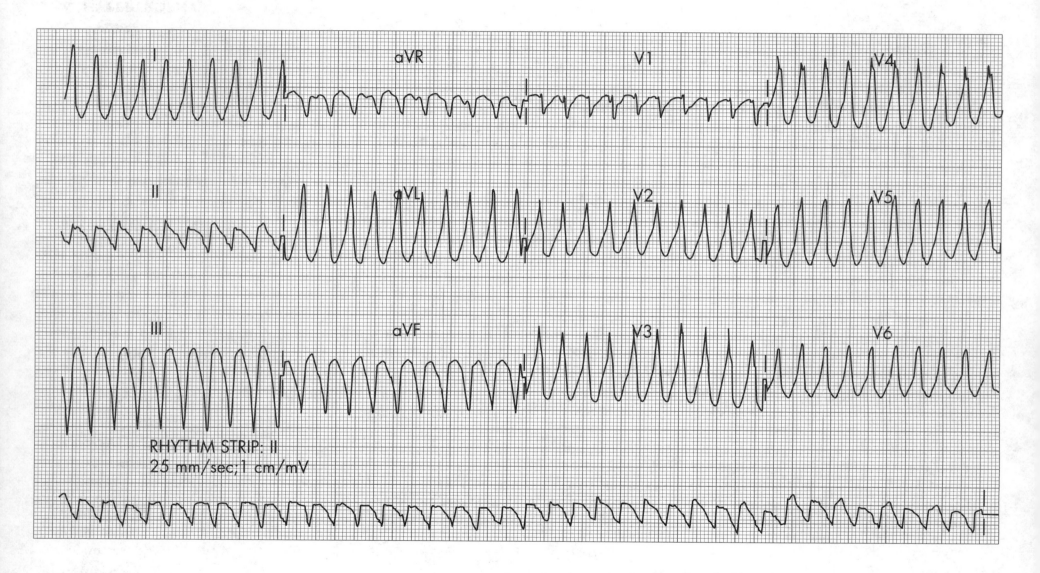

RHYTHM STRIP: II
25 mm/sec; 1 cm/mV

Figure 3-13
Resting 12-Lead ECG
140

1. **RATE**

   Atrial:

   Ventricular:

2. **RHYTHM**

   Atrial:

   Ventricular:

3. **WAVES**

   P waves present:

   　Appearance:

   　Consistent:

   　Relation to QRS:

   Q waves present:

   　Leads:

   　Pathological:

   T waves present:

   　Morphology:

4. **INTERVALS**

   P-R interval:

   　Consistent:

   QRS:

   　Appearance:

   　Consistent:

   Q-T interval:

5. **AXIS**

   Quadrant:

   Degrees:

6. **HYPERTROPHY**

   Atrial:

   Ventricular:

7. **MYOCARDIAL INFARCTION**

   Q waves:

   S-T displacement:

8. **ISCHEMIA**

   S-T displacement:

9. **POSSIBLE DRUG EFFECTS**

10. **ECG ANALYSIS**

11. **INTERPRETATION**

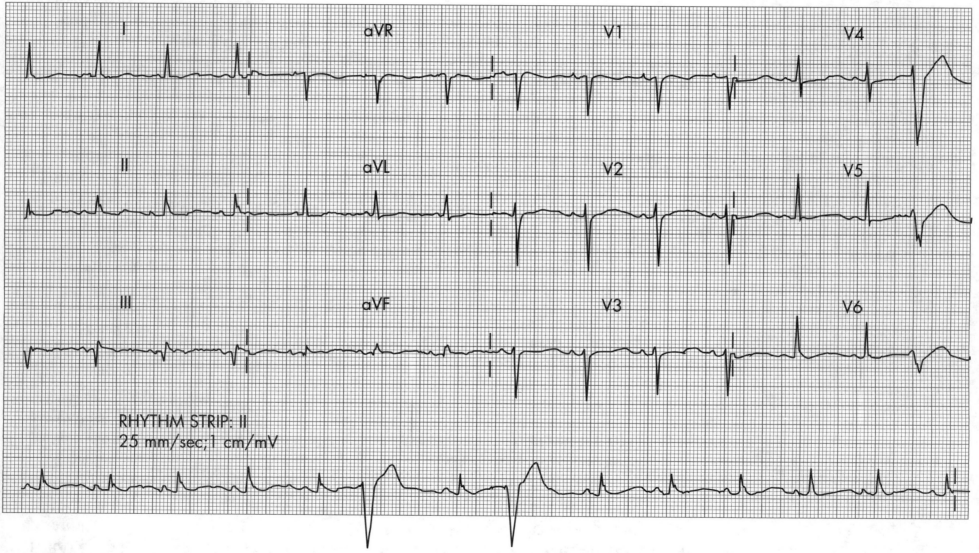

I aVR V1 V4

II aVL V2 V5

III aVF V3 V6

RHYTHM STRIP: II
25 mm/sec; 1 cm/mV

Figure 3-14
Resting 12-Lead ECG

142

1. RATE

Atrial:

Ventricular:

2. RHYTHM

Atrial:

Ventricular:

3. WAVES

P waves present:

    Appearance:

    Consistent:

    Relation to QRS:

Q waves present:

    Leads:

    Pathological:

T waves present:

    Morphology:

4. INTERVALS

P-R interval:

    Consistent:

QRS:

    Appearance:

    Consistent:

Q-T interval:

5. AXIS

Quadrant:

Degrees:

6. HYPERTROPHY

Atrial:

Ventricular:

7. MYOCARDIAL INFARCTION

Q waves:

S-T displacement:

8. ISCHEMIA

S-T displacement:

9. POSSIBLE DRUG EFFECTS

10. ECG ANALYSIS

11. INTERPRETATION

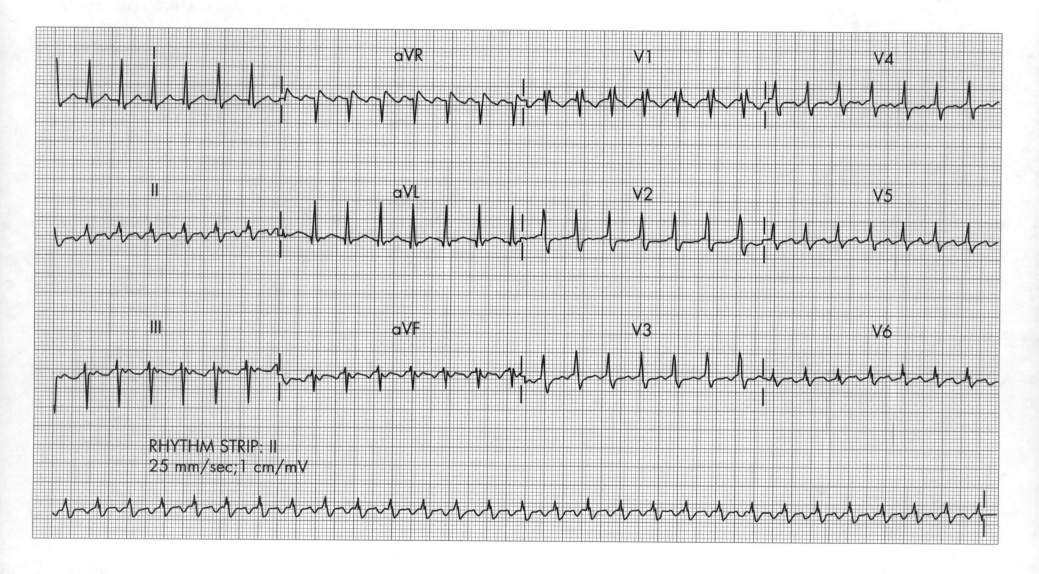

aVR   V1   V4

II   aVL   V2   V5

III   aVF   V3   V6

RHYTHM STRIP: II
25 mm/sec; 1 cm/mV

Figure 3-15
Resting 12-Lead ECG

1. RATE

Atrial:

Ventricular:

2. RHYTHM

Atrial:

Ventricular:

3. WAVES

P waves present:

Appearance:

Consistent:

Relation to QRS:

Q waves present:

Leads:

Pathological:

T waves present:

Morphology:

4. INTERVALS

P-R interval:

Consistent:

QRS:

Appearance:

Consistent:

Q-T interval:

5. AXIS

Quadrant:

Degrees:

6. HYPERTROPHY

Atrial:

Ventricular:

7. MYOCARDIAL INFARCTION

Q waves:

S-T displacement:

8. ISCHEMIA

S-T displacement:

9. POSSIBLE DRUG EFFECTS

10. ECG ANALYSIS

11. INTERPRETATION

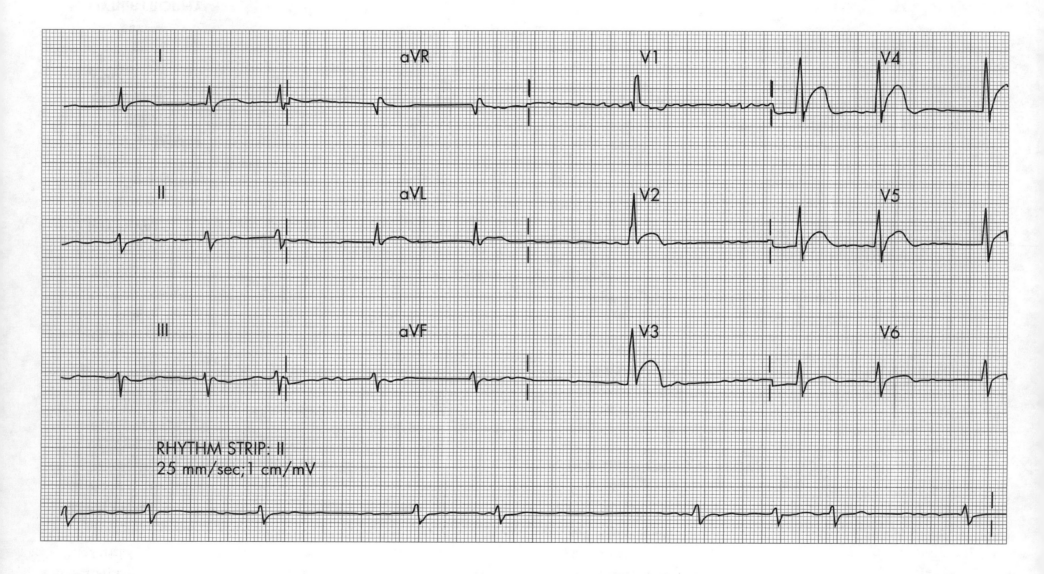

I aVR V1 V4

II aVL V2 V5

III aVF V3 V6

RHYTHM STRIP: II
25 mm/sec; 1 cm/mV

Figure 3-16
Resting 12-Lead ECG
146

1. RATE

Atrial:

Ventricular:

2. RHYTHM

Atrial:

Ventricular:

3. WAVES

P waves present:

Appearance:

Consistent:

Relation to QRS:

Q waves present:

Leads:

Pathological:

T waves present:

Morphology:

4. INTERVALS

P-R interval:

Consistent:

QRS:

Appearance:

Consistent:

Q-T interval:

5. AXIS

Quadrant:

Degrees:

6. HYPERTROPHY

Atrial:

Ventricular:

7. MYOCARDIAL INFARCTION

Q waves:

S-T displacement:

8. ISCHEMIA

S-T displacement:

9. POSSIBLE DRUG EFFECTS

10. ECG ANALYSIS

11. INTERPRETATION

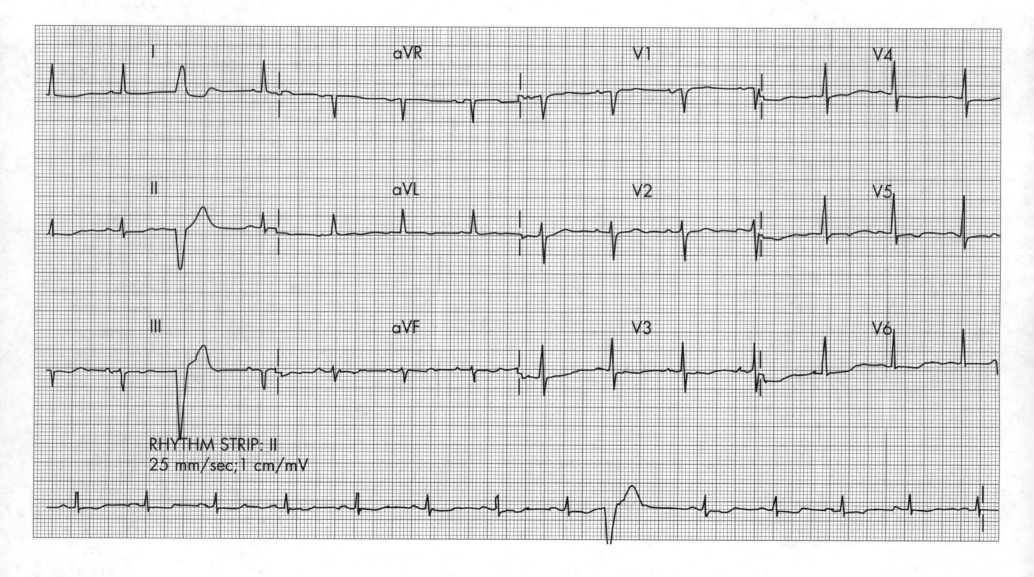

I aVR V1 V4

II aVL V2 V5

III aVF V3 V6

RHYTHM STRIP: II
25 mm/sec; 1 cm/mV

Figure 3-17
Resting 12-Lead ECG

148

1. **RATE**

   Atrial:

   Ventricular:

2. **RHYTHM**

   Atrial:

   Ventricular:

3. **WAVES**

   P waves present:

   Appearance:

   Consistent:

   Relation to QRS:

   Q waves present:

   Leads:

   Pathological:

   T waves present:

   Morphology:

4. **INTERVALS**

   P-R interval:

   Consistent:

   QRS:

   Appearance:

   Consistent:

   Q-T interval:

5. **AXIS**

   Quadrant:

   Degrees:

6. **HYPERTROPHY**

   Atrial:

   Ventricular:

7. **MYOCARDIAL INFARCTION**

   Q waves:

   S-T displacement:

8. **ISCHEMIA**

   S-T displacement:

9. **POSSIBLE DRUG EFFECTS**

10. **ECG ANALYSIS**

11. **INTERPRETATION**

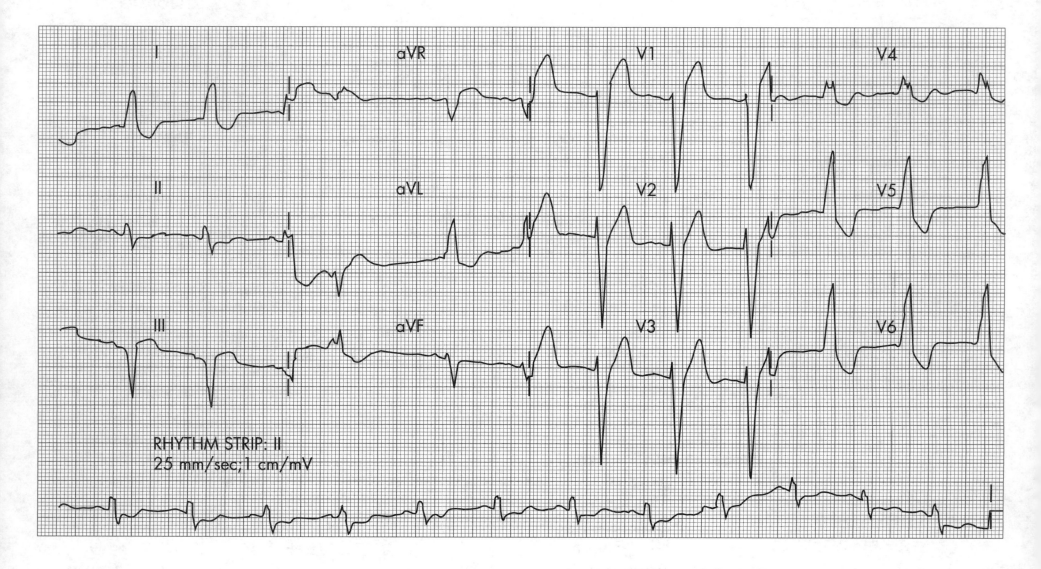

Figure 3-18
Resting 12-Lead ECG
150

I. RATE

Atrial:

Ventricular:

2. RHYTHM

Atrial:

Ventricular:

3. WAVES

P waves present:

Appearance:

Consistent:

Relation to QRS:

Q waves present:

Leads:

Pathological:

T waves present:

Morphology:

4. INTERVALS

P-R interval:

Consistent:

QRS:

Appearance:

Consistent:

Q-T interval:

5. AXIS

Quadrant:

Degrees:

6. HYPERTROPHY

Atrial:

Ventricular:

7. MYOCARDIAL INFARCTION

Q waves:

S-T displacement:

8. ISCHEMIA

S-T displacement:

9. POSSIBLE DRUG EFFECTS

10. ECG ANALYSIS

11. INTERPRETATION

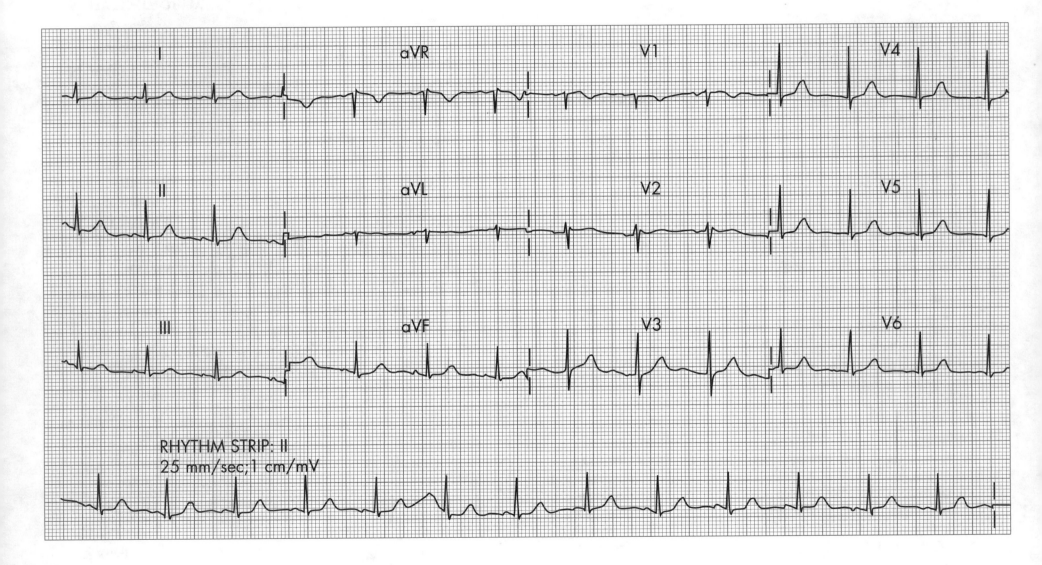

I   aVR   V1   V4

II   aVL   V2   V5

III   aVF   V3   V6

RHYTHM STRIP: II
25 mm/sec;1 cm/mV

Figure 3-19
Resting 12-Lead ECG

152

1. RATE

Atrial:

Ventricular:

2. RHYTHM

Atrial:

Ventricular:

3. WAVES

P waves present:

    Appearance:

    Consistent:

    Relation to QRS:

Q waves present:

    Leads:

    Pathological:

T waves present:

    Morphology:

4. INTERVALS

P-R interval:

    Consistent:

QRS:

    Appearance:

    Consistent:

Q-T interval:

5. AXIS

Quadrant:

Degrees:

6. HYPERTROPHY

Atrial:

Ventricular:

7. MYOCARDIAL INFARCTION

Q waves:

S-T displacement:

8. ISCHEMIA

S-T displacement:

9. POSSIBLE DRUG EFFECTS

10. ECG ANALYSIS

11. INTERPRETATION

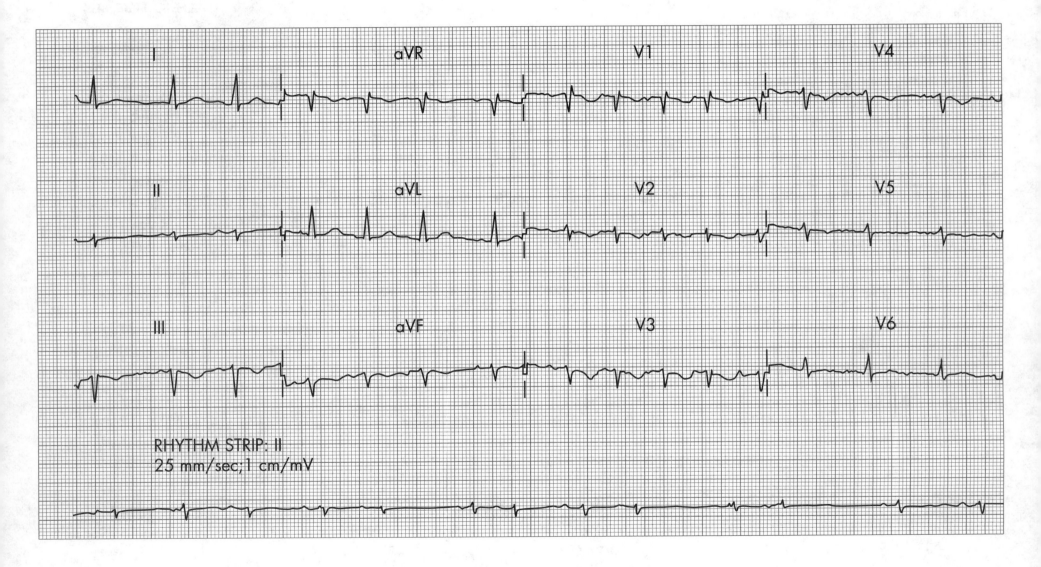

Figure 3-20
Resting 12-Lead ECG

154

1. **RATE**

   Atrial:

   Ventricular:

2. **RHYTHM**

   Atrial:

   Ventricular:

3. **WAVES**

   P waves present:

       Appearance:

       Consistent:

       Relation to QRS:

   Q waves present:

       Leads:

       Pathological:

   T waves present:

       Morphology:

4. **INTERVALS**

   P-R interval:

       Consistent:

   QRS:

       Appearance:

       Consistent:

   Q-T interval:

5. **AXIS**

   Quadrant:

   Degrees:

6. **HYPERTROPHY**

   Atrial:

   Ventricular:

7. **MYOCARDIAL INFARCTION**

   Q waves:

   S-T displacement:

8. **ISCHEMIA**

   S-T displacement:

9. **POSSIBLE DRUG EFFECTS**

10. **ECG ANALYSIS**

11. **INTERPRETATION**

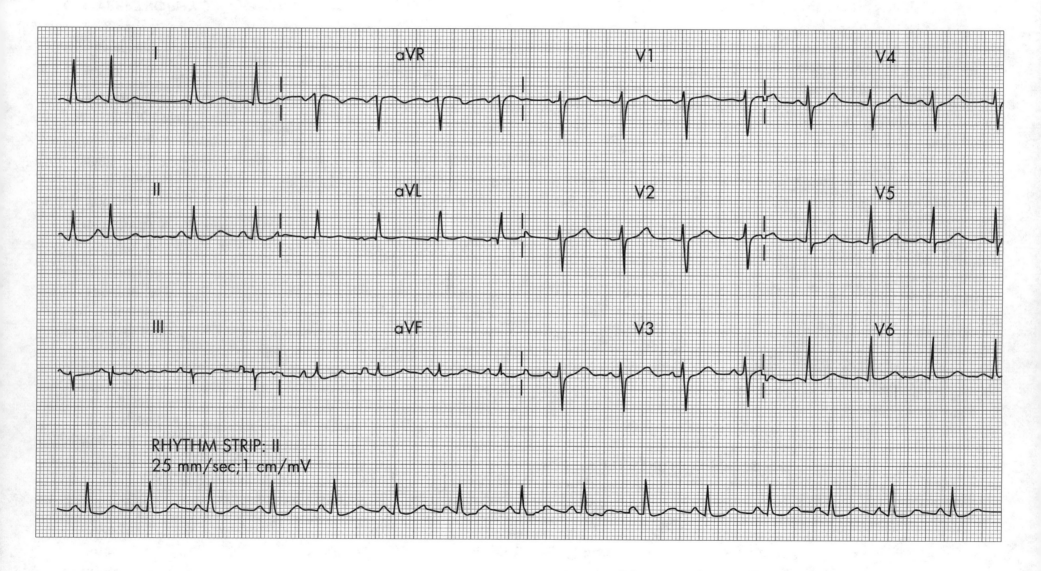

I aVR V1 V4

II aVL V2 V5

III aVF V3 V6

RHYTHM STRIP: II
25 mm/sec;1 cm/mV

Figure 3-21
Resting 12-Lead ECG
156

1. RATE

Atrial:

Ventricular:

2. RHYTHM

Atrial:

Ventricular:

3. WAVES

P waves present:

    Appearance:

    Consistent:

    Relation to QRS:

Q waves present:

    Leads:

    Pathological:

T waves present:

    Morphology:

4. INTERVALS

P-R interval:

    Consistent:

QRS:

    Appearance:

    Consistent:

Q-T interval:

5. AXIS

Quadrant:

Degrees:

6. HYPERTROPHY

Atrial:

Ventricular:

7. MYOCARDIAL INFARCTION

Q waves:

S-T displacement:

8. ISCHEMIA

S-T displacement:

9. POSSIBLE DRUG EFFECTS

10. ECG ANALYSIS

11. INTERPRETATION

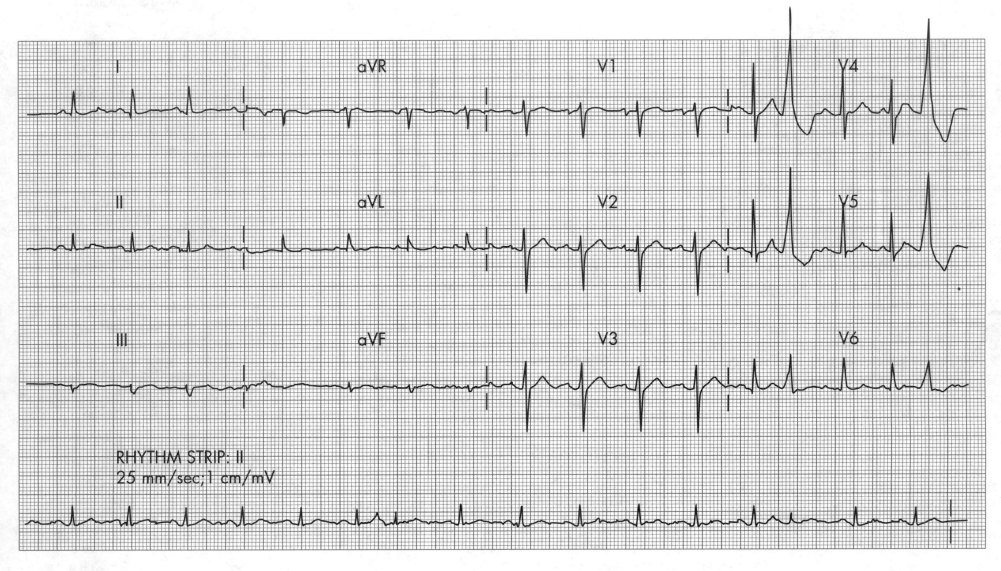

I

aVR

V1

V4

II

aVL

V2

V5

III

aVF

V3

V6

RHYTHM STRIP: II
25 mm/sec;1 cm/mV

Figure 3-22
Resting 12-Lead ECG

158

1. **RATE**

   Atrial:

   Ventricular:

2. **RHYTHM**

   Atrial:

   Ventricular:

3. **WAVES**

   P waves present:

       Appearance:

       Consistent:

       Relation to QRS:

   Q waves present:

       Leads:

       Pathological:

   T waves present:

       Morphology:

4. **INTERVALS**

   P-R interval:

       Consistent:

   QRS:

       Appearance:

       Consistent:

   Q-T interval:

5. **AXIS**

   Quadrant:

   Degrees:

6. **HYPERTROPHY**

   Atrial:

   Ventricular:

7. **MYOCARDIAL INFARCTION**

   Q waves:

   S-T displacement:

8. **ISCHEMIA**

   S-T displacement:

9. **POSSIBLE DRUG EFFECTS**

10. **ECG ANALYSIS**

11. **INTERPRETATION**

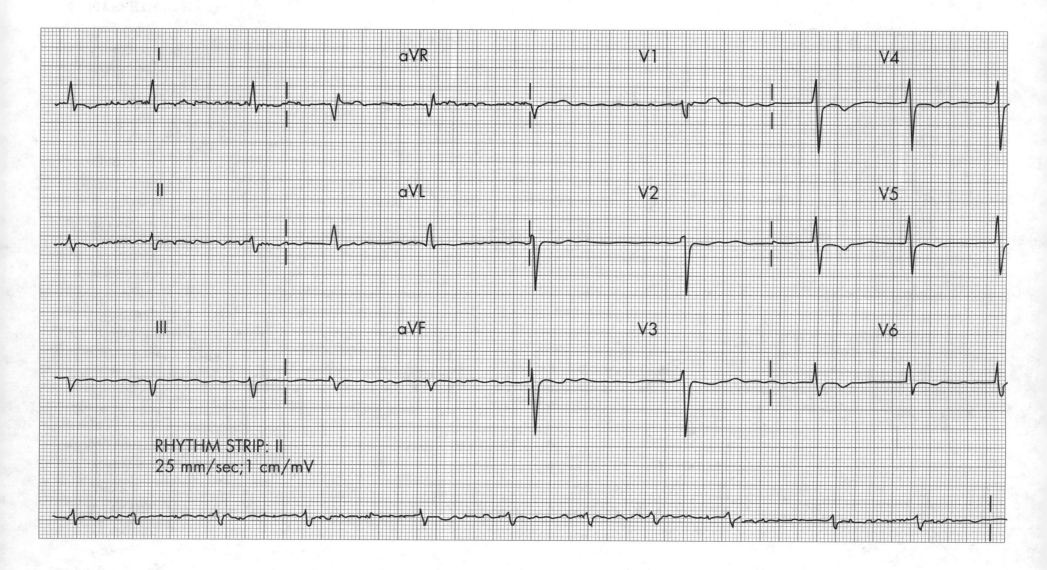

I aVR V1 V4

II aVL V2 V5

III aVF V3 V6

RHYTHM STRIP: II
25 mm/sec; 1 cm/mV

Figure 3-23
Resting 12-Lead ECG

1. **RATE**

   Atrial:

   Ventricular:

2. **RHYTHM**

   Atrial:

   Ventricular:

3. **WAVES**

   P waves present:

      Appearance:

      Consistent:

      Relation to QRS:

   Q waves present:

      Leads:

      Pathological:

   T waves present:

      Morphology:

4. **INTERVALS**

   P-R interval:

      Consistent:

   QRS:

      Appearance:

      Consistent:

   Q-T interval:

5. **AXIS**

   Quadrant:

   Degrees:

6. **HYPERTROPHY**

   Atrial:

   Ventricular:

7. **MYOCARDIAL INFARCTION**

   Q waves:

   S-T displacement:

8. **ISCHEMIA**

   S-T displacement:

9. **POSSIBLE DRUG EFFECTS**

10. **ECG ANALYSIS**

11. **INTERPRETATION**

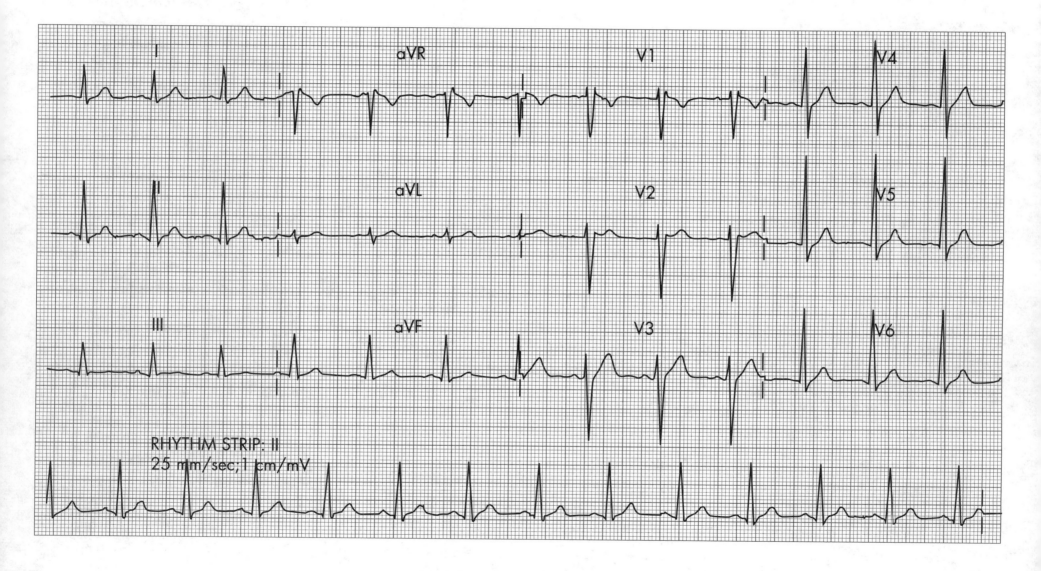

I aVR V1 V4

aVL V2 V5

III aVF V3 V6

RHYTHM STRIP: II
25 mm/sec; 1 cm/mV

Figure 3-24
Resting 12-Lead ECG

162

I. RATE

Atrial:

Ventricular:

2. RHYTHM

Atrial:

Ventricular:

3. WAVES

P waves present:

Appearance:

Consistent:

Relation to QRS:

Q waves present:

Leads:

Pathological:

T waves present:

Morphology:

4. INTERVALS

P-R interval:

Consistent:

QRS:

Appearance:

Consistent:

Q-T interval:

5. AXIS

Quadrant:

Degrees:

6. HYPERTROPHY

Atrial:

Ventricular:

7. MYOCARDIAL INFARCTION

Q waves:

S-T displacement:

8. ISCHEMIA

S-T displacement:

9. POSSIBLE DRUG EFFECTS

10. ECG ANALYSIS

11. INTERPRETATION

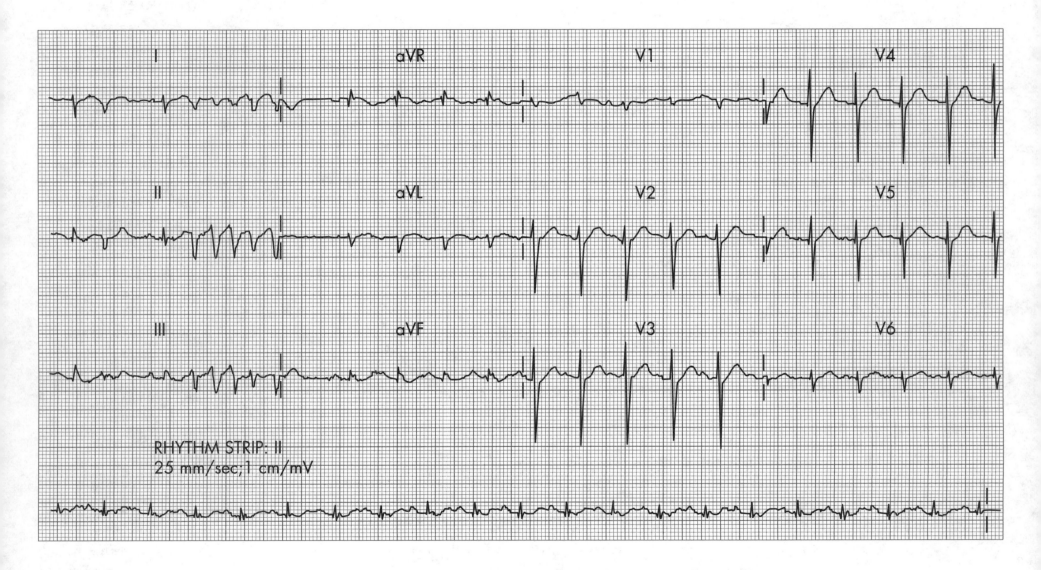

I	aVR	V1	V4
II	aVL	V2	V5
III	aVF	V3	V6

RHYTHM STRIP: II
25 mm/sec;1 cm/mV

Figure 3-25
Resting 12-Lead ECG

164

1. RATE

  Atrial:

  Ventricular:

2. RHYTHM

  Atrial:

  Ventricular:

3. WAVES

  P waves present:

    Appearance:

    Consistent:

    Relation to QRS:

  Q waves present:

    Leads:

    Pathological:

  T waves present:

    Morphology:

4. INTERVALS

  P-R interval:

    Consistent:

  QRS:

    Appearance:

    Consistent:

  Q-T interval:

5. AXIS

  Quadrant:

  Degrees:

6. HYPERTROPHY

  Atrial:

  Ventricular:

7. MYOCARDIAL INFARCTION

  Q waves:

  S-T displacement:

8. ISCHEMIA

  S-T displacement:

9. POSSIBLE DRUG EFFECTS

10. ECG ANALYSIS

11. INTERPRETATION

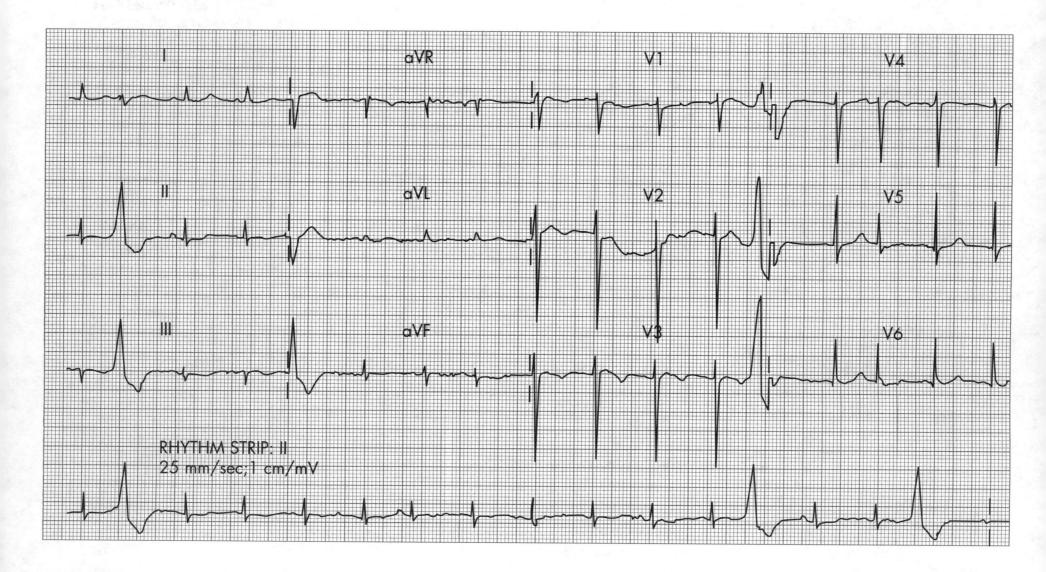

I aVR V1 V4

II aVL V2 V5

III aVF V3 V6

RHYTHM STRIP: II
25 mm/sec;1 cm/mV

Figure 3-26
Resting 12-Lead ECG
166

1. RATE

Atrial:

Ventricular:

2. RHYTHM

Atrial:

Ventricular:

3. WAVES

P waves present:

    Appearance:

    Consistent:

    Relation to QRS:

Q waves present:

    Leads:

    Pathological:

T waves present:

    Morphology:

4. INTERVALS

P-R interval:

    Consistent:

QRS:

    Appearance:

    Consistent:

Q-T interval:

5. AXIS

Quadrant:

Degrees:

6. HYPERTROPHY

Atrial:

Ventricular:

7. MYOCARDIAL INFARCTION

Q waves:

S-T displacement:

8. ISCHEMIA

S-T displacement:

9. POSSIBLE DRUG EFFECTS

10. ECG ANALYSIS

11. INTERPRETATION

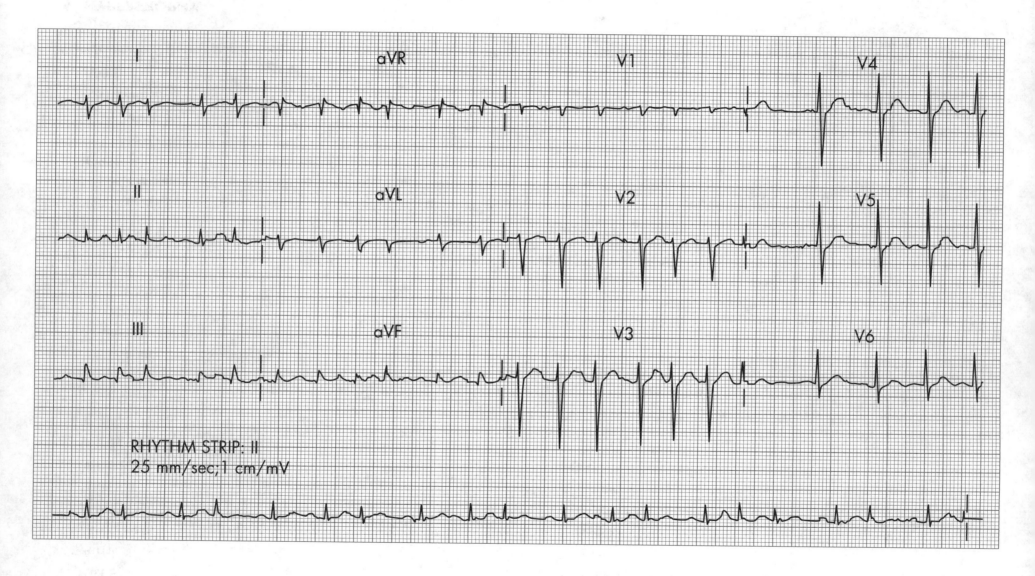

I aVR V1 V4

II aVL V2 V5

III aVF V3 V6

RHYTHM STRIP: II
25 mm/sec; 1 cm/mV

Figure 3-27
Resting 12-Lead ECG

1. **RATE**

   Atrial:

   Ventricular:

2. **RHYTHM**

   Atrial:

   Ventricular:

3. **WAVES**

   P waves present:

   Appearance:

   Consistent:

   Relation to QRS:

   Q waves present:

   Leads:

   Pathological:

   T waves present:

   Morphology:

4. **INTERVALS**

   P-R interval:

   Consistent:

   QRS:

   Appearance:

   Consistent:

   Q-T interval:

5. **AXIS**

   Quadrant:

   Degrees:

6. **HYPERTROPHY**

   Atrial:

   Ventricular:

7. **MYOCARDIAL INFARCTION**

   Q waves:

   S-T displacement:

8. **ISCHEMIA**

   S-T displacement:

9. **POSSIBLE DRUG EFFECTS**

10. **ECG ANALYSIS**

11. **INTERPRETATION**

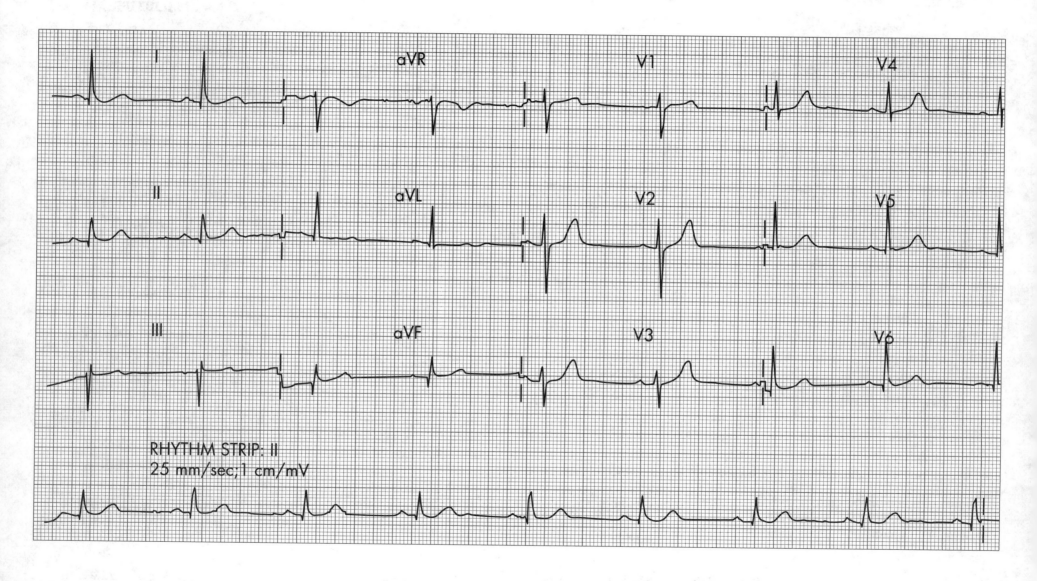

I   aVR   V1   V4

II   aVL   V2   V5

III   aVF   V3   V6

RHYTHM STRIP: II
25 mm/sec;1 cm/mV

Figure 3-28
Resting 12-Lead ECG

1. RATE

Atrial:

Ventricular:

2. RHYTHM

Atrial:

Ventricular:

3. WAVES

P waves present:

Appearance:

Consistent:

Relation to QRS:

Q waves present:

Leads:

Pathological:

T waves present:

Morphology:

4. INTERVALS

P-R interval:

Consistent:

QRS:

Appearance:

Consistent:

Q-T interval:

5. AXIS

Quadrant:

Degrees:

6. HYPERTROPHY

Atrial:

Ventricular:

7. MYOCARDIAL INFARCTION

Q waves:

S-T displacement:

8. ISCHEMIA

S-T displacement:

9. POSSIBLE DRUG EFFECTS

10. ECG ANALYSIS

11. INTERPRETATION

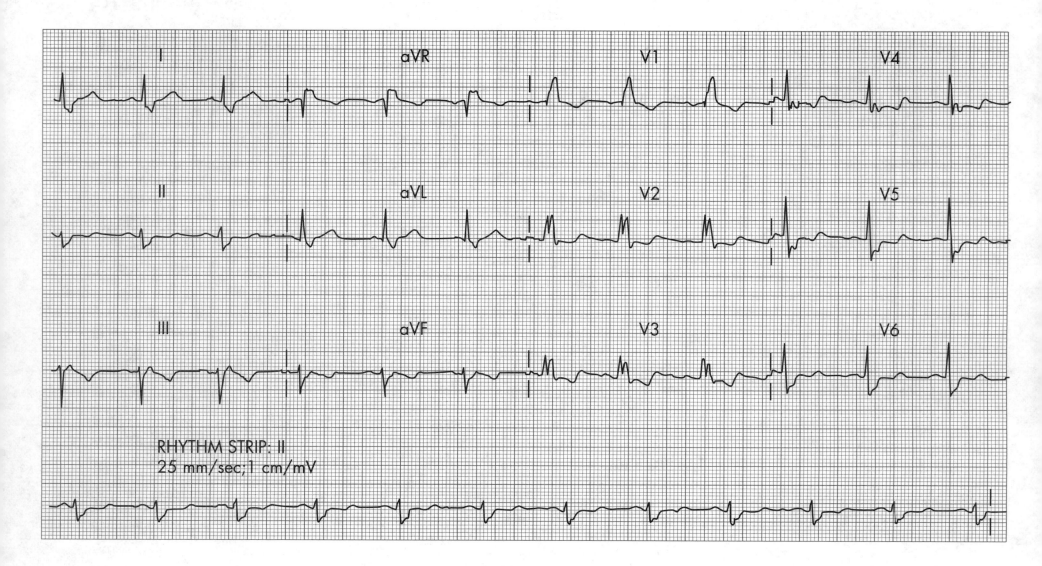

I   aVR   V1   V4

II   aVL   V2   V5

III   aVF   V3   V6

RHYTHM STRIP: II
25 mm/sec;1 cm/mV

Figure 3-29
Resting 12-Lead ECG

172

1. **RATE**

   Atrial:

   Ventricular:

2. **RHYTHM**

   Atrial:

   Ventricular:

3. **WAVES**

   P waves present:

   Appearance:

   Consistent:

   Relation to QRS:

   Q waves present:

   Leads:

   Pathological:

   T waves present:

   Morphology:

4. **INTERVALS**

   P-R interval:

   Consistent:

   QRS:

   Appearance:

   Consistent:

   Q-T interval:

5. **AXIS**

   Quadrant:

   Degrees:

6. **HYPERTROPHY**

   Atrial:

   Ventricular:

7. **MYOCARDIAL INFARCTION**

   Q waves:

   S-T displacement:

8. **ISCHEMIA**

   S-T displacement:

9. **POSSIBLE DRUG EFFECTS**

10. **ECG ANALYSIS**

11. **INTERPRETATION**

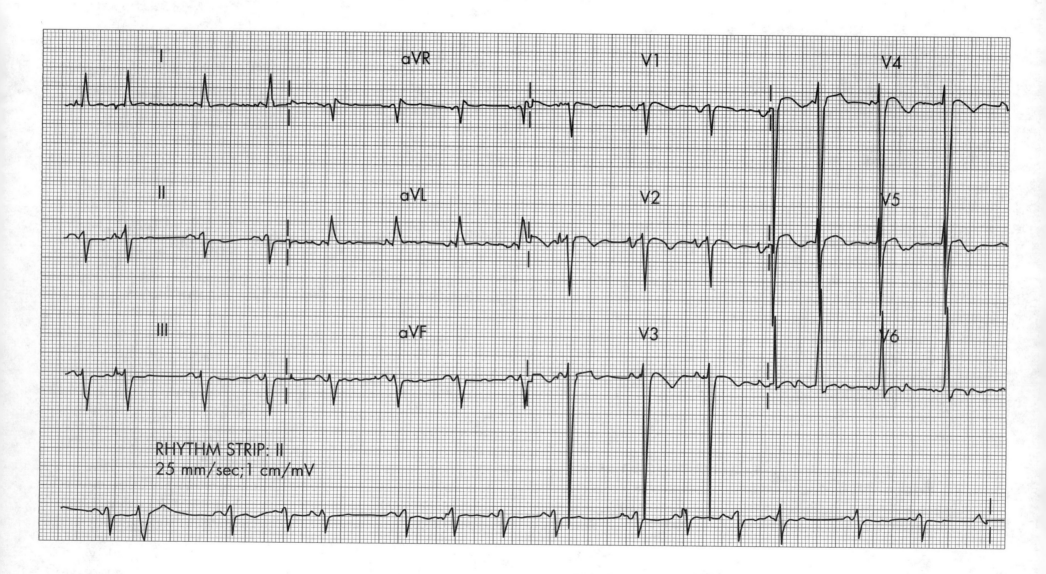

I aVR V1 V4

II aVL V2 V5

III aVF V3 V6

RHYTHM STRIP: II
25 mm/sec; 1 cm/mV

Figure 3-30
Resting 12-Lead ECG

1. **RATE**

   Atrial:

   Ventricular:

2. **RHYTHM**

   Atrial:

   Ventricular:

3. **WAVES**

   P waves present:

   Appearance:

   Consistent:

   Relation to QRS:

   Q waves present:

   Leads:

   Pathological:

   T waves present:

   Morphology:

4. **INTERVALS**

   P-R interval:

   Consistent:

   QRS:

   Appearance:

   Consistent:

   Q-T interval:

5. **AXIS**

   Quadrant:

   Degrees:

6. **HYPERTROPHY**

   Atrial:

   Ventricular:

7. **MYOCARDIAL INFARCTION**

   Q waves:

   S-T displacement:

8. **ISCHEMIA**

   S-T displacement:

9. **POSSIBLE DRUG EFFECTS**

10. **ECG ANALYSIS**

11. **INTERPRETATION**

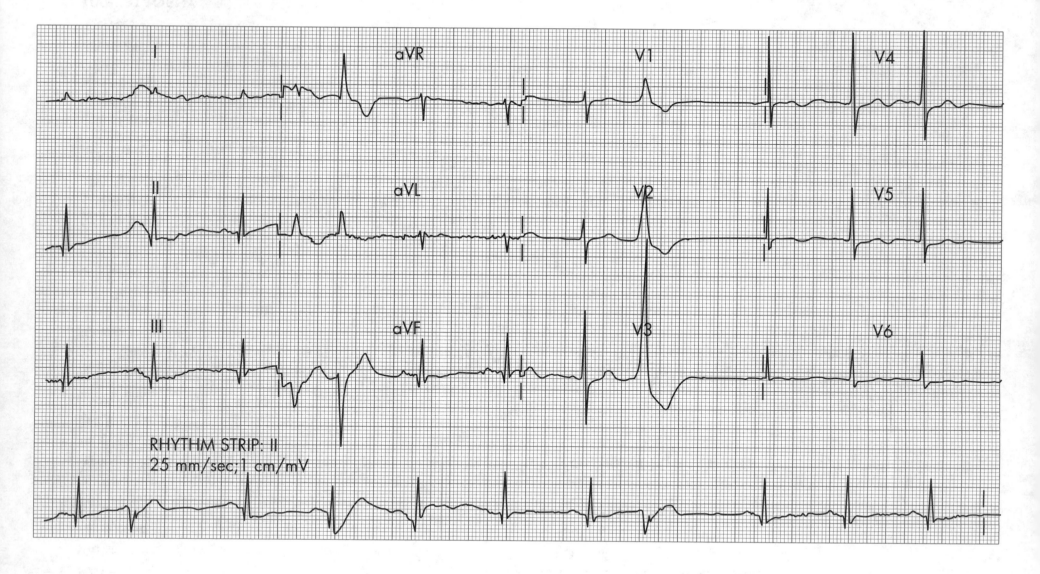

I   aVR   V1   V4

II   aVL   V2   V5

III   aVF   V3   V6

RHYTHM STRIP: II
25 mm/sec; 1 cm/mV

Figure 3-31
Resting 12-Lead ECG

1. **RATE**

   Atrial:

   Ventricular:

2. **RHYTHM**

   Atrial:

   Ventricular:

3. **WAVES**

   P waves present:

       Appearance:

       Consistent:

       Relation to QRS:

   Q waves present:

       Leads:

       Pathological:

   T waves present:

       Morphology:

4. **INTERVALS**

   P-R interval:

       Consistent:

   QRS:

       Appearance:

       Consistent:

   Q-T interval:

5. **AXIS**

   Quadrant:

   Degrees:

6. **HYPERTROPHY**

   Atrial:

   Ventricular:

7. **MYOCARDIAL INFARCTION**

   Q waves:

   S-T displacement:

8. **ISCHEMIA**

   S-T displacement:

9. **POSSIBLE DRUG EFFECTS**

10. **ECG ANALYSIS**

11. **INTERPRETATION**

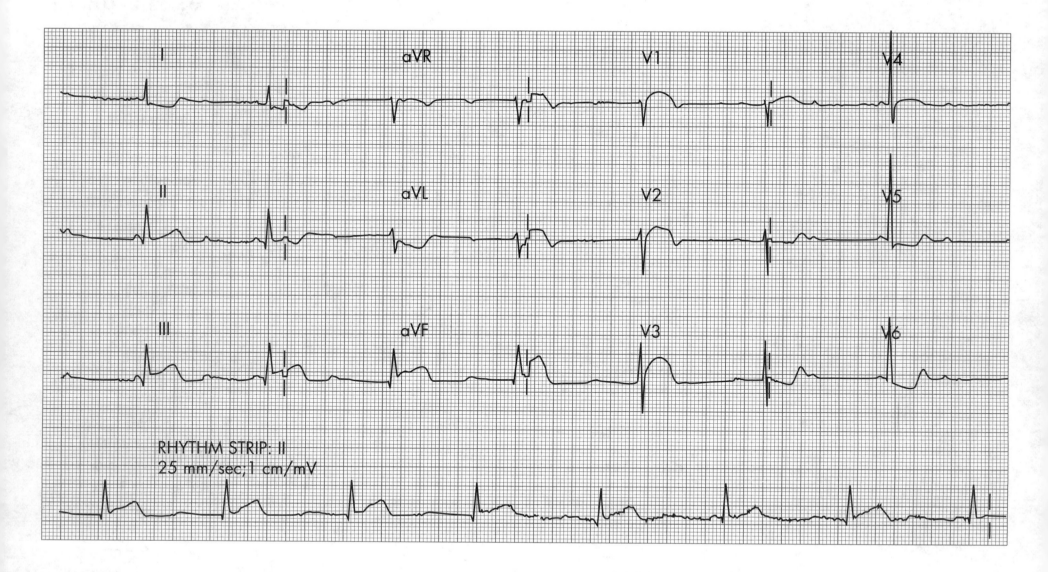

Figure 3-32
Resting 12-Lead ECG
178

1. **RATE**

   Atrial:

   Ventricular:

2. **RHYTHM**

   Atrial:

   Ventricular:

3. **WAVES**

   P waves present:

      Appearance:

      Consistent:

      Relation to QRS:

   Q waves present:

      Leads:

      Pathological:

   T waves present:

      Morphology:

4. **INTERVALS**

   P-R interval:

      Consistent:

   QRS:

      Appearance:

      Consistent:

   Q-T interval:

5. **AXIS**

   Quadrant:

   Degrees:

6. **HYPERTROPHY**

   Atrial:

   Ventricular:

7. **MYOCARDIAL INFARCTION**

   Q waves:

   S-T displacement:

8. **ISCHEMIA**

   S-T displacement:

9. **POSSIBLE DRUG EFFECTS**

10. **ECG ANALYSIS**

11. **INTERPRETATION**

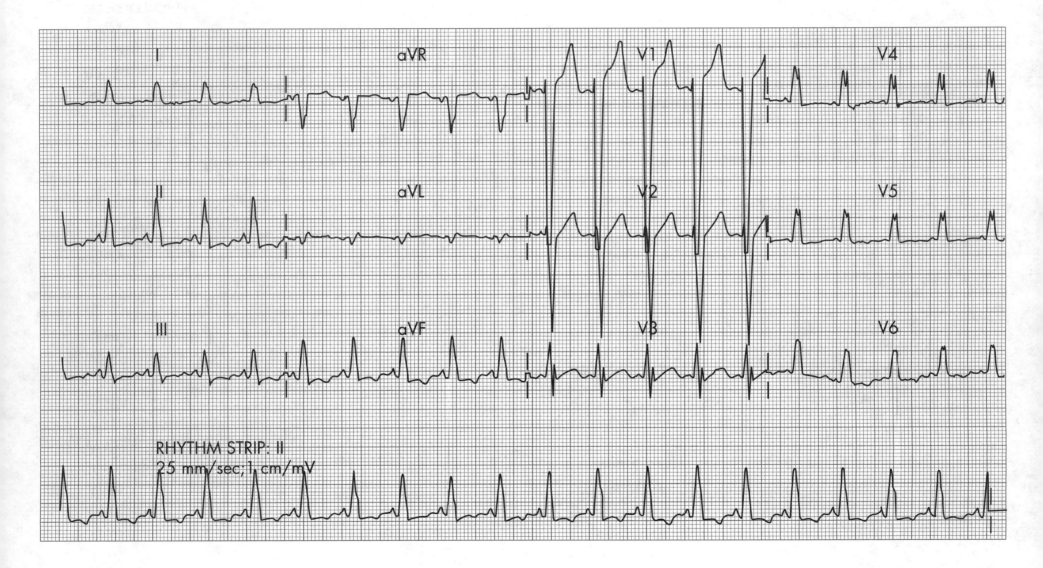

Figure 3-33
Resting 12-Lead ECG

180

I. RATE

   Atrial:

   Ventricular:

2. RHYTHM

   Atrial:

   Ventricular:

3. WAVES

   P waves present:

   　　Appearance:

   　　Consistent:

   　　Relation to QRS:

   Q waves present:

   　　Leads:

   　　Pathological:

   T waves present:

   　　Morphology:

4. INTERVALS

   P-R interval:

   　　Consistent:

   QRS:

   　　Appearance:

   　　Consistent:

   Q-T interval:

5. AXIS

   Quadrant:

   Degrees:

6. HYPERTROPHY

   Atrial:

   Ventricular:

7. MYOCARDIAL INFARCTION

   Q waves:

   S-T displacement:

8. ISCHEMIA

   S-T displacement:

9. POSSIBLE DRUG EFFECTS

10. ECG ANALYSIS

11. INTERPRETATION

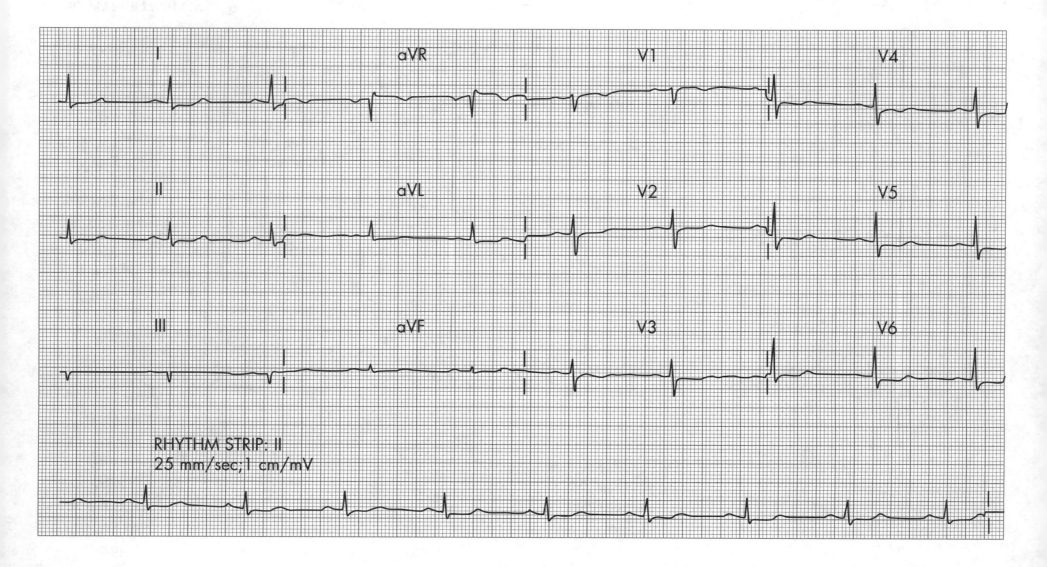

I aVR V1 V4

II aVL V2 V5

III aVF V3 V6

RHYTHM STRIP: II
25 mm/sec; 1 cm/mV

Figure 3-34
Resting 12-Lead ECG
182

1. **RATE**

   Atrial:

   Ventricular:

2. **RHYTHM**

   Atrial:

   Ventricular:

3. **WAVES**

   P waves present:

      Appearance:

      Consistent:

      Relation to QRS:

   Q waves present:

      Leads:

      Pathological:

   T waves present:

      Morphology:

4. **INTERVALS**

   P-R interval:

      Consistent:

   QRS:

      Appearance:

      Consistent:

   Q-T interval:

5. **AXIS**

   Quadrant:

   Degrees:

6. **HYPERTROPHY**

   Atrial:

   Ventricular:

7. **MYOCARDIAL INFARCTION**

   Q waves:

   S-T displacement:

8. **ISCHEMIA**

   S-T displacement:

9. **POSSIBLE DRUG EFFECTS**

10. **ECG ANALYSIS**

11. **INTERPRETATION**

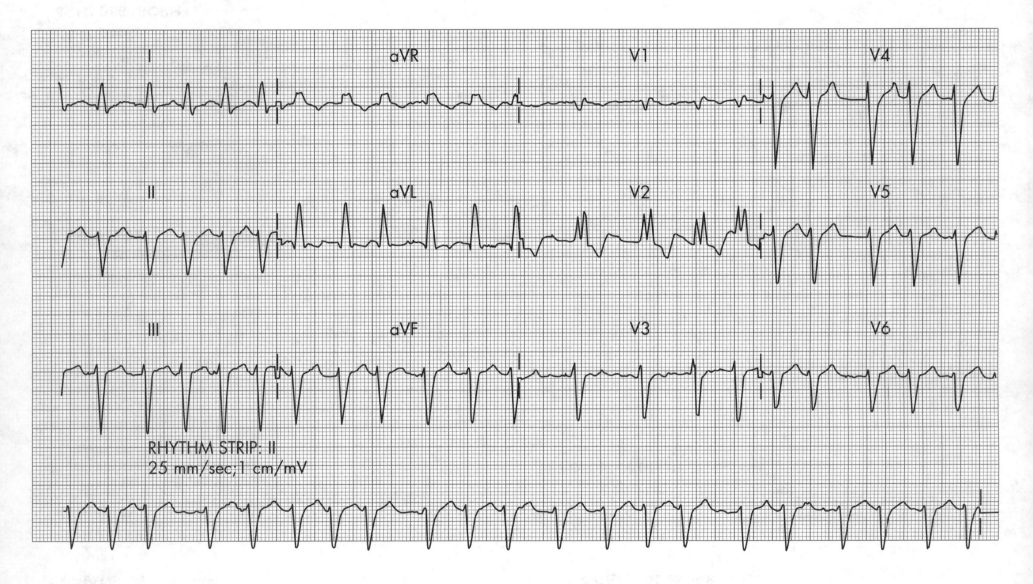

Figure 3-35
Resting 12-Lead ECG

I. RATE

    Atrial:

    Ventricular:

2. RHYTHM

    Atrial:

    Ventricular:

3. WAVES

    P waves present:

        Appearance:

        Consistent:

        Relation to QRS:

    Q waves present:

        Leads:

        Pathological:

    T waves present:

        Morphology:

4. INTERVALS

    P-R interval:

        Consistent:

    QRS:

        Appearance:

        Consistent:

    Q-T interval:

5. AXIS

    Quadrant:

    Degrees:

6. HYPERTROPHY

    Atrial:

    Ventricular:

7. MYOCARDIAL INFARCTION

    Q waves:

    S-T displacement:

8. ISCHEMIA

    S-T displacement:

9. POSSIBLE DRUG EFFECTS

10. ECG ANALYSIS

11. INTERPRETATION

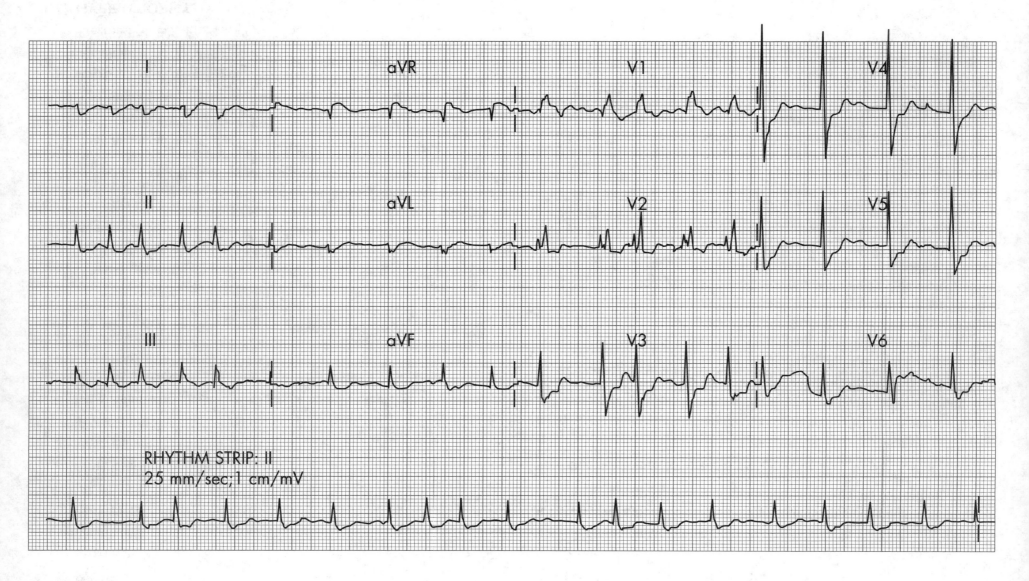

I   aVR   V1   V4

II   aVL   V2   V5

III   aVF   V3   V6

RHYTHM STRIP: II
25 mm/sec; 1 cm/mV

Figure 3-36
Resting 12-Lead ECG

1. RATE

Atrial:

Ventricular:

2. RHYTHM

Atrial:

Ventricular:

3. WAVES

P waves present:

Appearance:

Consistent:

Relation to QRS:

Q waves present:

Leads:

Pathological:

T waves present:

Morphology:

4. INTERVALS

P-R interval:

Consistent:

QRS:

Appearance:

Consistent:

Q-T interval:

5. AXIS

Quadrant:

Degrees:

6. HYPERTROPHY

Atrial:

Ventricular:

7. MYOCARDIAL INFARCTION

Q waves:

S-T displacement:

8. ISCHEMIA

S-T displacement:

9. POSSIBLE DRUG EFFECTS

10. ECG ANALYSIS

11. INTERPRETATION

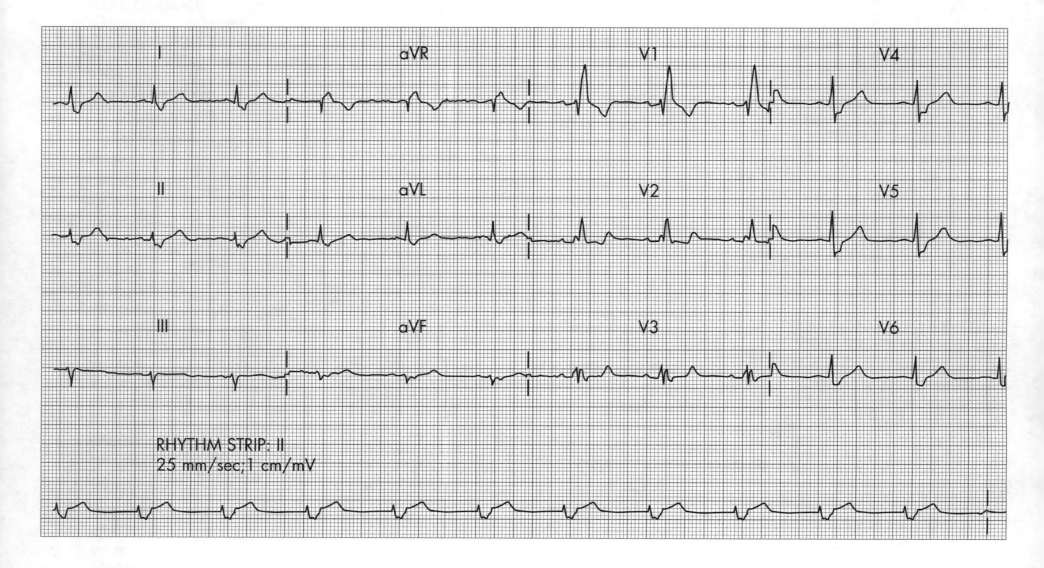

I aVR V1 V4

II aVL V2 V5

III aVF V3 V6

RHYTHM STRIP: II
25 mm/sec; 1 cm/mV

Figure 3-37
Resting 12-Lead ECG

1. **RATE**

   Atrial:

   Ventricular:

2. **RHYTHM**

   Atrial:

   Ventricular:

3. **WAVES**

   P waves present:

       Appearance:

       Consistent:

       Relation to QRS:

   Q waves present:

       Leads:

       Pathological:

   T waves present:

       Morphology:

4. **INTERVALS**

   P-R interval:

       Consistent:

   QRS:

       Appearance:

       Consistent:

   Q-T interval:

5. **AXIS**

   Quadrant:

   Degrees:

6. **HYPERTROPHY**

   Atrial:

   Ventricular:

7. **MYOCARDIAL INFARCTION**

   Q waves:

   S-T displacement:

8. **ISCHEMIA**

   S-T displacement:

9. **POSSIBLE DRUG EFFECTS**

10. **ECG ANALYSIS**

11. **INTERPRETATION**

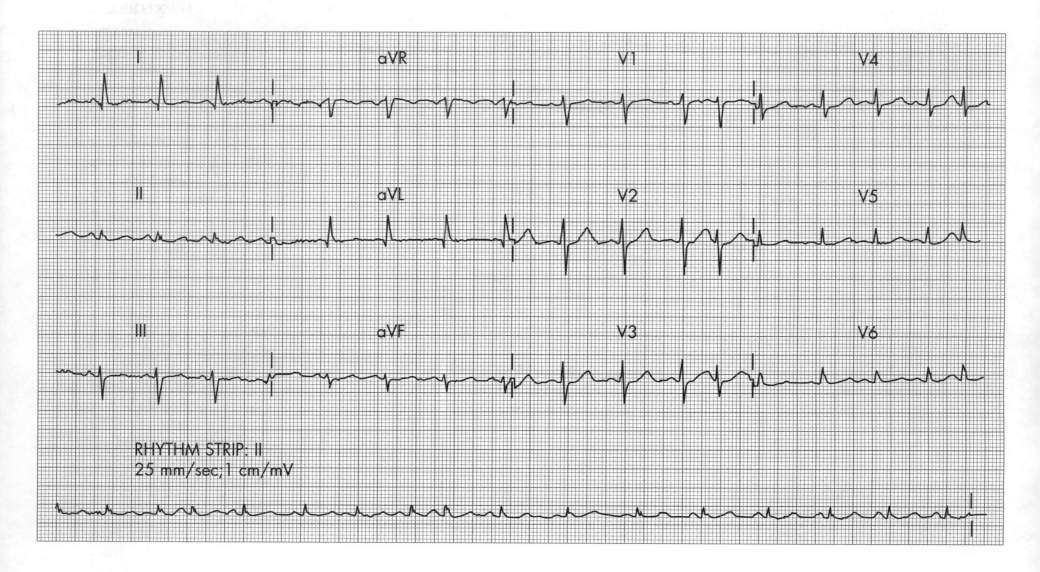

Figure 3-38
Resting 12-Lead ECG
190

1. RATE

Atrial:

Ventricular:

2. RHYTHM

Atrial:

Ventricular:

3. WAVES

P waves present:

Appearance:

Consistent:

Relation to QRS:

Q waves present:

Leads:

Pathological:

T waves present:

Morphology:

4. INTERVALS

P-R interval:

Consistent:

QRS:

Appearance:

Consistent:

Q-T interval:

5. AXIS

Quadrant:

Degrees:

6. HYPERTROPHY

Atrial:

Ventricular:

7. MYOCARDIAL INFARCTION

Q waves:

S-T displacement:

8. ISCHEMIA

S-T displacement:

9. POSSIBLE DRUG EFFECTS

10. ECG ANALYSIS

11. INTERPRETATION

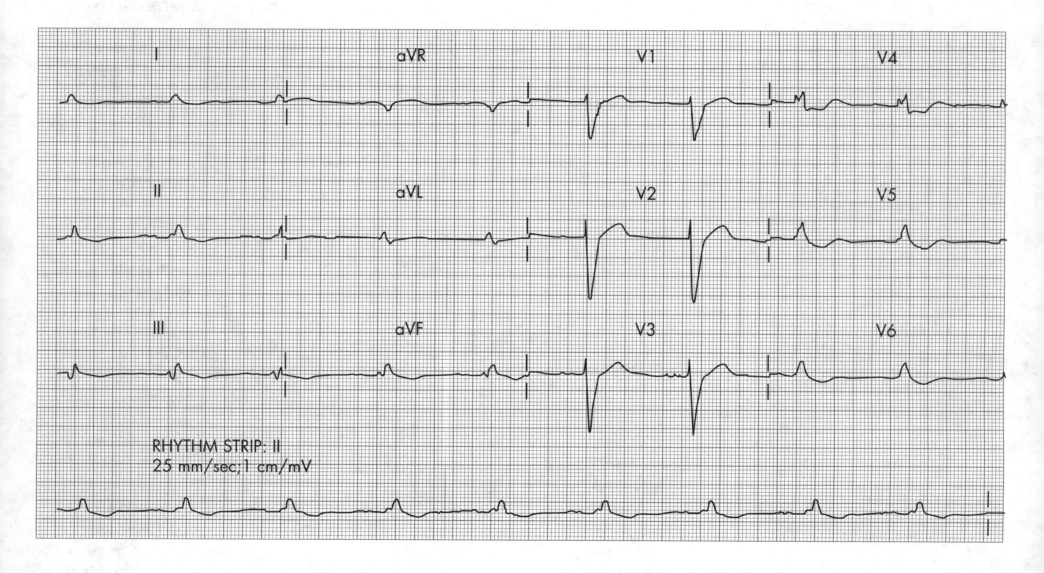

I aVR V1 V4

II aVL V2 V5

III aVF V3 V6

RHYTHM STRIP: II
25 mm/sec; 1 cm/mV

Figure 3-39
Resting 12-Lead ECG

192

1. **RATE**

   Atrial:

   Ventricular:

2. **RHYTHM**

   Atrial:

   Ventricular:

3. **WAVES**

   P waves present:

       Appearance:

       Consistent:

       Relation to QRS:

   Q waves present:

       Leads:

       Pathological:

   T waves present:

       Morphology:

4. **INTERVALS**

   P-R interval:

       Consistent:

   QRS:

       Appearance:

       Consistent:

   Q-T interval:

5. **AXIS**

   Quadrant:

   Degrees:

6. **HYPERTROPHY**

   Atrial:

   Ventricular:

7. **MYOCARDIAL INFARCTION**

   Q waves:

   S-T displacement:

8. **ISCHEMIA**

   S-T displacement:

9. **POSSIBLE DRUG EFFECTS**

10. **ECG ANALYSIS**

11. **INTERPRETATION**

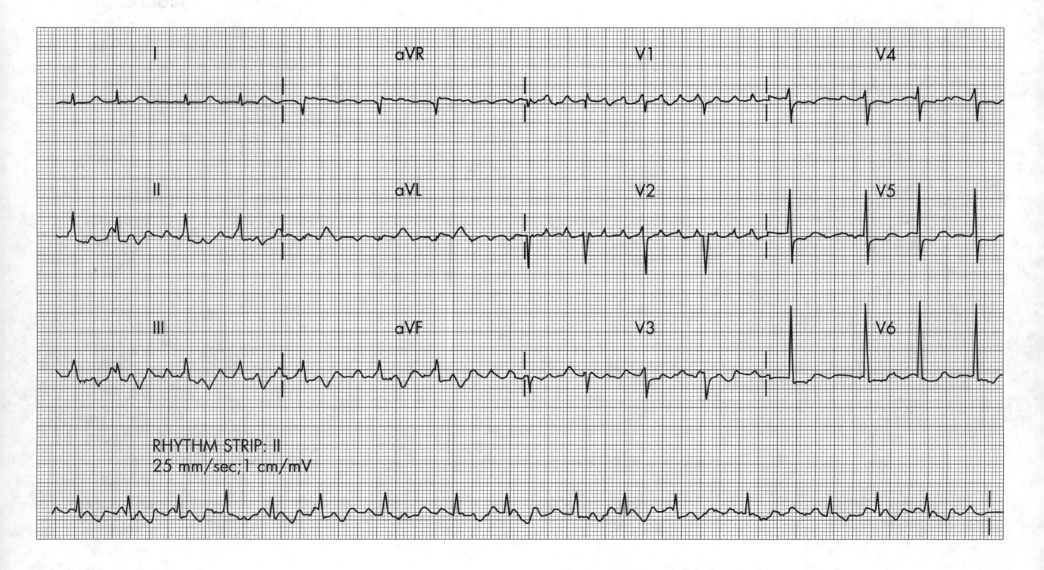

I aVR V1 V4

II aVL V2 V5

III aVF V3 V6

RHYTHM STRIP: II
25 mm/sec;1 cm/mV

Figure 3-40
Resting 12-Lead ECG
194

1. RATE

Atrial:

Ventricular:

2. RHYTHM

Atrial:

Ventricular:

3. WAVES

P waves present:

   Appearance:

   Consistent:

   Relation to QRS:

Q waves present:

   Leads:

   Pathological:

T waves present:

   Morphology:

4. INTERVALS

P-R interval:

   Consistent:

QRS:

   Appearance:

   Consistent:

Q-T interval:

5. AXIS

Quadrant:

Degrees:

6. HYPERTROPHY

Atrial:

Ventricular:

7. MYOCARDIAL INFARCTION

Q waves:

S-T displacement:

8. ISCHEMIA

S-T displacement:

9. POSSIBLE DRUG EFFECTS

10. ECG ANALYSIS

11. INTERPRETATION

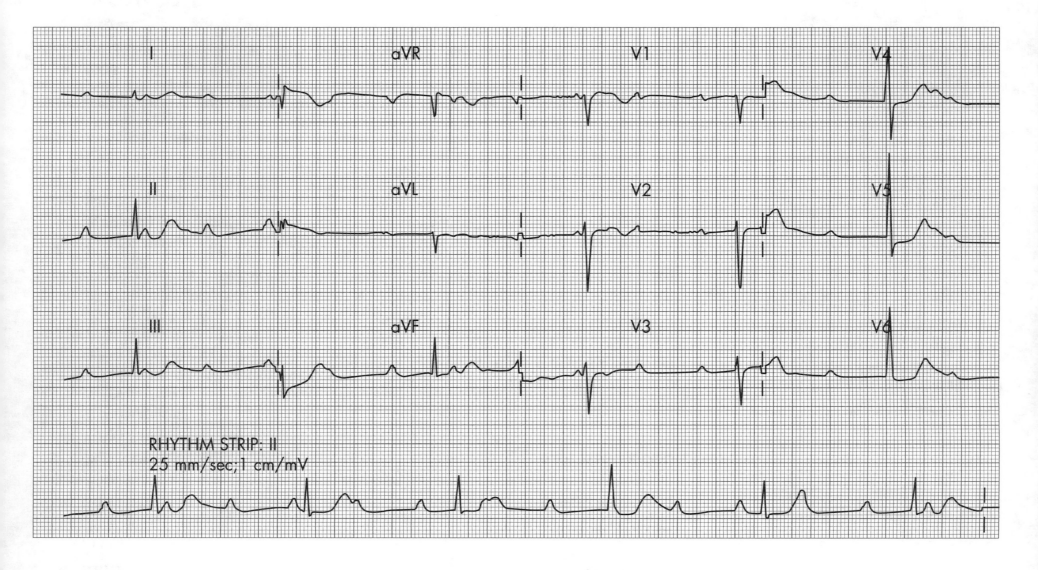

RHYTHM STRIP: II
25 mm/sec;1 cm/mV

Figure 3-41
Resting 12-Lead ECG
196

1. RATE

Atrial:

Ventricular:

2. RHYTHM

Atrial:

Ventricular:

3. WAVES

P waves present:

Appearance:

Consistent:

Relation to QRS:

Q waves present:

Leads:

Pathological:

T waves present:

Morphology:

4. INTERVALS

P-R interval:

Consistent:

QRS:

Appearance:

Consistent:

Q-T interval:

5. AXIS

Quadrant:

Degrees:

6. HYPERTROPHY

Atrial:

Ventricular:

7. MYOCARDIAL INFARCTION

Q waves:

S-T displacement:

8. ISCHEMIA

S-T displacement:

9. POSSIBLE DRUG EFFECTS

10. ECG ANALYSIS

11. INTERPRETATION

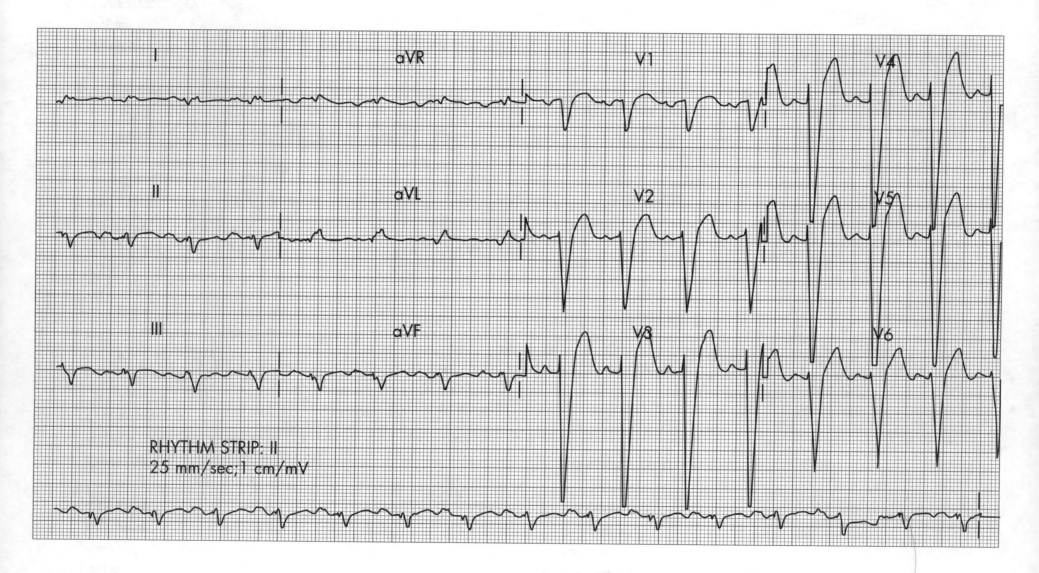

I aVR V1 V4

II aVL V2 V5

III aVF V3 V6

RHYTHM STRIP: II
25 mm/sec; 1 cm/mV

Figure 3-42
Resting 12-Lead ECG
198

I. RATE

Atrial:

Ventricular:

2. RHYTHM

Atrial:

Ventricular:

3. WAVES

P waves present:

Appearance:

Consistent:

Relation to QRS:

Q waves present:

Leads:

Pathological:

T waves present:

Morphology:

4. INTERVALS

P-R interval:

Consistent:

QRS:

Appearance:

Consistent:

Q-T interval:

5. AXIS

Quadrant:

Degrees:

6. HYPERTROPHY

Atrial:

Ventricular:

7. MYOCARDIAL INFARCTION

Q waves:

S-T displacement:

8. ISCHEMIA

S-T displacement:

9. POSSIBLE DRUG EFFECTS

10. ECG ANALYSIS

11. INTERPRETATION

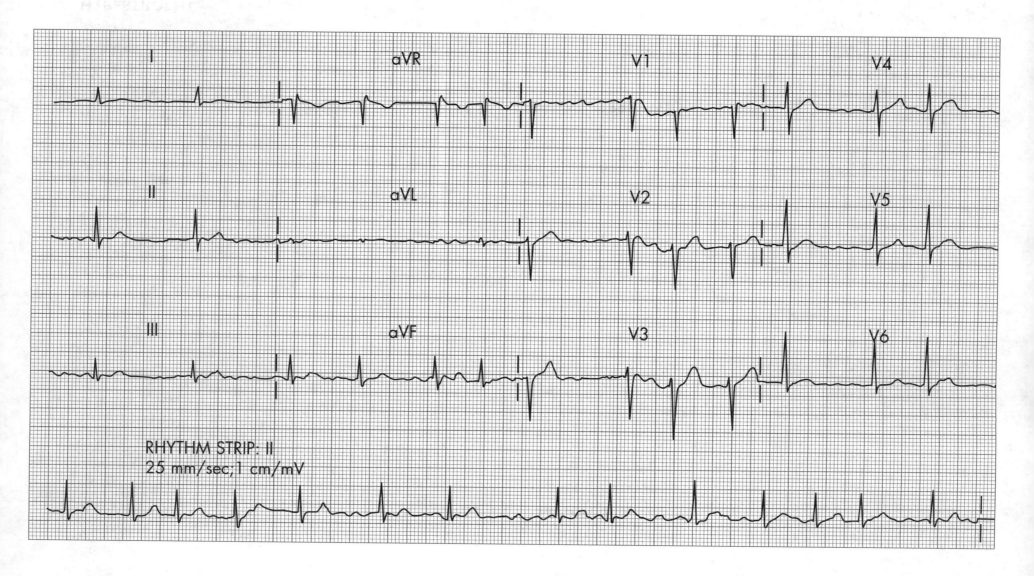

I

aVR

V1

V4

II

aVL

V2

V5

III

aVF

V3

V6

RHYTHM STRIP: II
25 mm/sec; 1 cm/mV

Figure 3-43
Resting 12-Lead ECG
200

1. RATE

Atrial:

Ventricular:

2. RHYTHM

Atrial:

Ventricular:

3. WAVES

P waves present:

Appearance:

Consistent:

Relation to QRS:

Q waves present:

Leads:

Pathological:

T waves present:

Morphology:

4. INTERVALS

P-R interval:

Consistent:

QRS:

Appearance:

Consistent:

Q-T interval:

5. AXIS

Quadrant:

Degrees:

6. HYPERTROPHY

Atrial:

Ventricular:

7. MYOCARDIAL INFARCTION

Q waves:

S-T displacement:

8. ISCHEMIA

S-T displacement:

9. POSSIBLE DRUG EFFECTS

10. ECG ANALYSIS

11. INTERPRETATION

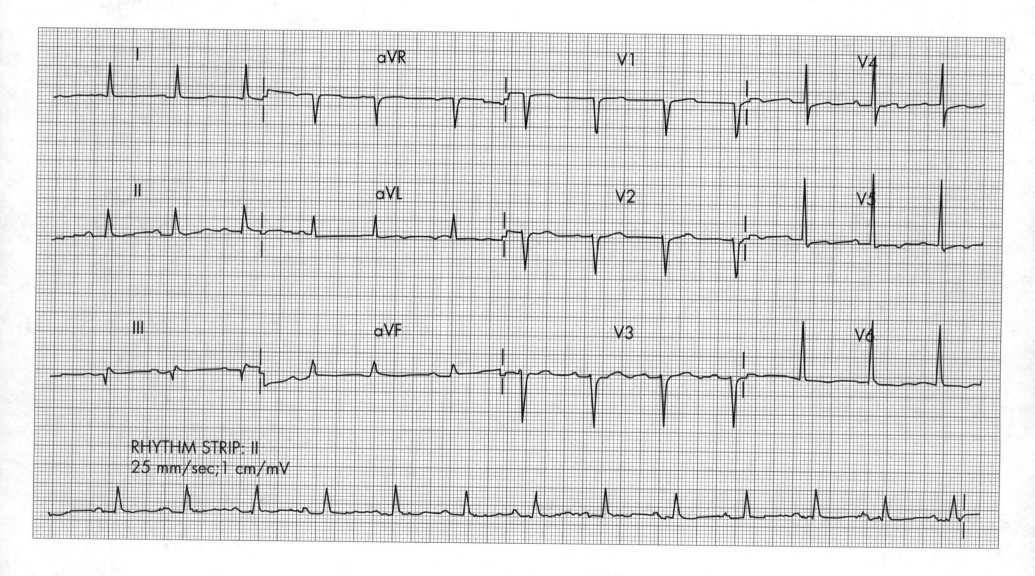

RHYTHM STRIP: II
25 mm/sec;1 cm/mV

Figure 3-44
Resting 12-Lead ECG
202

1. RATE

Atrial:

Ventricular:

2. RHYTHM

Atrial:

Ventricular:

3. WAVES

P waves present:

Appearance:

Consistent:

Relation to QRS:

Q waves present:

Leads:

Pathological:

T waves present:

Morphology:

4. INTERVALS

P-R interval:

Consistent:

QRS:

Appearance:

Consistent:

Q-T interval:

5. AXIS

Quadrant:

Degrees:

6. HYPERTROPHY

Atrial:

Ventricular:

7. MYOCARDIAL INFARCTION

Q waves:

S-T displacement:

8. ISCHEMIA

S-T displacement:

9. POSSIBLE DRUG EFFECTS

10. ECG ANALYSIS

11. INTERPRETATION

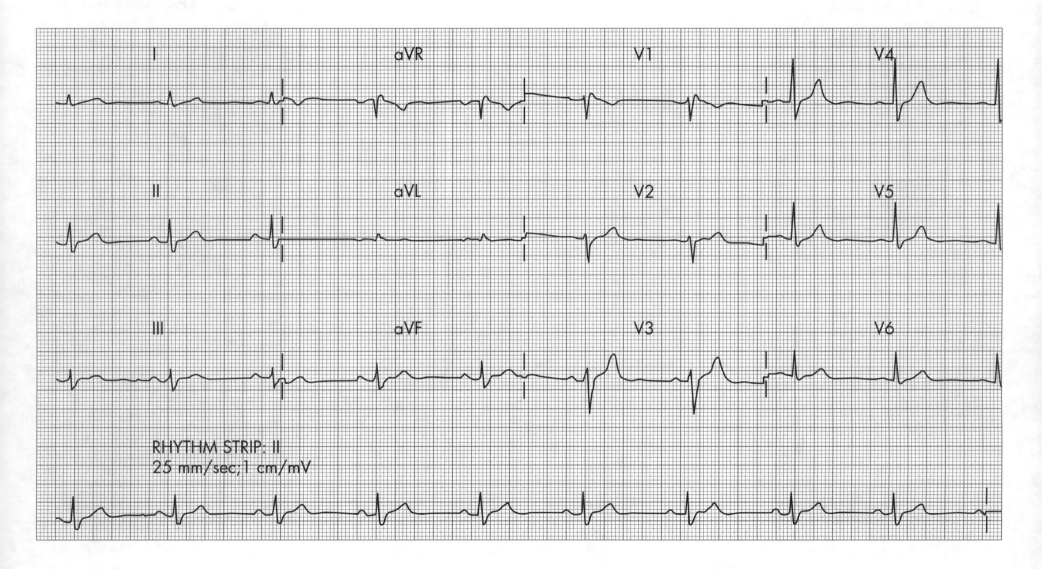

RHYTHM STRIP: II
25 mm/sec;1 cm/mV

Figure 3-45
Resting 12-Lead ECG
204

1. RATE

Atrial:

Ventricular:

2. RHYTHM

Atrial:

Ventricular:

3. WAVES

P waves present:

    Appearance:

    Consistent:

    Relation to QRS:

Q waves present:

    Leads:

    Pathological:

T waves present:

    Morphology:

4. INTERVALS

P-R interval:

    Consistent:

QRS:

    Appearance:

    Consistent:

Q-T interval:

5. AXIS

Quadrant:

Degrees:

6. HYPERTROPHY

Atrial:

Ventricular:

7. MYOCARDIAL INFARCTION

Q waves:

S-T displacement:

8. ISCHEMIA

S-T displacement:

9. POSSIBLE DRUG EFFECTS

10. ECG ANALYSIS

11. INTERPRETATION

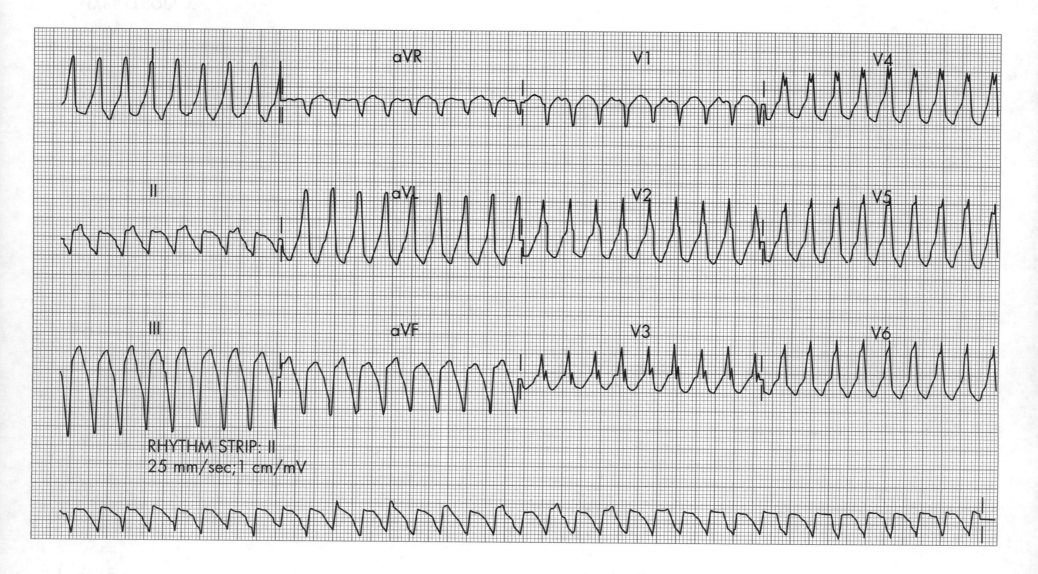

Figure 3-46
Resting 12-Lead ECG

206

1. **RATE**
   Atrial:
   Ventricular:

2. **RHYTHM**
   Atrial:
   Ventricular:

3. **WAVES**
   P waves present:
      Appearance:
      Consistent:
      Relation to QRS:
   Q waves present:
      Leads:
      Pathological:
   T waves present:
      Morphology:

4. **INTERVALS**
   P-R interval:
      Consistent:
   QRS:
      Appearance:
      Consistent:
   Q-T interval:

5. **AXIS**
   Quadrant:
   Degrees:

6. **HYPERTROPHY**
   Atrial:
   Ventricular:

7. **MYOCARDIAL INFARCTION**
   Q waves:
   S-T displacement:

8. **ISCHEMIA**
   S-T displacement:

9. **POSSIBLE DRUG EFFECTS**

10. **ECG ANALYSIS**

11. **INTERPRETATION**

Part IV
Atrial and Ventricular Hypertrophy

ECG CRITERIA

Atrial Enlargement

Right Atrial Enlargement (RAE)
- P wave in lead II is tall and peaked (greater than or equal to 2.5 mm)

Leads III and aVF may also have tall peaked P waves
- Supporting evidence: Biphasic P in V_1 with a more prominent initial deflection

Left Atrial Enlargement (LAE)
- P wave in lead II broad "M" shaped and greater than or equal to 0.12 seconds

Leads III, aVF, and V_{5-6} may also have broad P waves
- Supporting evidence: Biphasic P in V_1 with prominent terminal deflection

Ventricular Hypertrophy

Right Ventricular Hypertrophy (RVH)
RVH is often associated with pulmonary disease, therefore the ECG criteria for chronic pulmonary disease is essentially the same as for RVH.
- R greater than S in V_1

Other suggestive ECG findings include the following:
- Right axis deviation or indeterminate axis
- rSR' in V_1 (incomplete right bundle branch block)
- Right ventricular strain pattern (S-T depression)
- S greater than R in V_6
- Low QRS voltage

Left Ventricular Hypertrophy (LVH)
- S wave in V_1 or V_2 added to R in V_5 or V_6 is greater than or equal to 35 mm
- Left axis deviation
- Left ventricular strain pattern (S-T depression)
- R in lead aVL greater than or equal to 12 mm
- Left atrial involvement

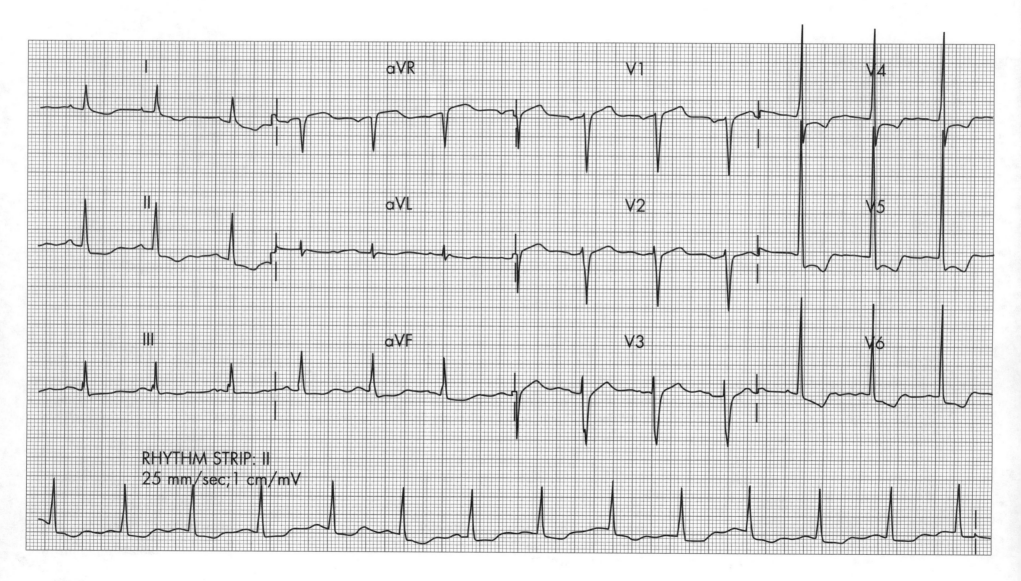

RHYTHM STRIP: II
25 mm/sec; 1 cm/mV

Figure 4-1
Resting 12-Lead ECG
212

1. **RATE**

   Atrial:

   Ventricular:

2. **RHYTHM**

   Atrial:

   Ventricular:

3. **WAVES**

   P waves present:

       Appearance:

       Consistent:

       Relation to QRS:

   Q waves present:

       Leads:

       Pathological:

   T waves present:

       Morphology:

4. **INTERVALS**

   P-R interval:

       Consistent:

   QRS:

       Appearance:

       Consistent:

   Q-T interval:

5. **AXIS**

   Quadrant:

   Degrees:

6. **HYPERTROPHY**

   Atrial:

   Ventricular:

7. **MYOCARDIAL INFARCTION**

   Q waves:

   S-T displacement:

8. **ISCHEMIA**

   S-T displacement:

9. **POSSIBLE DRUG EFFECTS**

10. **ECG ANALYSIS**

11. **INTERPRETATION**

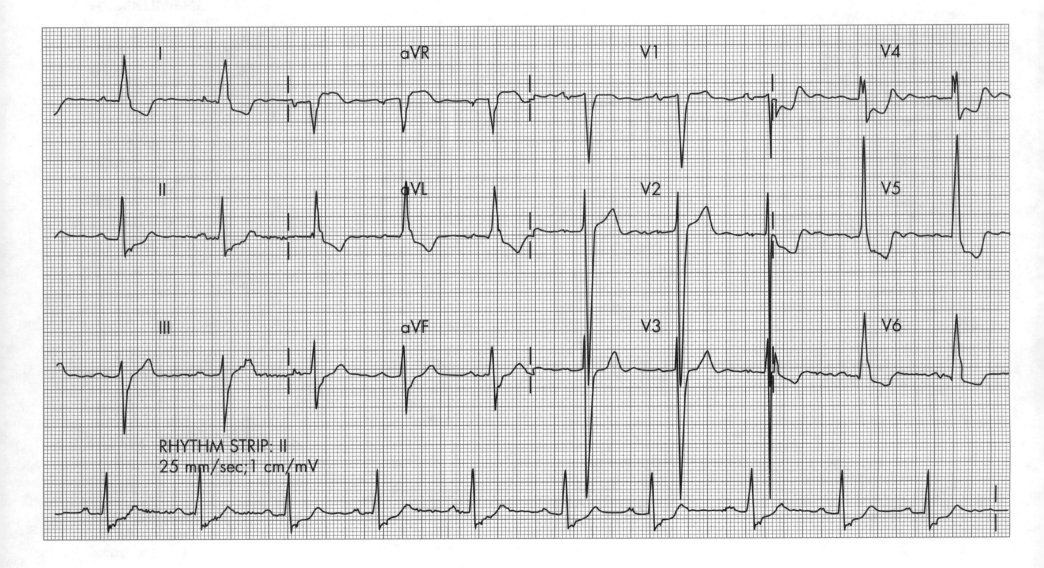

I aVR V1 V4

II aVL V2 V5

III aVF V3 V6

RHYTHM STRIP: II
25 mm/sec; 1 cm/mV

Figure 4-2
Resting 12-Lead ECG
214

ANALYSIS 4-2

I. RATE

    Atrial:

    Ventricular:

2. RHYTHM

    Atrial:

    Ventricular:

3. WAVES

    P waves present:

        Appearance:

        Consistent:

        Relation to QRS:

    Q waves present:

        Leads:

        Pathological:

    T waves present:

        Morphology:

4. INTERVALS

    P-R interval:

        Consistent:

    QRS:

        Appearance:

        Consistent:

    Q-T interval:

5. AXIS

    Quadrant:

    Degrees:

6. HYPERTROPHY

    Atrial:

    Ventricular:

7. MYOCARDIAL INFARCTION

    Q waves:

    S-T displacement:

8. ISCHEMIA

    S-T displacement:

9. POSSIBLE DRUG EFFECTS

10. ECG ANALYSIS

11. INTERPRETATION

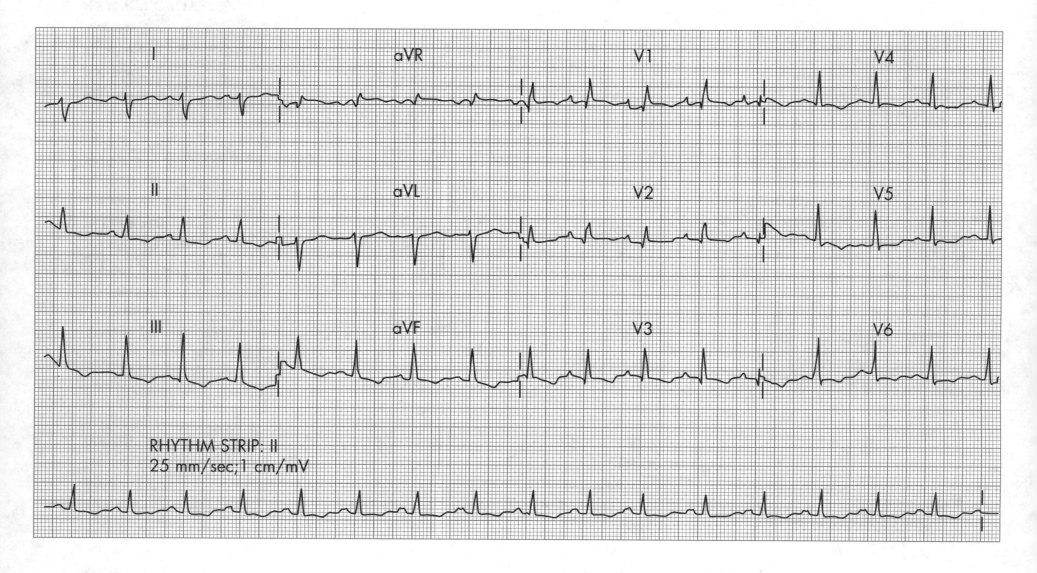

Figure 4-3
Resting 12-Lead ECG
216

I. RATE

Atrial:

Ventricular:

2. RHYTHM

Atrial:

Ventricular:

3. WAVES

P waves present:

   Appearance:

   Consistent:

   Relation to QRS:

Q waves present:

   Leads:

   Pathological:

T waves present:

   Morphology:

4. INTERVALS

P-R interval:

   Consistent:

QRS:

   Appearance:

   Consistent:

Q-T interval:

5. AXIS

Quadrant:

Degrees:

6. HYPERTROPHY

Atrial:

Ventricular:

7. MYOCARDIAL INFARCTION

Q waves:

S-T displacement:

8. ISCHEMIA

S-T displacement:

9. POSSIBLE DRUG EFFECTS

10. ECG ANALYSIS

11. INTERPRETATION

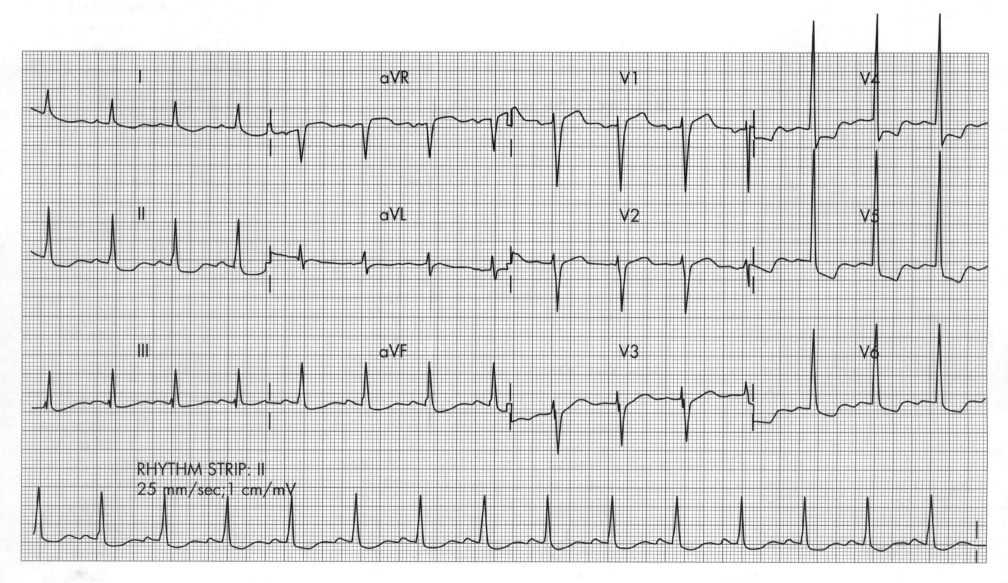

I aVR V1 V4

II aVL V2 V5

III aVF V3 V6

RHYTHM STRIP: II
25 mm/sec; 1 cm/mV

Figure 4-4
Resting 12-Lead ECG
218

1. RATE

Atrial:

Ventricular:

2. RHYTHM

Atrial:

Ventricular:

3. WAVES

P waves present:

Appearance:

Consistent:

Relation to QRS:

Q waves present:

Leads:

Pathological:

T waves present:

Morphology:

4. INTERVALS

P-R interval:

Consistent:

QRS:

Appearance:

Consistent:

Q-T interval:

5. AXIS

Quadrant:

Degrees:

6. HYPERTROPHY

Atrial:

Ventricular:

7. MYOCARDIAL INFARCTION

Q waves:

S-T displacement:

8. ISCHEMIA

S-T displacement:

9. POSSIBLE DRUG EFFECTS

10. ECG ANALYSIS

11. INTERPRETATION

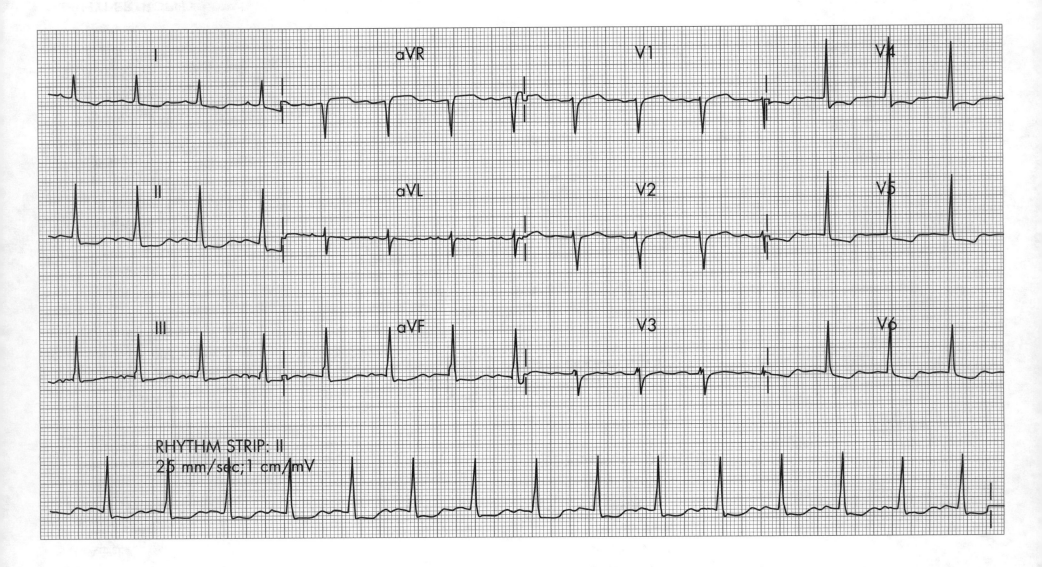

I	aVR	V1	V4
II	aVL	V2	V5
III	aVF	V3	V6

RHYTHM STRIP: II
25 mm/sec; 1 cm/mV

Figure 4-5
Resting 12-Lead ECG
220

I. RATE

Atrial:

Ventricular:

2. RHYTHM

Atrial:

Ventricular:

3. WAVES

P waves present:

Appearance:

Consistent:

Relation to QRS:

Q waves present:

Leads:

Pathological:

T waves present:

Morphology:

4. INTERVALS

P-R interval:

Consistent:

QRS:

Appearance:

Consistent:

Q-T interval:

5. AXIS

Quadrant:

Degrees:

6. HYPERTROPHY

Atrial:

Ventricular:

7. MYOCARDIAL INFARCTION

Q waves:

S-T displacement:

8. ISCHEMIA

S-T displacement:

9. POSSIBLE DRUG EFFECTS

10. ECG ANALYSIS

11. INTERPRETATION

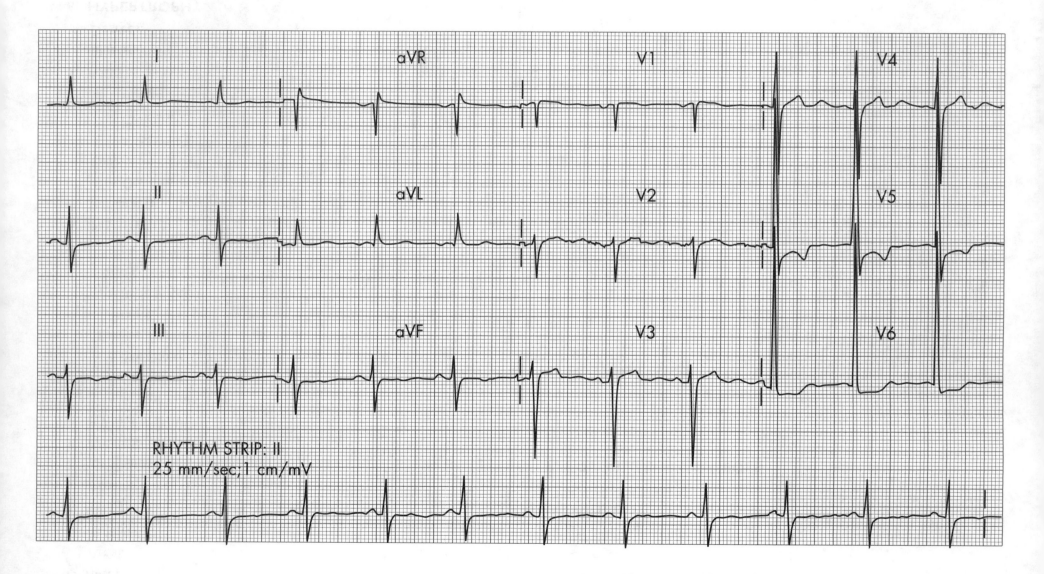

RHYTHM STRIP: II
25 mm/sec; 1 cm/mV

Figure 4-6
Resting 12-Lead ECG

1. RATE

Atrial:

Ventricular:

2. RHYTHM

Atrial:

Ventricular:

3. WAVES

P waves present:

Appearance:

Consistent:

Relation to QRS:

Q waves present:

Leads:

Pathological:

T waves present:

Morphology:

4. INTERVALS

P-R interval:

Consistent:

QRS:

Appearance:

Consistent:

Q-T interval:

5. AXIS

Quadrant:

Degrees:

6. HYPERTROPHY

Atrial:

Ventricular:

7. MYOCARDIAL INFARCTION

Q waves:

S-T displacement:

8. ISCHEMIA

S-T displacement:

9. POSSIBLE DRUG EFFECTS

10. ECG ANALYSIS

11. INTERPRETATION

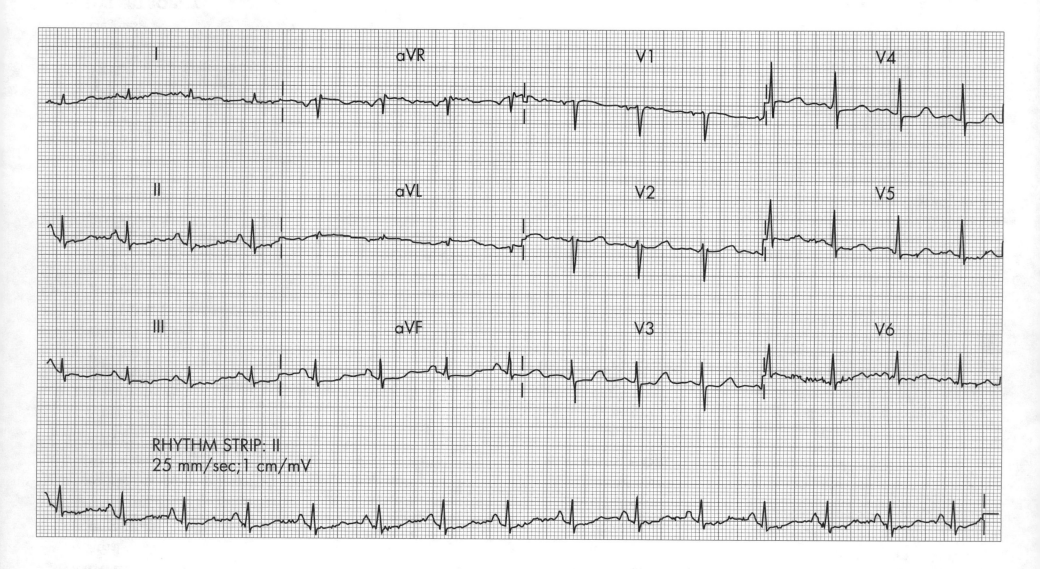

I   aVR   V1   V4

II   aVL   V2   V5

III   aVF   V3   V6

RHYTHM STRIP: II
25 mm/sec; 1 cm/mV

Figure 4-7
Resting 12-Lead ECG

1. RATE

Atrial:

Ventricular:

2. RHYTHM

Atrial:

Ventricular:

3. WAVES

P waves present:

Appearance:

Consistent:

Relation to QRS:

Q waves present:

Leads:

Pathological:

T waves present:

Morphology:

4. INTERVALS

P-R interval:

Consistent:

QRS:

Appearance:

Consistent:

Q-T interval:

5. AXIS

Quadrant:

Degrees:

6. HYPERTROPHY

Atrial:

Ventricular:

7. MYOCARDIAL INFARCTION

Q waves:

S-T displacement:

8. ISCHEMIA

S-T displacement:

9. POSSIBLE DRUG EFFECTS

10. ECG ANALYSIS

11. INTERPRETATION

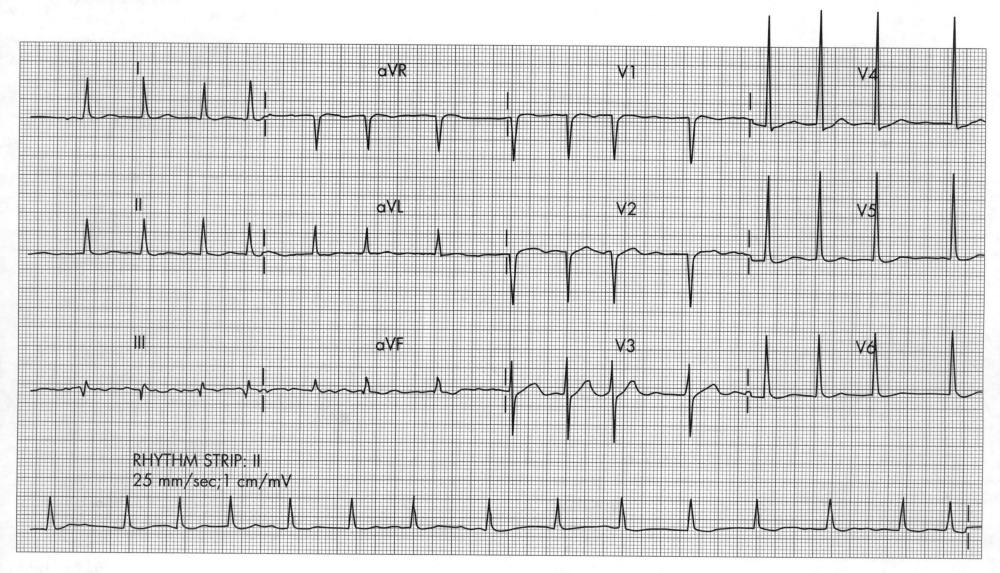

RHYTHM STRIP: II
25 mm/sec; 1 cm/mV

Figure 4-8
Resting 12-Lead ECG

1. RATE

Atrial:

Ventricular:

2. RHYTHM

Atrial:

Ventricular:

3. WAVES

P waves present:

    Appearance:

    Consistent:

    Relation to QRS:

Q waves present:

    Leads:

    Pathological:

T waves present:

    Morphology:

4. INTERVALS

P-R interval:

    Consistent:

QRS:

    Appearance:

    Consistent:

Q-T interval:

5. AXIS

Quadrant:

Degrees:

6. HYPERTROPHY

Atrial:

Ventricular:

7. MYOCARDIAL INFARCTION

Q waves:

S-T displacement:

8. ISCHEMIA

S-T displacement:

9. POSSIBLE DRUG EFFECTS

10. ECG ANALYSIS

11. INTERPRETATION

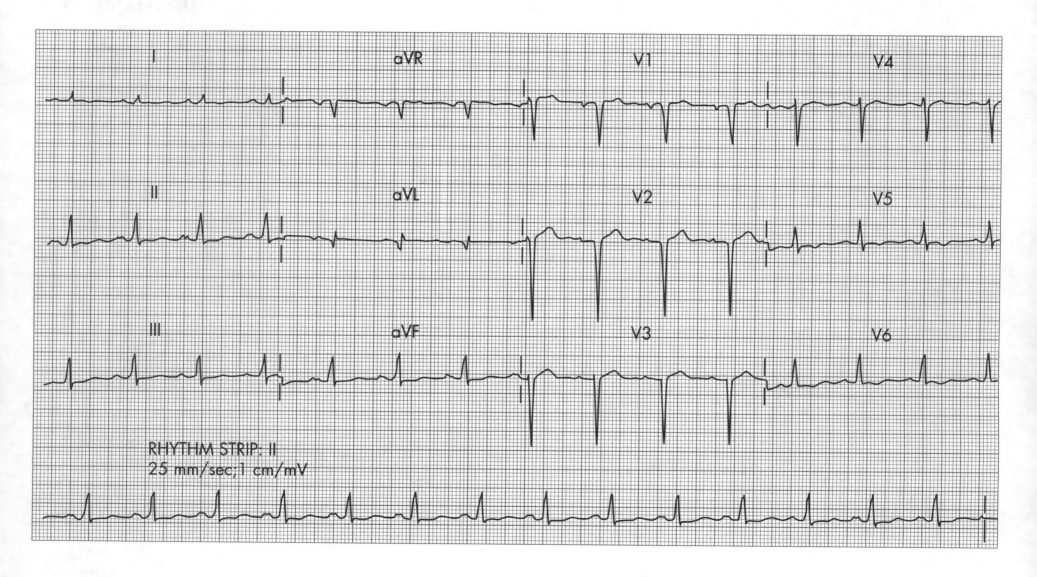

I aVR V1 V4

II aVL V2 V5

III aVF V3 V6

RHYTHM STRIP: II
25 mm/sec; 1 cm/mV

Figure 4-9
Resting 12-Lead ECG

228

1. RATE

    Atrial:

    Ventricular:

2. RHYTHM

    Atrial:

    Ventricular:

3. WAVES

    P waves present:

        Appearance:

        Consistent:

        Relation to QRS:

    Q waves present:

        Leads:

        Pathological:

    T waves present:

        Morphology:

4. INTERVALS

    P-R interval:

        Consistent:

    QRS:

        Appearance:

        Consistent:

    Q-T interval:

5. AXIS

    Quadrant:

    Degrees:

6. HYPERTROPHY

    Atrial:

    Ventricular:

7. MYOCARDIAL INFARCTION

    Q waves:

    S-T displacement:

8. ISCHEMIA

    S-T displacement:

9. POSSIBLE DRUG EFFECTS

10. ECG ANALYSIS

11. INTERPRETATION

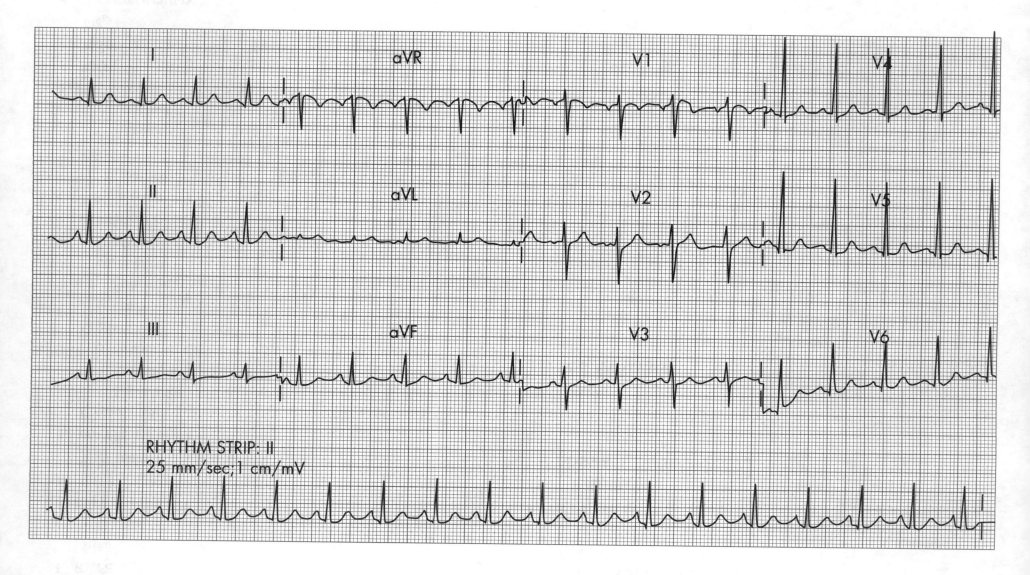

Figure 4-10
Resting 12-Lead ECG

1. RATE

Atrial:

Ventricular:

2. RHYTHM

Atrial:

Ventricular:

3. WAVES

P waves present:

Appearance:

Consistent:

Relation to QRS:

Q waves present:

Leads:

Pathological:

T waves present:

Morphology:

4. INTERVALS

P-R interval:

Consistent:

QRS:

Appearance:

Consistent:

Q-T interval:

5. AXIS

Quadrant:

Degrees:

6. HYPERTROPHY

Atrial:

Ventricular:

7. MYOCARDIAL INFARCTION

Q waves:

S-T displacement:

8. ISCHEMIA

S-T displacement:

9. POSSIBLE DRUG EFFECTS

10. ECG ANALYSIS

11. INTERPRETATION

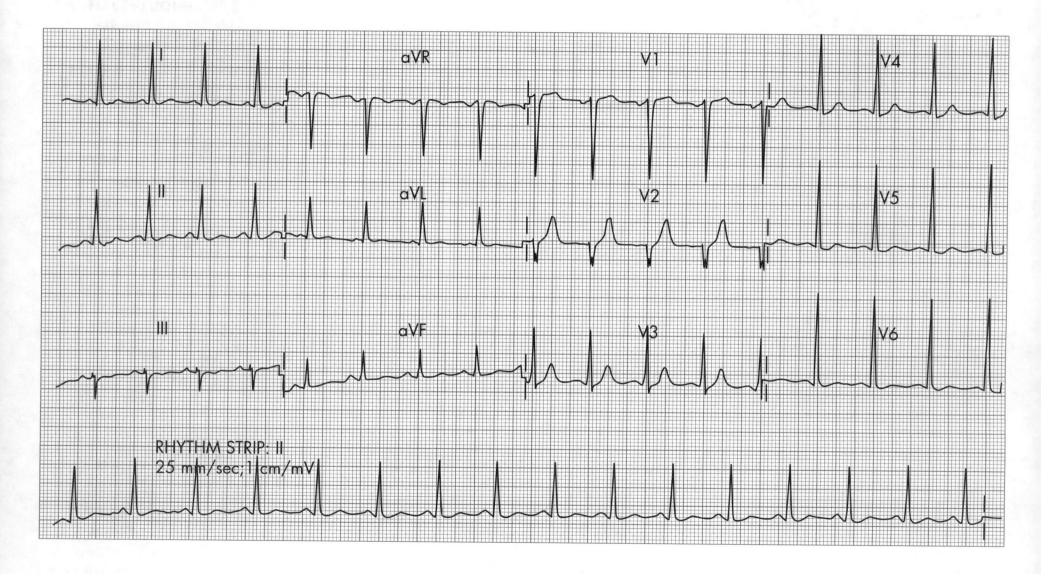

RHYTHM STRIP: II
25 mm/sec; 1 cm/mV

Figure 4-11
Resting 12-Lead ECG

232

1. RATE
Atrial:

Ventricular:

2. RHYTHM
Atrial:

Ventricular:

3. WAVES
P waves present:

    Appearance:

    Consistent:

    Relation to QRS:

Q waves present:

    Leads:

    Pathological:

T waves present:

    Morphology:

4. INTERVALS
P-R interval:

    Consistent:

QRS:

    Appearance:

    Consistent:

Q-T interval:

5. AXIS
Quadrant:

Degrees:

6. HYPERTROPHY
Atrial:

Ventricular:

7. MYOCARDIAL INFARCTION
Q waves:

S-T displacement:

8. ISCHEMIA
S-T displacement:

9. POSSIBLE DRUG EFFECTS

10. ECG ANALYSIS

11. INTERPRETATION

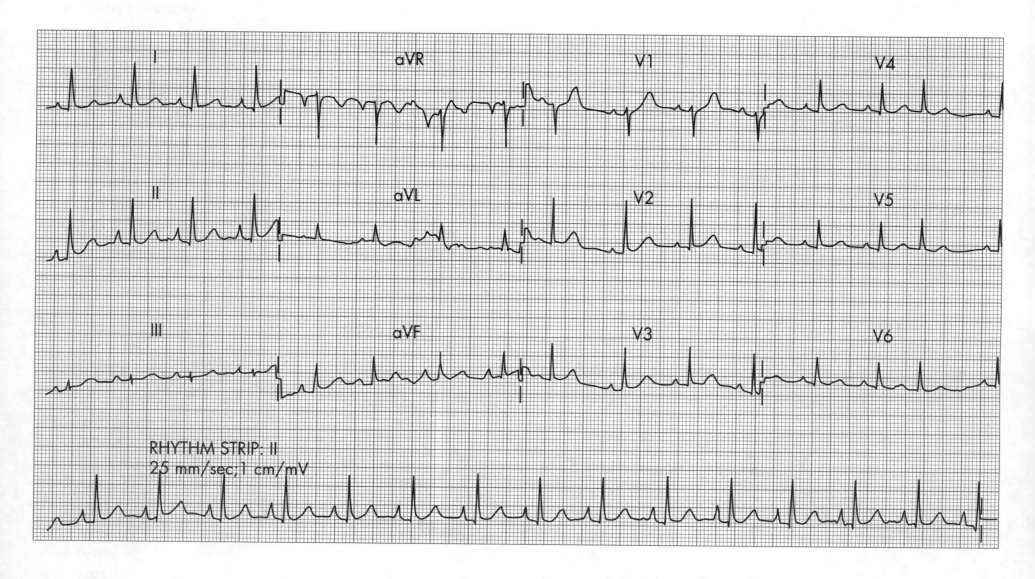

I   aVR   V1   V4

II   aVL   V2   V5

III   aVF   V3   V6

RHYTHM STRIP: II
25 mm/sec; 1 cm/mV

Figure 4-12
Resting 12-Lead ECG

234

1. **RATE**

   Atrial:

   Ventricular:

2. **RHYTHM**

   Atrial:

   Ventricular:

3. **WAVES**

   P waves present:

      Appearance:

      Consistent:

      Relation to QRS:

   Q waves present:

      Leads:

      Pathological:

   T waves present:

      Morphology:

4. **INTERVALS**

   P-R interval:

      Consistent:

   QRS:

      Appearance:

      Consistent:

   Q-T interval:

5. **AXIS**

   Quadrant:

   Degrees:

6. **HYPERTROPHY**

   Atrial:

   Ventricular:

7. **MYOCARDIAL INFARCTION**

   Q waves:

   S-T displacement:

8. **ISCHEMIA**

   S-T displacement:

9. **POSSIBLE DRUG EFFECTS**

10. **ECG ANALYSIS**

11. **INTERPRETATION**

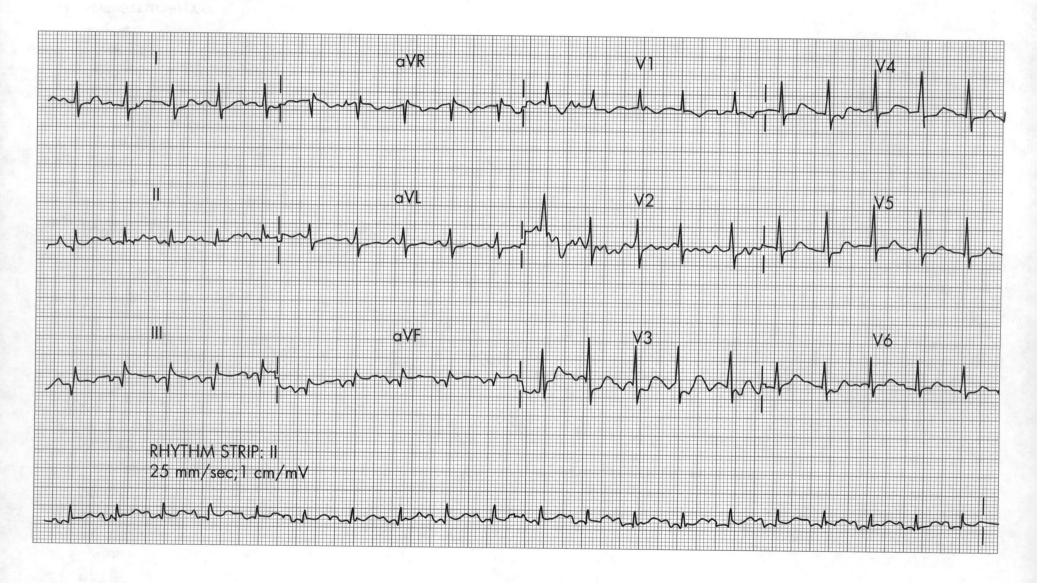

I aVR V1 V4

II aVL V2 V5

III aVF V3 V6

RHYTHM STRIP: II
25 mm/sec; 1 cm/mV

Figure 4-13
Resting 12-Lead ECG

1. RATE

Atrial:

Ventricular:

2. RHYTHM

Atrial:

Ventricular:

3. WAVES

P waves present:

    Appearance:

    Consistent:

    Relation to QRS:

Q waves present:

    Leads:

    Pathological:

T waves present:

    Morphology:

4. INTERVALS

P-R interval:

    Consistent:

QRS:

    Appearance:

    Consistent:

Q-T interval:

5. AXIS

Quadrant:

Degrees:

6. HYPERTROPHY

Atrial:

Ventricular:

7. MYOCARDIAL INFARCTION

Q waves:

S-T displacement:

8. ISCHEMIA

S-T displacement:

9. POSSIBLE DRUG EFFECTS

10. ECG ANALYSIS

11. INTERPRETATION

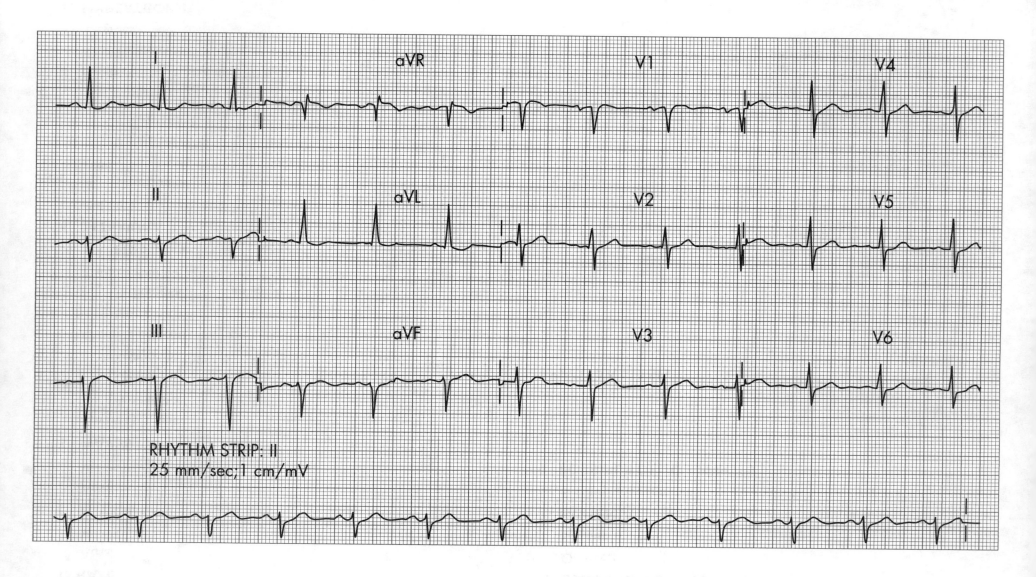

RHYTHM STRIP: II
25 mm/sec;1 cm/mV

Figure 4-14
Resting 12-Lead ECG
238

1. RATE

Atrial:

Ventricular:

2. RHYTHM

Atrial:

Ventricular:

3. WAVES

P waves present:

Appearance:

Consistent:

Relation to QRS:

Q waves present:

Leads:

Pathological:

T waves present:

Morphology:

4. INTERVALS

P-R interval:

Consistent:

QRS:

Appearance:

Consistent:

Q-T interval:

5. AXIS

Quadrant:

Degrees:

6. HYPERTROPHY

Atrial:

Ventricular:

7. MYOCARDIAL INFARCTION

Q waves:

S-T displacement:

8. ISCHEMIA

S-T displacement:

9. POSSIBLE DRUG EFFECTS

10. ECG ANALYSIS

11. INTERPRETATION

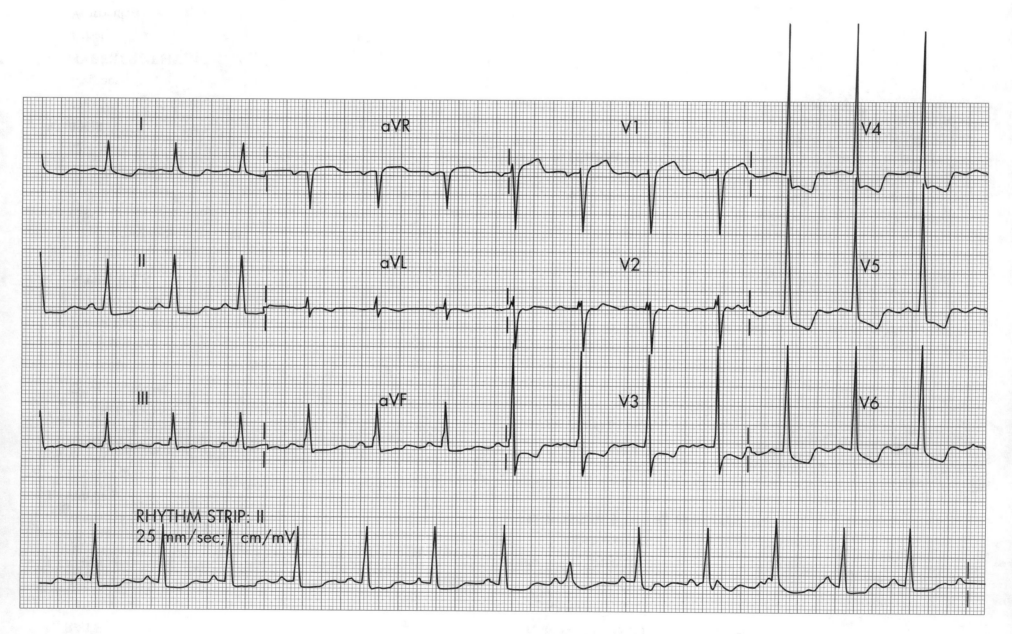

I aVR V1 V4

II aVL V2 V5

III aVF V3 V6

RHYTHM STRIP: II
25 mm/sec; 1 cm/mV

Figure 4-15
Resting 12-Lead ECG
240

1. RATE

    Atrial:

    Ventricular:

2. RHYTHM

    Atrial:

    Ventricular:

3. WAVES

    P waves present:

        Appearance:

        Consistent:

        Relation to QRS:

    Q waves present:

        Leads:

        Pathological:

    T waves present:

        Morphology:

4. INTERVALS

    P-R interval:

        Consistent:

    QRS:

        Appearance:

        Consistent:

    Q-T interval:

5. AXIS

    Quadrant:

    Degrees:

6. HYPERTROPHY

    Atrial:

    Ventricular:

7. MYOCARDIAL INFARCTION

    Q waves:

    S-T displacement:

8. ISCHEMIA

    S-T displacement:

9. POSSIBLE DRUG EFFECTS

10. ECG ANALYSIS

11. INTERPRETATION

Part V
Myocardial Infarctions and Ischemia

Myocardial Infarctions

Subendocardial Infarction (non-Q wave infarction)

Acute (minutes to days)
ECG Criteria
- S-T depression and T wave inversion

Nonacute (days to months)
ECG Criteria
- T wave inversion or possibly no ECG effects

Transmural Infarction (Q wave infarction)

Hyperacute (minutes to hours)
ECG Criteria
- S-T elevation with high peaked T waves
- Reciprocal S-T depression and T wave inversion

Acute (hours)
ECG Criteria
- S-T elevation decreases somewhat, T wave inversion
- Development of Q waves

Recent/Evolving/Resolving (weeks to months)
ECG Criteria
- S-T returns to baseline
- T waves may remain inverted
- Q waves remain

Nonacute (old—months to years)
ECG Criteria
- Q waves remain

Myocardial Ischemia
S-T segment depression and/or T wave inversion

Area of Infarction/Involvement (Diagnostic Leads)

Inferior	II, III, aVF
Septal*	V_1, V_2
Anterior**	V_3, V_4
Low Lateral	V_5, V_6
High Lateral	I, aVL
Posterior	(R greater than S) V_1

* Often leads V_{1-3} are referred to as "anteroseptal."
** Leads V_{4-6} are termed "anterolateral."

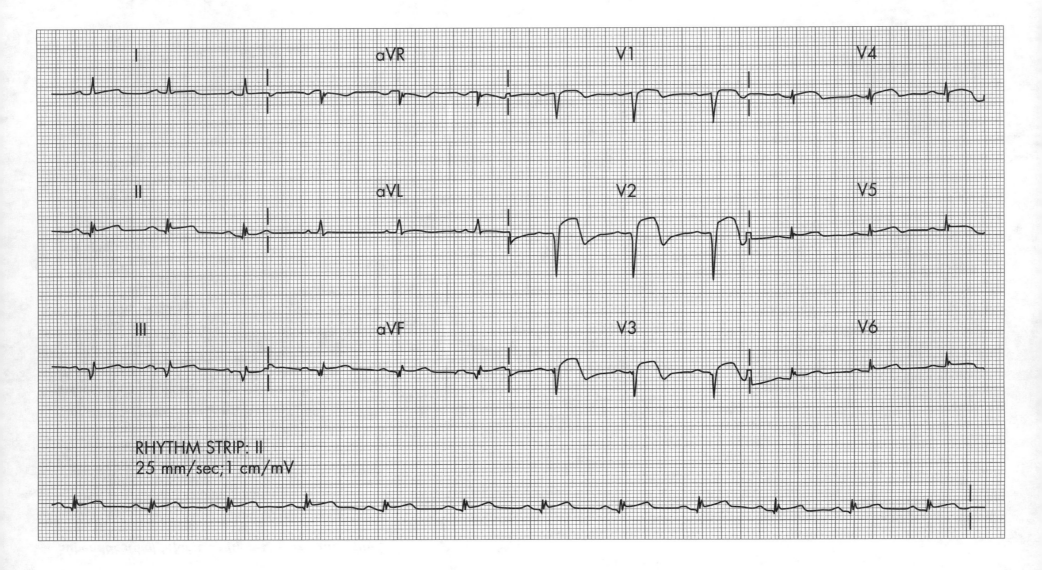

Figure 5-1
Resting 12-Lead ECG

246

1. RATE

Atrial:

Ventricular:

2. RHYTHM

Atrial:

Ventricular:

3. WAVES

P waves present:

Appearance:

Consistent:

Relation to QRS:

Q waves present:

Leads:

Pathological:

T waves present:

Morphology:

4. INTERVALS

P-R interval:

Consistent:

QRS:

Appearance:

Consistent:

Q-T interval:

5. AXIS

Quadrant:

Degrees:

6. HYPERTROPHY

Atrial:

Ventricular:

7. MYOCARDIAL INFARCTION

Q waves:

S-T displacement:

8. ISCHEMIA

S-T displacement:

9. POSSIBLE DRUG EFFECTS

10. ECG ANALYSIS

11. INTERPRETATION

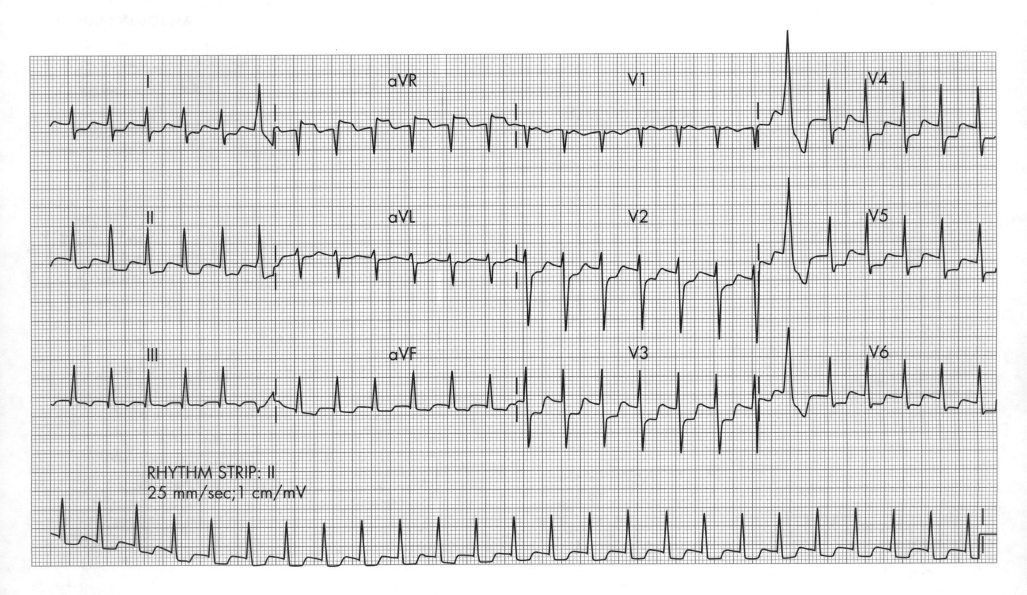

I   aVR   V1   V4

II   aVL   V2   V5

III   aVF   V3   V6

RHYTHM STRIP: II
25 mm/sec; 1 cm/mV

Figure 5-2
Resting 12-Lead ECG
248

1. RATE

Atrial:

Ventricular:

2. RHYTHM

Atrial:

Ventricular:

3. WAVES

P waves present:

Appearance:

Consistent:

Relation to QRS:

Q waves present:

Leads:

Pathological:

T waves present:

Morphology:

4. INTERVALS

P-R interval:

Consistent:

QRS:

Appearance:

Consistent:

Q-T interval:

5. AXIS

Quadrant:

Degrees:

6. HYPERTROPHY

Atrial:

Ventricular:

7. MYOCARDIAL INFARCTION

Q waves:

S-T displacement:

8. ISCHEMIA

S-T displacement:

9. POSSIBLE DRUG EFFECTS

10. ECG ANALYSIS

11. INTERPRETATION

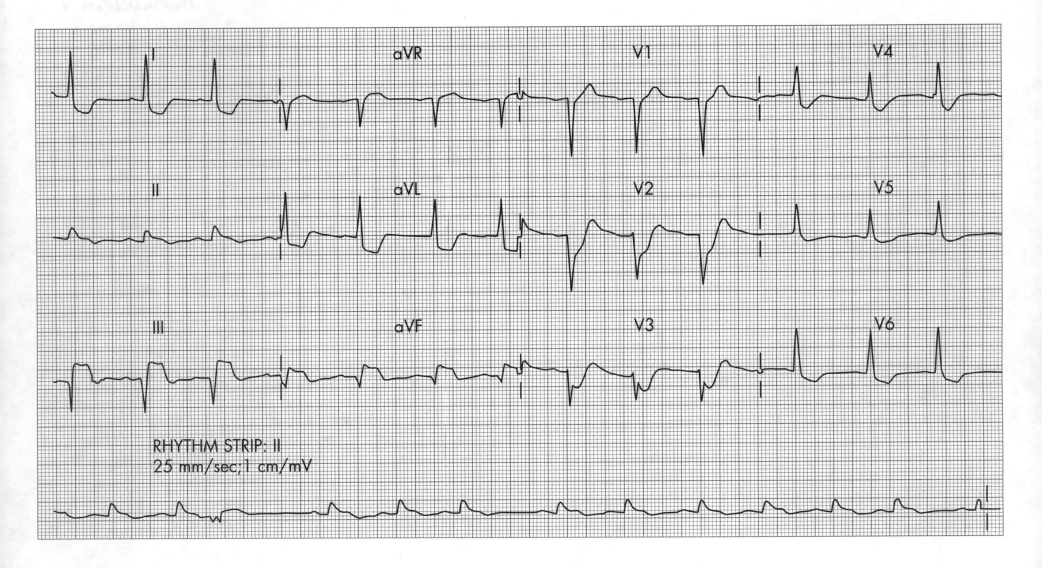

RHYTHM STRIP: II
25 mm/sec; 1 cm/mV

Figure 5-3
Resting 12-Lead ECG
250

1. **RATE**

   Atrial:

   Ventricular:

2. **RHYTHM**

   Atrial:

   Ventricular:

3. **WAVES**

   P waves present:

   Appearance:

   Consistent:

   Relation to QRS:

   Q waves present:

   Leads:

   Pathological:

   T waves present:

   Morphology:

4. **INTERVALS**

   P-R interval:

   Consistent:

   QRS:

   Appearance:

   Consistent:

   Q-T interval:

5. **AXIS**

   Quadrant:

   Degrees:

6. **HYPERTROPHY**

   Atrial:

   Ventricular:

7. **MYOCARDIAL INFARCTION**

   Q waves:

   S-T displacement:

8. **ISCHEMIA**

   S-T displacement:

9. **POSSIBLE DRUG EFFECTS**

10. **ECG ANALYSIS**

11. **INTERPRETATION**

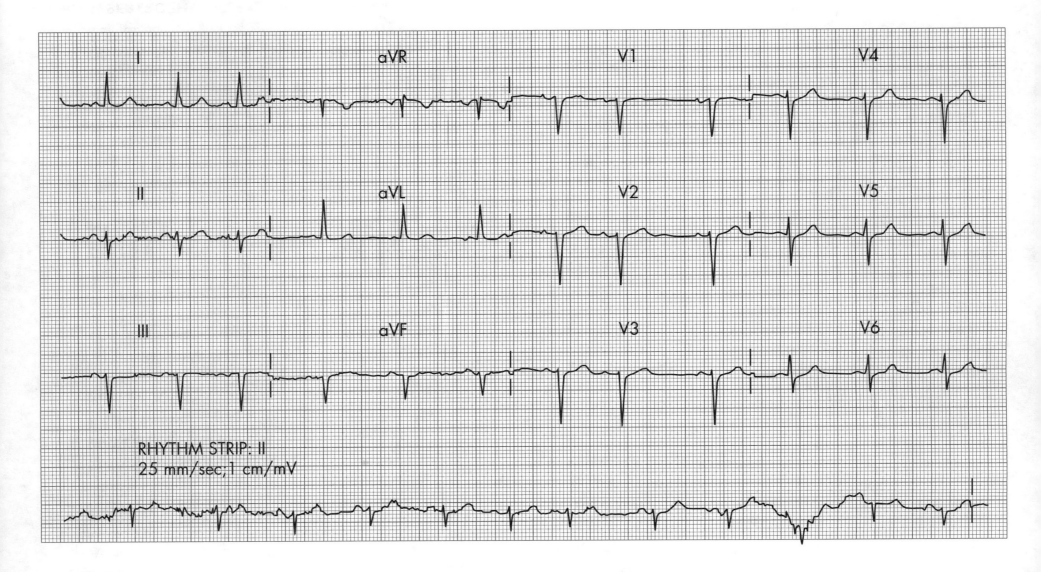

RHYTHM STRIP: II
25 mm/sec; 1 cm/mV

Figure 5-4
Resting 12-Lead ECG
252

1. RATE

  Atrial:

  Ventricular:

2. RHYTHM

  Atrial:

  Ventricular:

3. WAVES

  P waves present:

    Appearance:

    Consistent:

    Relation to QRS:

  Q waves present:

    Leads:

    Pathological:

  T waves present:

    Morphology:

4. INTERVALS

  P-R interval:

    Consistent:

  QRS:

    Appearance:

    Consistent:

  Q-T interval:

5. AXIS

  Quadrant:

  Degrees:

6. HYPERTROPHY

  Atrial:

  Ventricular:

7. MYOCARDIAL INFARCTION

  Q waves:

  S-T displacement:

8. ISCHEMIA

  S-T displacement:

9. POSSIBLE DRUG EFFECTS

10. ECG ANALYSIS

11. INTERPRETATION

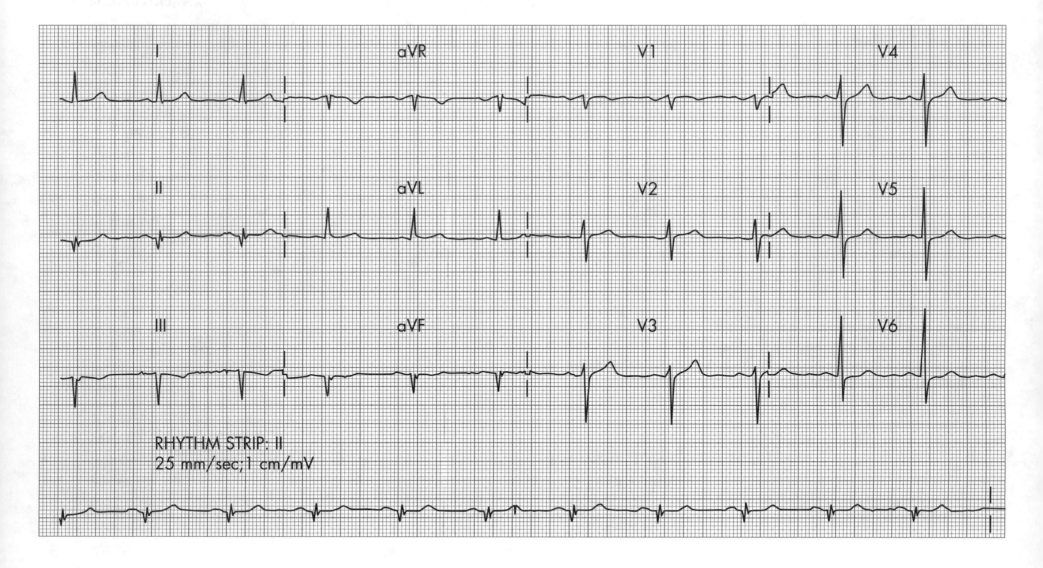

I aVR V1 V4

II aVL V2 V5

III aVF V3 V6

RHYTHM STRIP: II
25 mm/sec;1 cm/mV

Figure 5-5
Resting 12-Lead ECG

1. RATE

Atrial:

Ventricular:

2. RHYTHM

Atrial:

Ventricular:

3. WAVES

P waves present:

   Appearance:

   Consistent:

   Relation to QRS:

Q waves present:

   Leads:

   Pathological:

T waves present:

   Morphology:

4. INTERVALS

P-R interval:

   Consistent:

QRS:

   Appearance:

   Consistent:

Q-T interval:

5. AXIS

Quadrant:

Degrees:

6. HYPERTROPHY

Atrial:

Ventricular:

7. MYOCARDIAL INFARCTION

Q waves:

S-T displacement:

8. ISCHEMIA

S-T displacement:

9. POSSIBLE DRUG EFFECTS

10. ECG ANALYSIS

11. INTERPRETATION

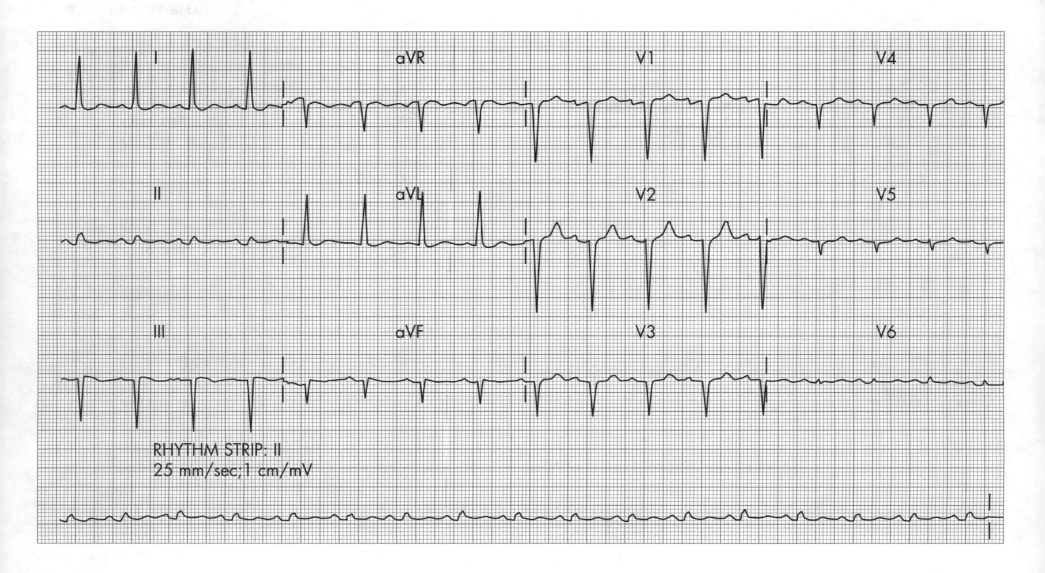

RHYTHM STRIP: II
25 mm/sec;1 cm/mV

Figure5-6
Resting 12-Lead ECG
256

1. **RATE**

    Atrial:

    Ventricular:

2. **RHYTHM**

    Atrial:

    Ventricular:

3. **WAVES**

    P waves present:

    Appearance:

    Consistent:

    Relation to QRS:

    Q waves present:

    Leads:

    Pathological:

    T waves present:

    Morphology:

4. **INTERVALS**

    P-R interval:

    Consistent:

    QRS:

    Appearance:

    Consistent:

    Q-T interval:

5. **AXIS**

    Quadrant:

    Degrees:

6. **HYPERTROPHY**

    Atrial:

    Ventricular:

7. **MYOCARDIAL INFARCTION**

    Q waves:

    S-T displacement:

8. **ISCHEMIA**

    S-T displacement:

9. **POSSIBLE DRUG EFFECTS**

10. **ECG ANALYSIS**

11. **INTERPRETATION**

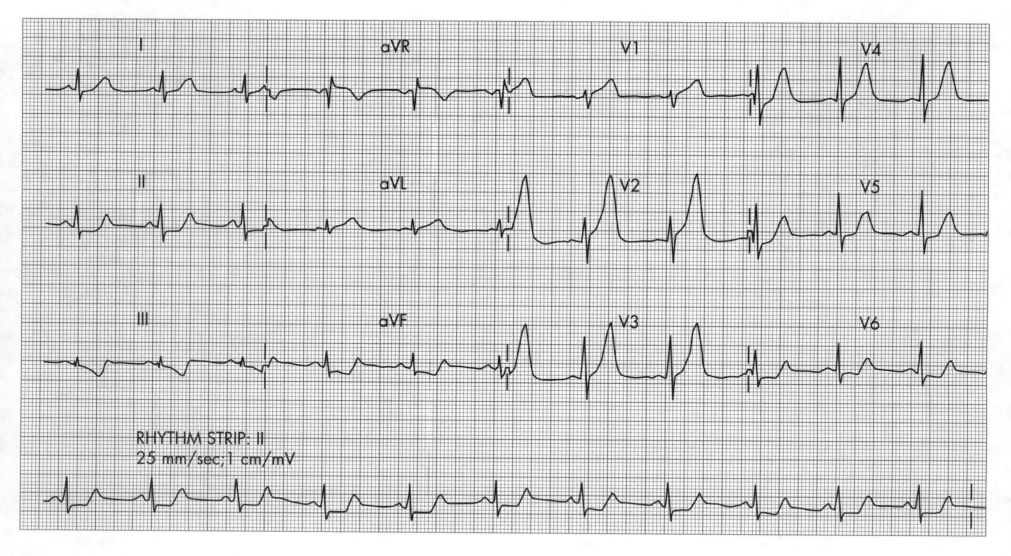

I aVR V1 V4

II aVL V2 V5

III aVF V3 V6

RHYTHM STRIP: II
25 mm/sec; 1 cm/mV

Figure 5-7
Resting 12-Lead ECG
ECG #1 of 2
258

1. RATE

Atrial:

Ventricular:

2. RHYTHM

Atrial:

Ventricular:

3. WAVES

P waves present:

Appearance:

Consistent:

Relation to QRS:

Q waves present:

Leads:

Pathological:

T waves present:

Morphology:

4. INTERVALS

P-R interval:

Consistent:

QRS:

Appearance:

Consistent:

Q-T interval:

5. AXIS

Quadrant:

Degrees:

6. HYPERTROPHY

Atrial:

Ventricular:

7. MYOCARDIAL INFARCTION

Q waves:

S-T displacement:

8. ISCHEMIA

S-T displacement:

9. POSSIBLE DRUG EFFECTS

10. ECG ANALYSIS

11. INTERPRETATION

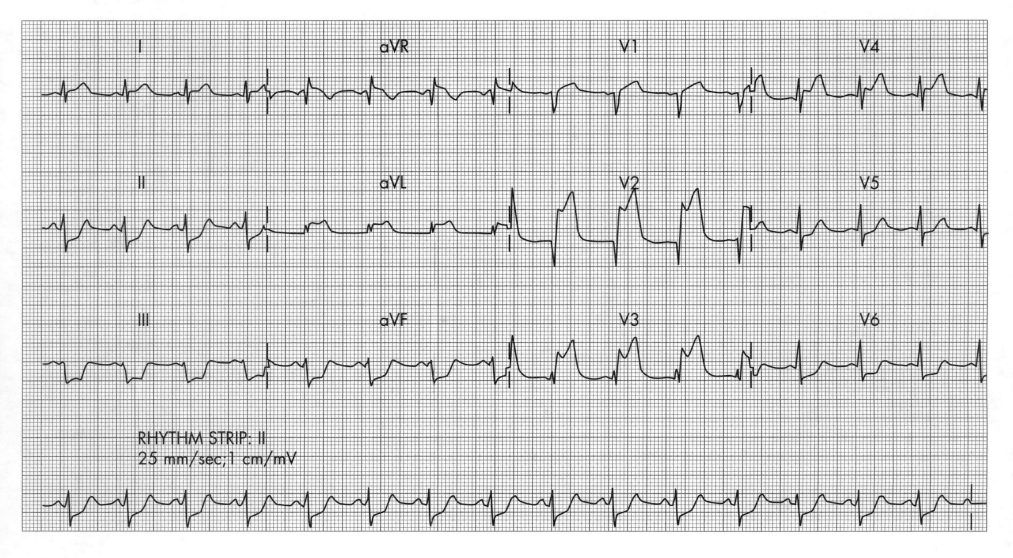

Figure 5-8
Resting 12-Lead ECG
ECG #2 of 2
260

1. RATE

Atrial:

Ventricular:

2. RHYTHM

Atrial:

Ventricular:

3. WAVES

P waves present:

Appearance:

Consistent:

Relation to QRS:

Q waves present:

Leads:

Pathological:

T waves present:

Morphology:

4. INTERVALS

P-R interval:

Consistent:

QRS:

Appearance:

Consistent:

Q-T interval:

5. AXIS

Quadrant:

Degrees:

6. HYPERTROPHY

Atrial:

Ventricular:

7. MYOCARDIAL INFARCTION

Q waves:

S-T displacement:

8. ISCHEMIA

S-T displacement:

9. POSSIBLE DRUG EFFECTS

10. ECG ANALYSIS

11. INTERPRETATION

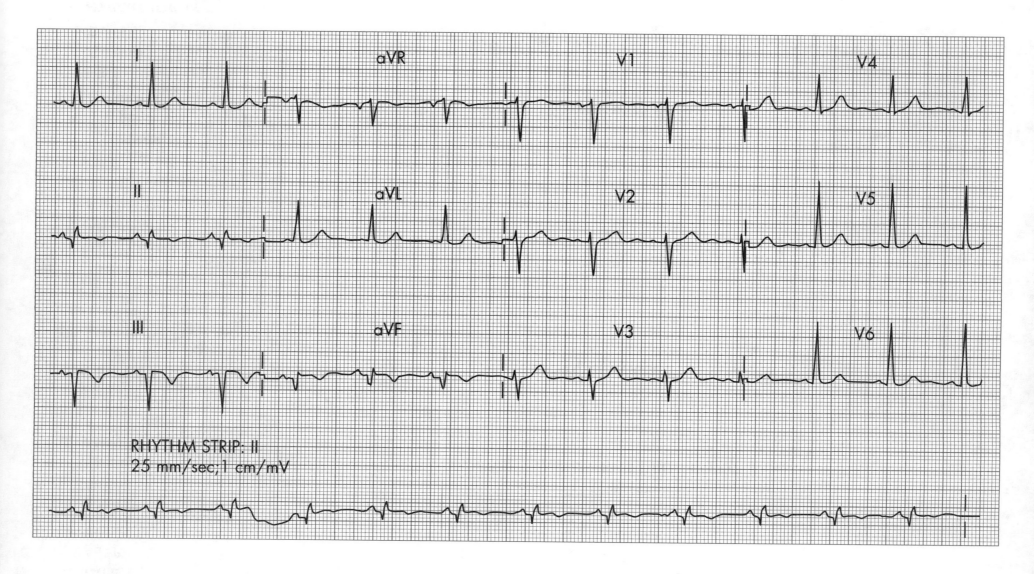

Figure 5-9
Resting 12-Lead ECG
262

1. RATE

    Atrial:

    Ventricular:

2. RHYTHM

    Atrial:

    Ventricular:

3. WAVES

    P waves present:

        Appearance:

        Consistent:

        Relation to QRS:

    Q waves present:

        Leads:

        Pathological:

    T waves present:

        Morphology:

4. INTERVALS

    P-R interval:

        Consistent:

    QRS:

        Appearance:

        Consistent:

    Q-T interval:

5. AXIS

    Quadrant:

    Degrees:

6. HYPERTROPHY

    Atrial:

    Ventricular:

7. MYOCARDIAL INFARCTION

    Q waves:

    S-T displacement:

8. ISCHEMIA

    S-T displacement:

9. POSSIBLE DRUG EFFECTS

10. ECG ANALYSIS

11. INTERPRETATION

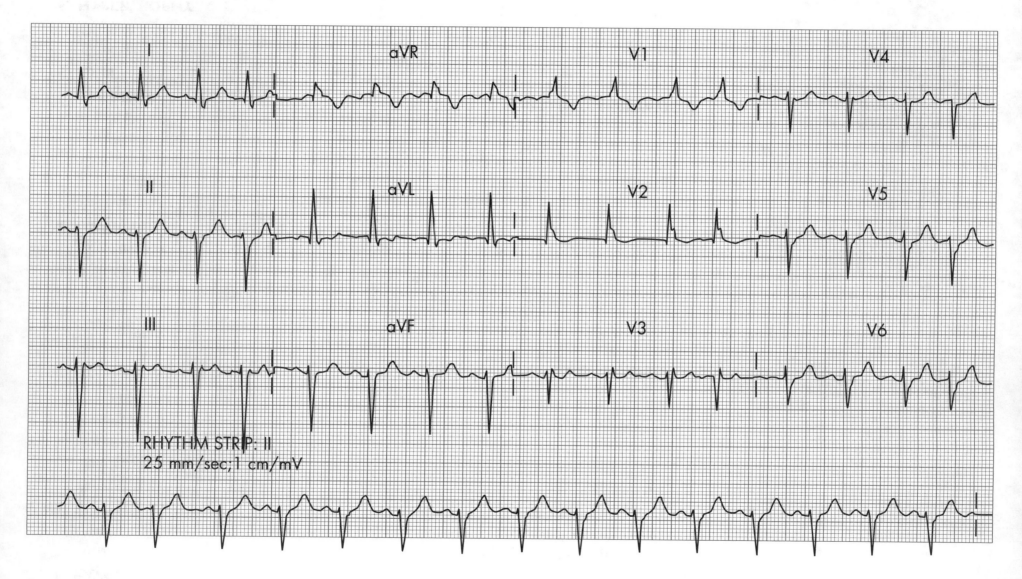

I	aVR	V1	V4
II	aVL	V2	V5
III	aVF	V3	V6

RHYTHM STRIP: II
25 mm/sec;1 cm/mV

Figure 5-10
Resting 12-Lead ECG
264

I. RATE

    Atrial:

    Ventricular:

2. RHYTHM

    Atrial:

    Ventricular:

3. WAVES

    P waves present:

        Appearance:

        Consistent:

        Relation to QRS:

    Q waves present:

        Leads:

        Pathological:

    T waves present:

        Morphology:

4. INTERVALS

    P-R interval:

        Consistent:

    QRS:

        Appearance:

        Consistent:

    Q-T interval:

5. AXIS

    Quadrant:

    Degrees:

6. HYPERTROPHY

    Atrial:

    Ventricular:

7. MYOCARDIAL INFARCTION

    Q waves:

    S-T displacement:

8. ISCHEMIA

    S-T displacement:

9. POSSIBLE DRUG EFFECTS

10. ECG ANALYSIS

11. INTERPRETATION

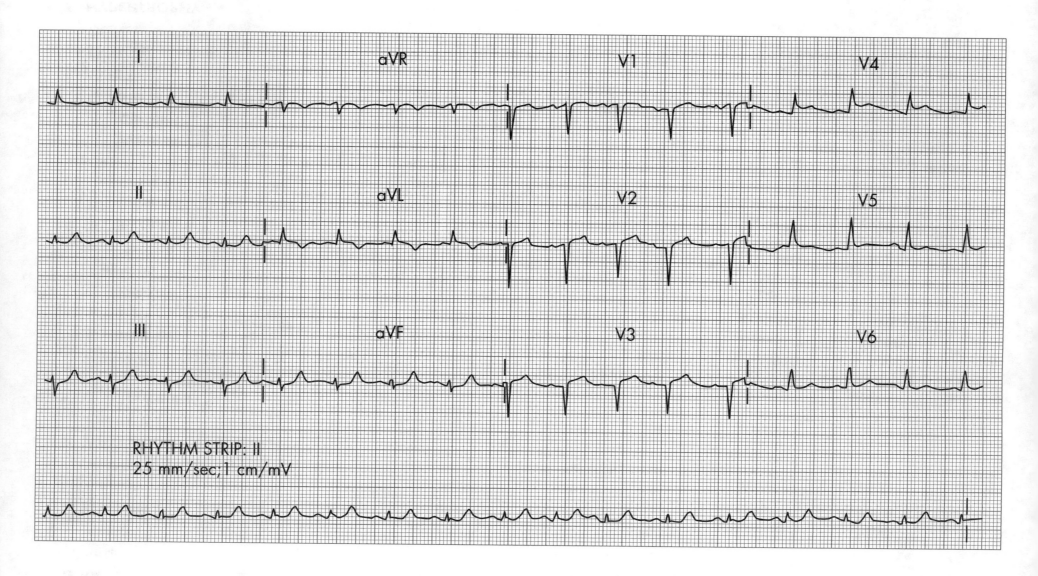

I   aVR   V1   V4

II   aVL   V2   V5

III   aVF   V3   V6

RHYTHM STRIP: II
25 mm/sec; 1 cm/mV

Figure 5-11
Resting 12-Lead ECG

1. RATE
Atrial:

Ventricular:

2. RHYTHM
Atrial:

Ventricular:

3. WAVES
P waves present:

Appearance:

Consistent:

Relation to QRS:

Q waves present:

Leads:

Pathological:

T waves present:

Morphology:

4. INTERVALS
P-R interval:

Consistent:

QRS:

Appearance:

Consistent:

Q-T interval:

5. AXIS
Quadrant:

Degrees:

6. HYPERTROPHY
Atrial:

Ventricular:

7. MYOCARDIAL INFARCTION
Q waves:

S-T displacement:

8. ISCHEMIA
S-T displacement:

9. POSSIBLE DRUG EFFECTS

10. ECG ANALYSIS

11. INTERPRETATION

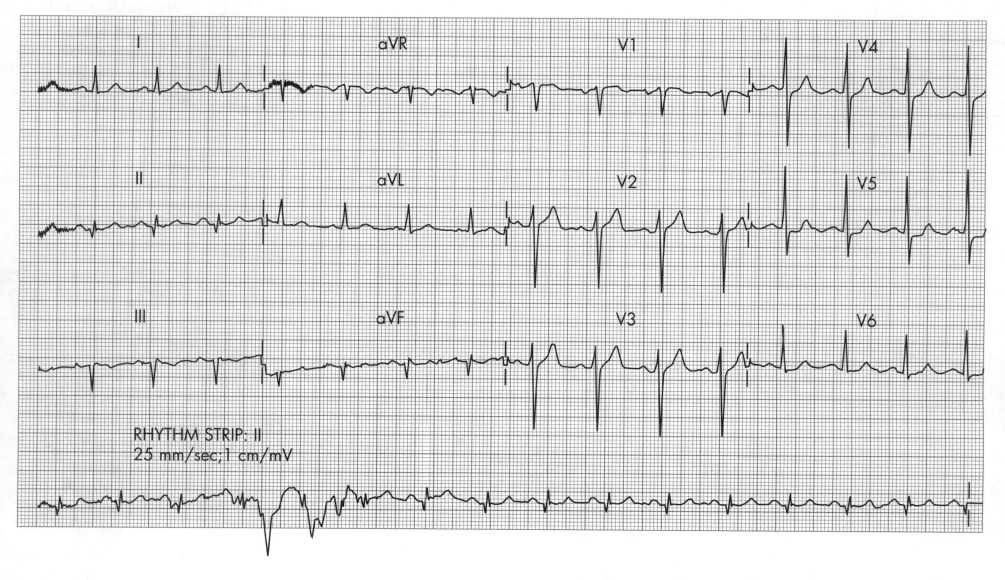

I　　　　aVR　　　　V1　　　　V4

II　　　　aVL　　　　V2　　　　V5

III　　　　aVF　　　　V3　　　　V6

RHYTHM STRIP: II
25 mm/sec;1 cm/mV

Figure 5-12
Resting 12-Lead ECG

1. RATE

    Atrial:

    Ventricular:

2. RHYTHM

    Atrial:

    Ventricular:

3. WAVES

    P waves present:

        Appearance:

        Consistent:

        Relation to QRS:

    Q waves present:

        Leads:

        Pathological:

    T waves present:

        Morphology:

4. INTERVALS

    P-R interval:

        Consistent:

    QRS:

        Appearance:

        Consistent:

    Q-T interval:

5. AXIS

    Quadrant:

    Degrees:

6. HYPERTROPHY

    Atrial:

    Ventricular:

7. MYOCARDIAL INFARCTION

    Q waves:

    S-T displacement:

8. ISCHEMIA

    S-T displacement:

9. POSSIBLE DRUG EFFECTS

10. ECG ANALYSIS

11. INTERPRETATION

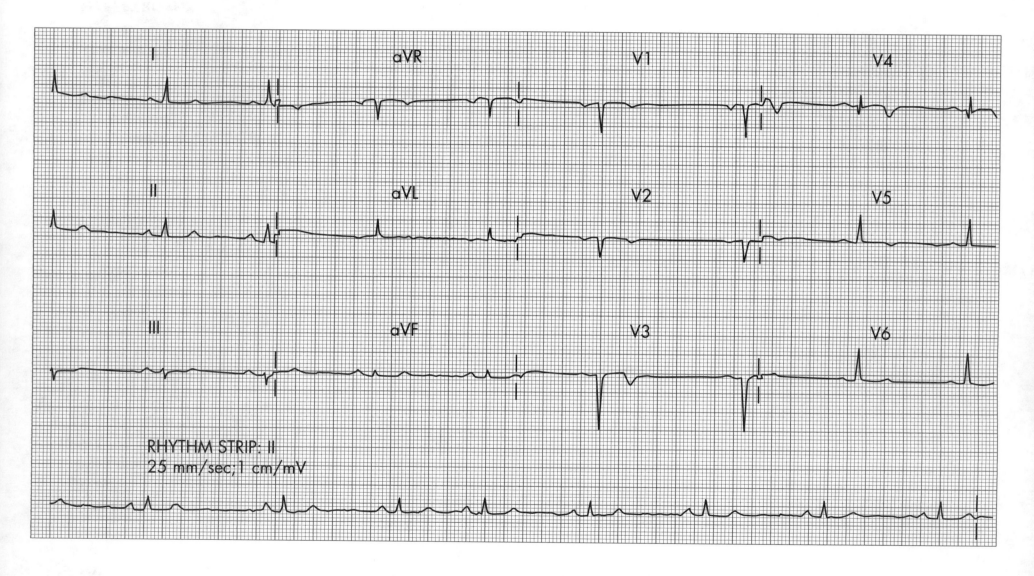

RHYTHM STRIP: II
25 mm/sec;1 cm/mV

Figure 5-13
Resting 12-Lead ECG
270

1. RATE

Atrial:

Ventricular:

2. RHYTHM

Atrial:

Ventricular:

3. WAVES

P waves present:

    Appearance:

    Consistent:

    Relation to QRS:

Q waves present:

    Leads:

    Pathological:

T waves present:

    Morphology:

4. INTERVALS

P-R interval:

    Consistent:

QRS:

    Appearance:

    Consistent:

Q-T interval:

5. AXIS

Quadrant:

Degrees:

6. HYPERTROPHY

Atrial:

Ventricular:

7. MYOCARDIAL INFARCTION

Q waves:

S-T displacement:

8. ISCHEMIA

S-T displacement:

9. POSSIBLE DRUG EFFECTS

10. ECG ANALYSIS

11. INTERPRETATION

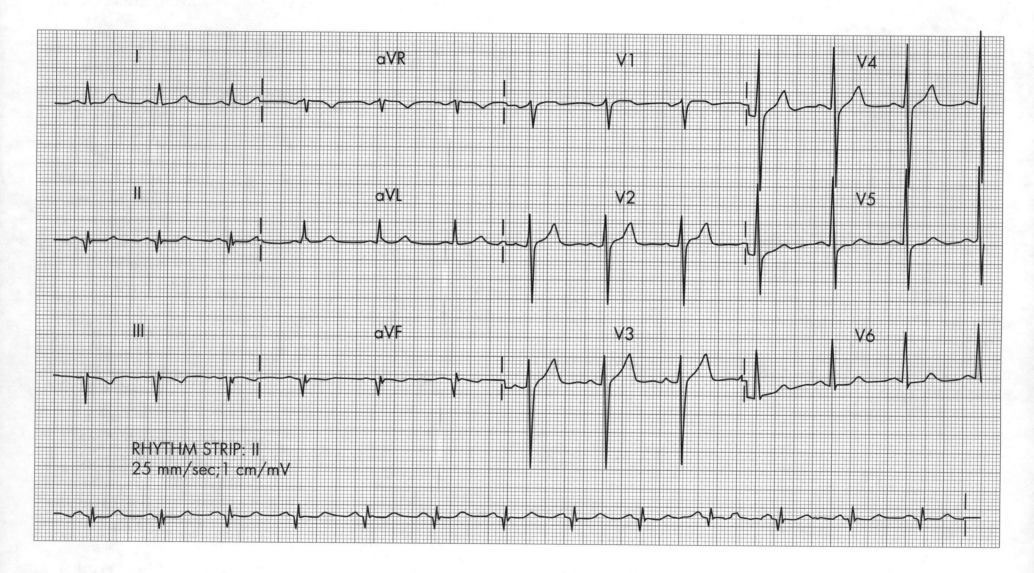

I   aVR   V1   V4

II   aVL   V2   V5

III   aVF   V3   V6

RHYTHM STRIP: II
25 mm/sec;1 cm/mV

Figure 5-14
Resting 12-Lead ECG
272

1. **RATE**

   Atrial:

   Ventricular:

2. **RHYTHM**

   Atrial:

   Ventricular:

3. **WAVES**

   P waves present:

       Appearance:

       Consistent:

       Relation to QRS:

   Q waves present:

       Leads:

       Pathological:

   T waves present:

       Morphology:

4. **INTERVALS**

   P-R interval:

       Consistent:

   QRS:

       Appearance:

       Consistent:

   Q-T interval:

5. **AXIS**

   Quadrant:

   Degrees:

6. **HYPERTROPHY**

   Atrial:

   Ventricular:

7. **MYOCARDIAL INFARCTION**

   Q waves:

   S-T displacement:

8. **ISCHEMIA**

   S-T displacement:

9. **POSSIBLE DRUG EFFECTS**

10. **ECG ANALYSIS**

11. **INTERPRETATION**

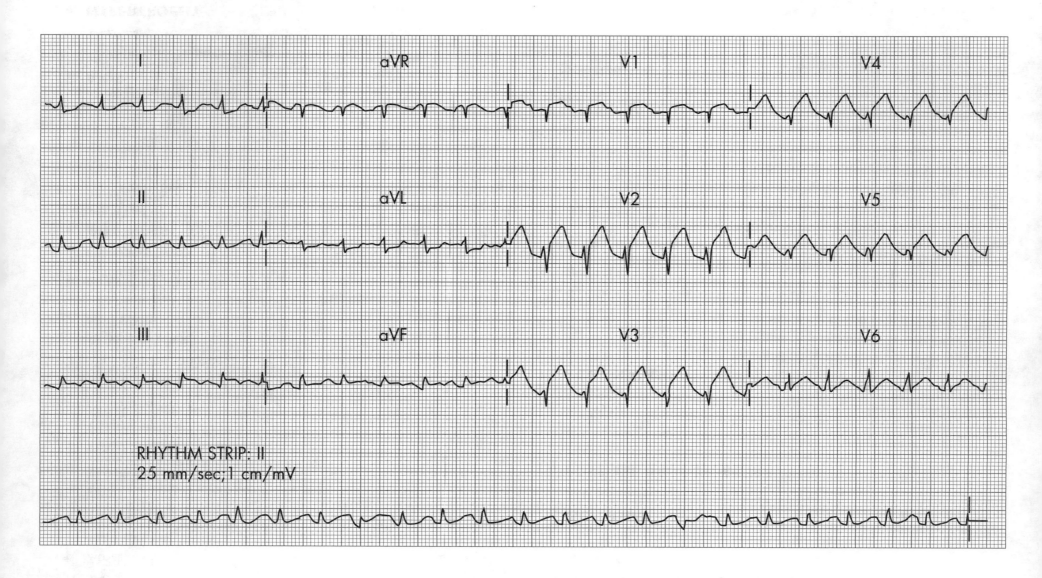

I aVR V1 V4

II aVL V2 V5

III aVF V3 V6

RHYTHM STRIP: II
25 mm/sec; 1 cm/mV

Figure 5-15
Resting 12-Lead ECG
274

1. RATE

    Atrial:

    Ventricular:

2. RHYTHM

    Atrial:

    Ventricular:

3. WAVES

    P waves present:

        Appearance:

        Consistent:

        Relation to QRS:

    Q waves present:

        Leads:

        Pathological:

    T waves present:

        Morphology:

4. INTERVALS

    P-R interval:

        Consistent:

    QRS:

        Appearance:

        Consistent:

    Q-T interval:

5. AXIS

    Quadrant:

    Degrees:

6. HYPERTROPHY

    Atrial:

    Ventricular:

7. MYOCARDIAL INFARCTION

    Q waves:

    S-T displacement:

8. ISCHEMIA

    S-T displacement:

9. POSSIBLE DRUG EFFECTS

10. ECG ANALYSIS

11. INTERPRETATION

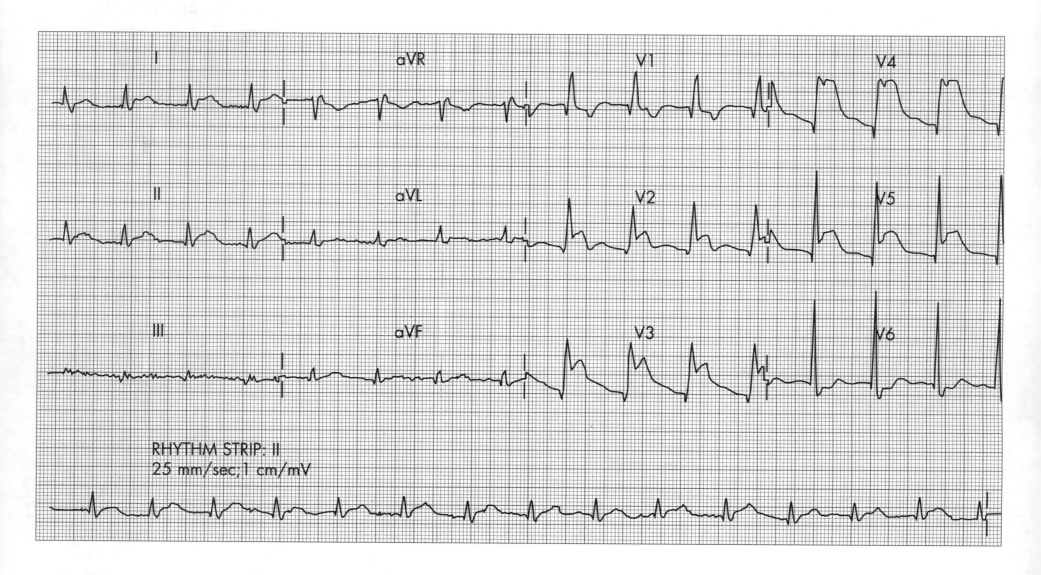

I aVR V1 V4

II aVL V2 V5

III aVF V3 V6

RHYTHM STRIP: II
25 mm/sec;1 cm/mV

Figure 5-16
Resting 12-Lead ECG
276

I. RATE

    Atrial:

    Ventricular:

2. RHYTHM

    Atrial:

    Ventricular:

3. WAVES

    P waves present:

        Appearance:

        Consistent:

        Relation to QRS:

    Q waves present:

        Leads:

        Pathological:

    T waves present:

        Morphology:

4. INTERVALS

    P-R interval:

        Consistent:

    QRS:

        Appearance:

        Consistent:

    Q-T interval:

5. AXIS

    Quadrant:

    Degrees:

6. HYPERTROPHY

    Atrial:

    Ventricular:

7. MYOCARDIAL INFARCTION

    Q waves:

    S-T displacement:

8. ISCHEMIA

    S-T displacement:

9. POSSIBLE DRUG EFFECTS

10. ECG ANALYSIS

11. INTERPRETATION

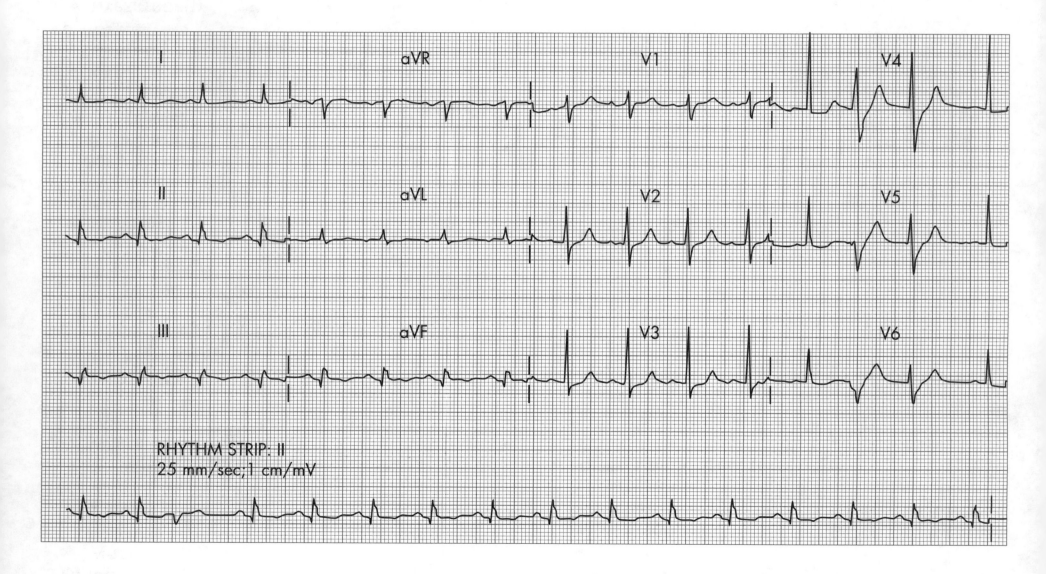

RHYTHM STRIP: II
25 mm/sec; 1 cm/mV

Figure 5-17
Resting 12-Lead ECG

1. **RATE**

   Atrial:

   Ventricular:

2. **RHYTHM**

   Atrial:

   Ventricular:

3. **WAVES**

   P waves present:

       Appearance:

       Consistent:

       Relation to QRS:

   Q waves present:

       Leads:

       Pathological:

   T waves present:

       Morphology:

4. **INTERVALS**

   P-R interval:

       Consistent:

   QRS:

       Appearance:

       Consistent:

   Q-T interval:

5. **AXIS**

   Quadrant:

   Degrees:

6. **HYPERTROPHY**

   Atrial:

   Ventricular:

7. **MYOCARDIAL INFARCTION**

   Q waves:

   S-T displacement:

8. **ISCHEMIA**

   S-T displacement:

9. **POSSIBLE DRUG EFFECTS**

10. **ECG ANALYSIS**

11. **INTERPRETATION**

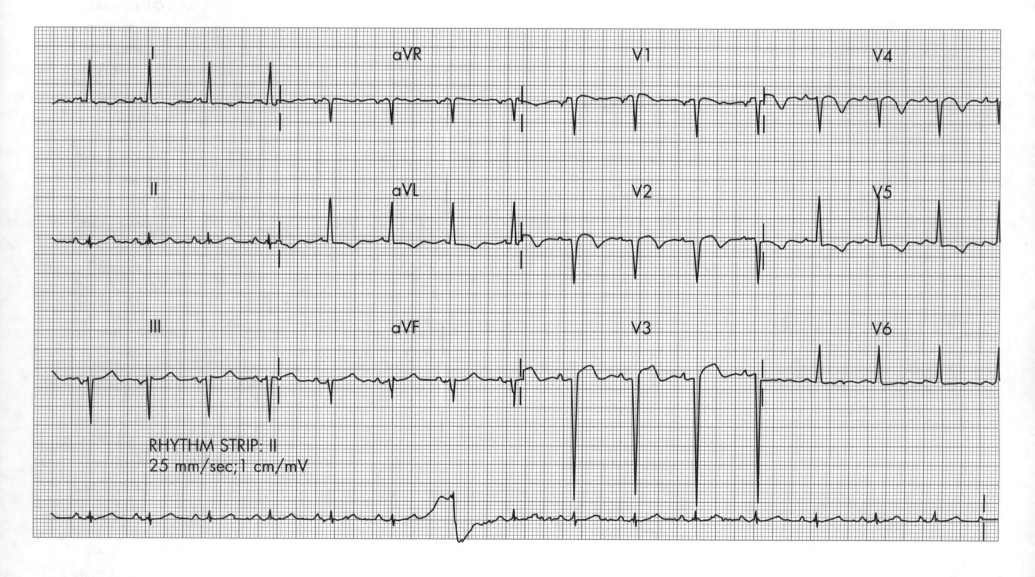

II   aVR   V1   V4

II   aVL   V2   V5

III   aVF   V3   V6

RHYTHM STRIP: II
25 mm/sec; 1 cm/mV

Figure 5-18
Resting 12-Lead ECG

1. RATE

    Atrial:

    Ventricular:

2. RHYTHM

    Atrial:

    Ventricular:

3. WAVES

    P waves present:

        Appearance:

        Consistent:

        Relation to QRS:

    Q waves present:

        Leads:

        Pathological:

    T waves present:

        Morphology:

4. INTERVALS

    P-R interval:

        Consistent:

    QRS:

        Appearance:

        Consistent:

    Q-T interval:

5. AXIS

    Quadrant:

    Degrees:

6. HYPERTROPHY

    Atrial:

    Ventricular:

7. MYOCARDIAL INFARCTION

    Q waves:

    S-T displacement:

8. ISCHEMIA

    S-T displacement:

9. POSSIBLE DRUG EFFECTS

10. ECG ANALYSIS

11. INTERPRETATION

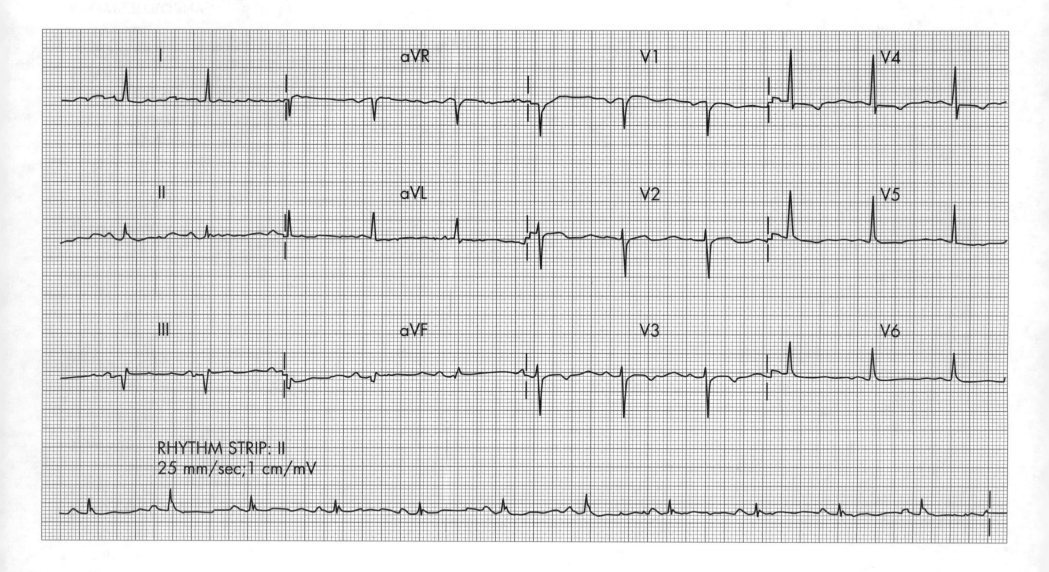

I aVR V1 V4

II aVL V2 V5

III aVF V3 V6

RHYTHM STRIP: II
25 mm/sec; 1 cm/mV

Figure 5-19
Resting 12-Lead ECG
282

1. **RATE**

   Atrial:

   Ventricular:

2. **RHYTHM**

   Atrial:

   Ventricular:

3. **WAVES**

   P waves present:

       Appearance:

       Consistent:

       Relation to QRS:

   Q waves present:

       Leads:

       Pathological:

   T waves present:

       Morphology:

4. **INTERVALS**

   P-R interval:

       Consistent:

   QRS:

       Appearance:

       Consistent:

   Q-T interval:

5. **AXIS**

   Quadrant:

   Degrees:

6. **HYPERTROPHY**

   Atrial:

   Ventricular:

7. **MYOCARDIAL INFARCTION**

   Q waves:

   S-T displacement:

8. **ISCHEMIA**

   S-T displacement:

9. **POSSIBLE DRUG EFFECTS**

10. **ECG ANALYSIS**

11. **INTERPRETATION**

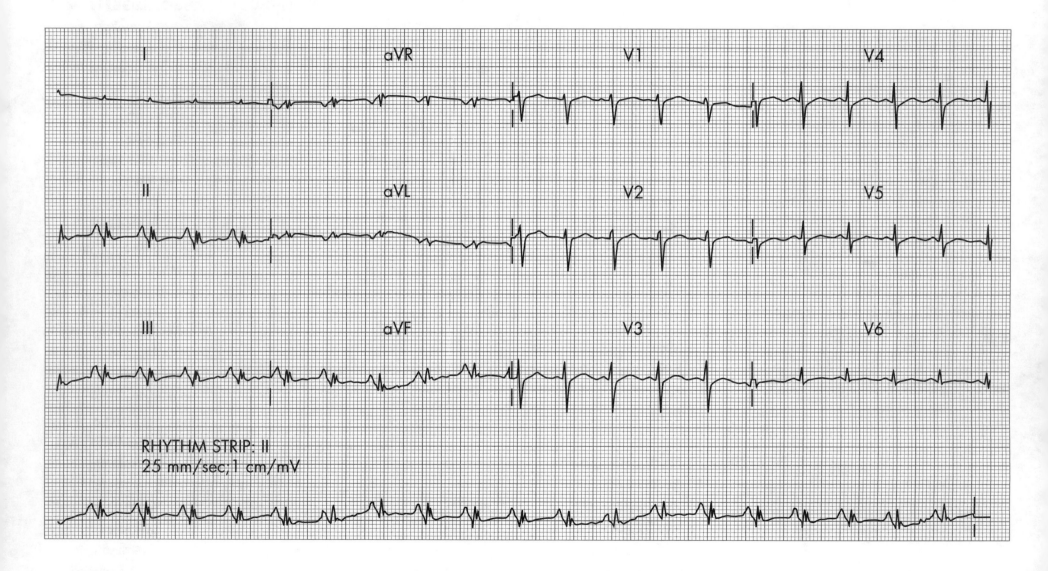

I aVR V1 V4

II aVL V2 V5

III aVF V3 V6

RHYTHM STRIP: II
25 mm/sec; 1 cm/mV

Figure 5-20
Resting 12-Lead ECG

1. RATE

Atrial:

Ventricular:

2. RHYTHM

Atrial:

Ventricular:

3. WAVES

P waves present:

Appearance:

Consistent:

Relation to QRS:

Q waves present:

Leads:

Pathological:

T waves present:

Morphology:

4. INTERVALS

P-R interval:

Consistent:

QRS:

Appearance:

Consistent:

Q-T interval:

5. AXIS

Quadrant:

Degrees:

6. HYPERTROPHY

Atrial:

Ventricular:

7. MYOCARDIAL INFARCTION

Q waves:

S-T displacement:

8. ISCHEMIA

S-T displacement:

9. POSSIBLE DRUG EFFECTS

10. ECG ANALYSIS

11. INTERPRETATION

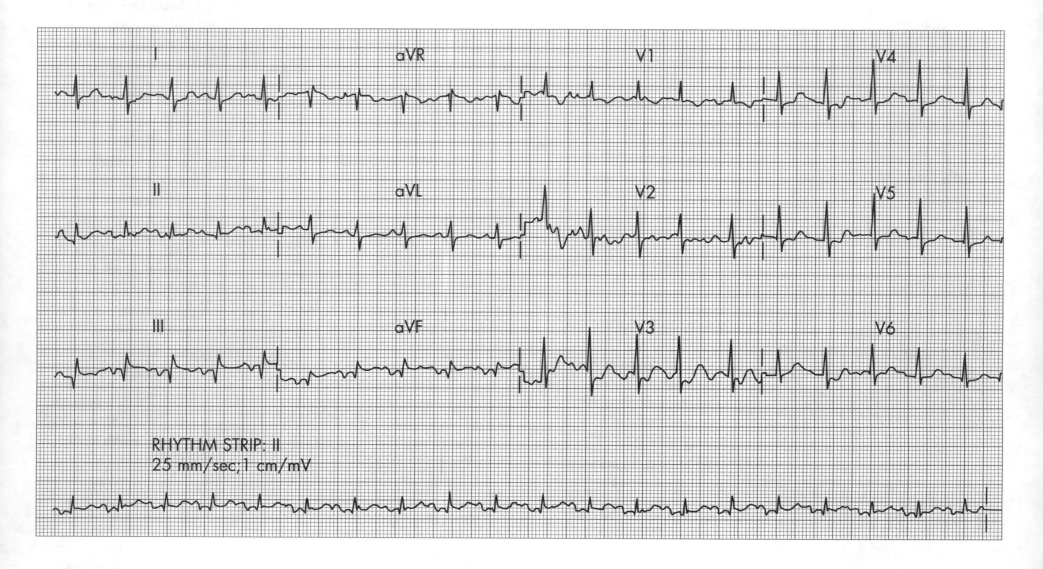

I aVR V1 V4

II aVL V2 V5

III aVF V3 V6

RHYTHM STRIP: II
25 mm/sec; 1 cm/mV

Figure 5-21
Resting 12-Lead ECG

1. RATE

    Atrial:

    Ventricular:

2. RHYTHM

    Atrial:

    Ventricular:

3. WAVES

    P waves present:

        Appearance:

        Consistent:

        Relation to QRS:

    Q waves present:

        Leads:

        Pathological:

    T waves present:

        Morphology:

4. INTERVALS

    P-R interval:

        Consistent:

    QRS:

        Appearance:

        Consistent:

    Q-T interval:

5. AXIS

    Quadrant:

    Degrees:

6. HYPERTROPHY

    Atrial:

    Ventricular:

7. MYOCARDIAL INFARCTION

    Q waves:

    S-T displacement:

8. ISCHEMIA

    S-T displacement:

9. POSSIBLE DRUG EFFECTS

10. ECG ANALYSIS

11. INTERPRETATION

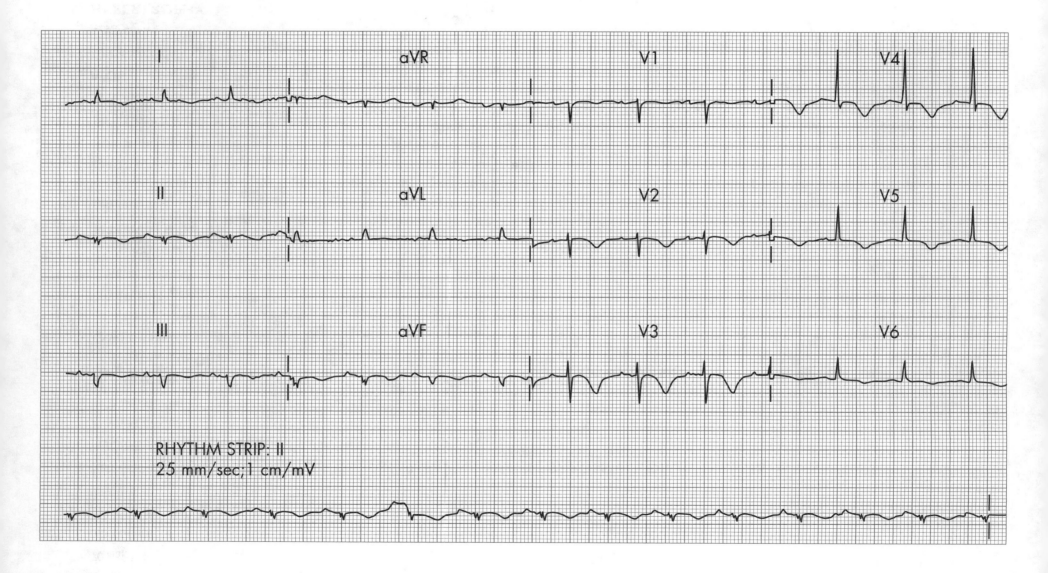

I aVR V1 V4

II aVL V2 V5

III aVF V3 V6

RHYTHM STRIP: II
25 mm/sec; 1 cm/mV

Figure 5-22
Resting 12-Lead ECG

1. **RATE**

   Atrial:

   Ventricular:

2. **RHYTHM**

   Atrial:

   Ventricular:

3. **WAVES**

   P waves present:

       Appearance:

       Consistent:

       Relation to QRS:

   Q waves present:

       Leads:

       Pathological:

   T waves present:

       Morphology:

4. **INTERVALS**

   P-R interval:

       Consistent:

   QRS:

       Appearance:

       Consistent:

   Q-T interval:

5. **AXIS**

   Quadrant:

   Degrees:

6. **HYPERTROPHY**

   Atrial:

   Ventricular:

7. **MYOCARDIAL INFARCTION**

   Q waves:

   S-T displacement:

8. **ISCHEMIA**

   S-T displacement:

9. **POSSIBLE DRUG EFFECTS**

10. **ECG ANALYSIS**

11. **INTERPRETATION**

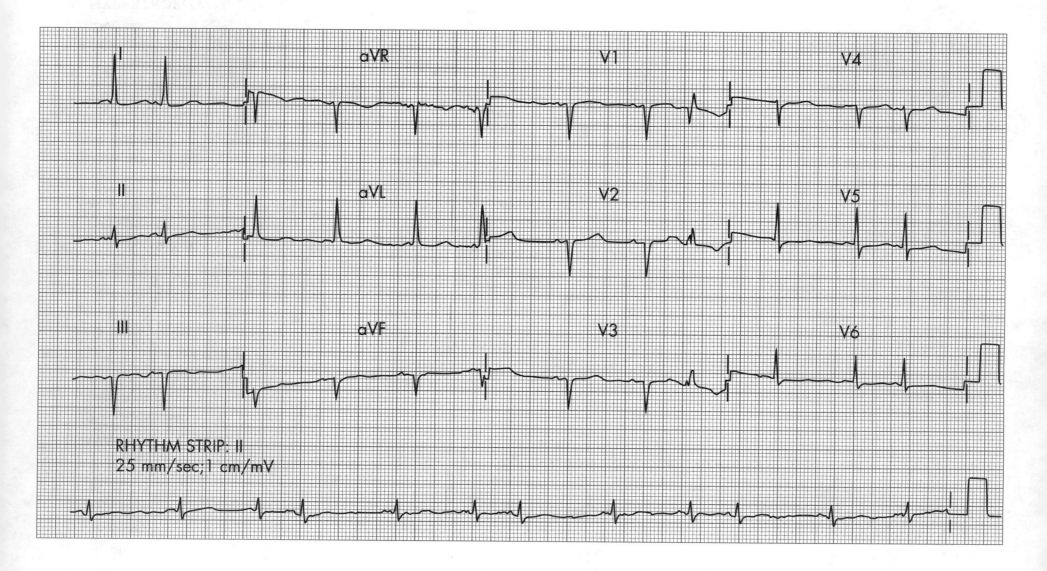

RHYTHM STRIP: II
25 mm/sec; 1 cm/mV

Figure 5-23
Resting 12-Lead ECG
290

I. RATE

Atrial:

Ventricular:

2. RHYTHM

Atrial:

Ventricular:

3. WAVES

P waves present:

    Appearance:

    Consistent:

    Relation to QRS:

Q waves present:

    Leads:

    Pathological:

T waves present:

    Morphology:

4. INTERVALS

P-R interval:

    Consistent:

QRS:

    Appearance:

    Consistent:

Q-T interval:

5. AXIS

Quadrant:

Degrees:

6. HYPERTROPHY

Atrial:

Ventricular:

7. MYOCARDIAL INFARCTION

Q waves:

S-T displacement:

8. ISCHEMIA

S-T displacement:

9. POSSIBLE DRUG EFFECTS

10. ECG ANALYSIS

11. INTERPRETATION

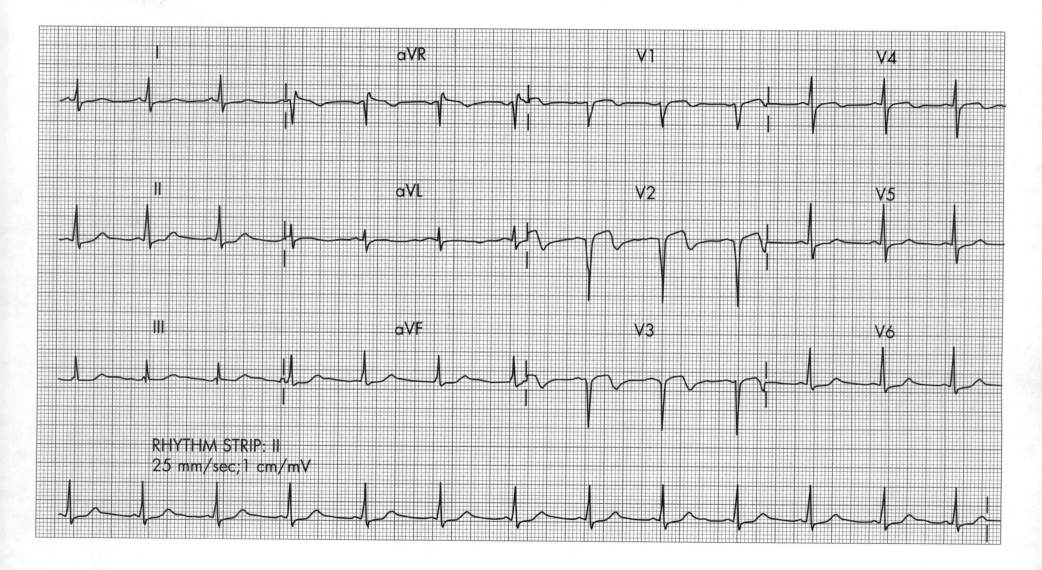

RHYTHM STRIP: II
25 mm/sec;1 cm/mV

Figure 5-24
Resting 12-Lead ECG

292

1. RATE

Atrial:

Ventricular:

2. RHYTHM

Atrial:

Ventricular:

3. WAVES

P waves present:

    Appearance:

    Consistent:

    Relation to QRS:

Q waves present:

    Leads:

    Pathological:

T waves present:

    Morphology:

4. INTERVALS

P-R interval:

    Consistent:

QRS:

    Appearance:

    Consistent:

Q-T interval:

5. AXIS

Quadrant:

Degrees:

6. HYPERTROPHY

Atrial:

Ventricular:

7. MYOCARDIAL INFARCTION

Q waves:

S-T displacement:

8. ISCHEMIA

S-T displacement:

9. POSSIBLE DRUG EFFECTS

10. ECG ANALYSIS

11. INTERPRETATION

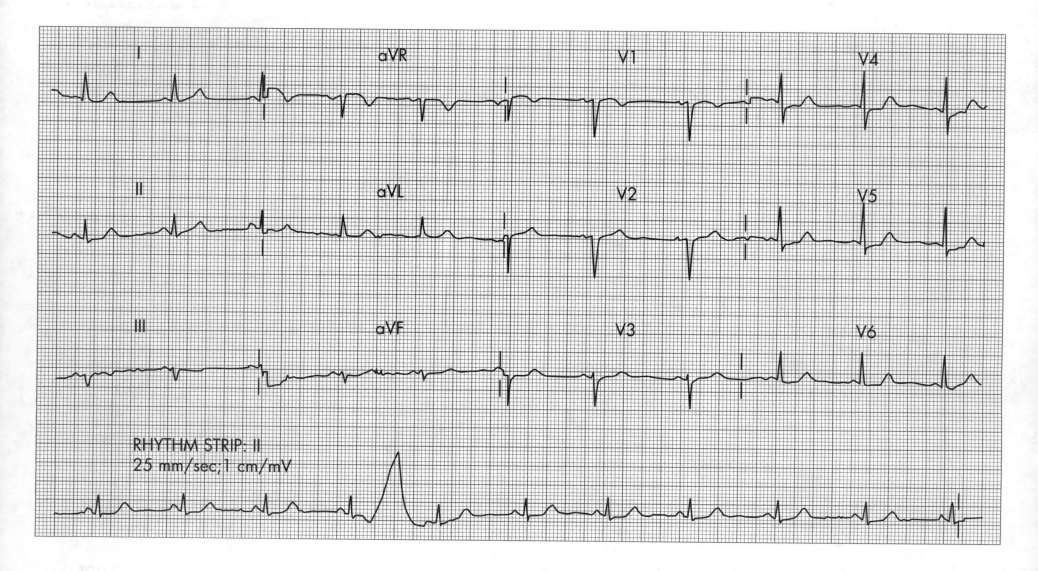

I aVR V1 V4

II aVL V2 V5

III aVF V3 V6

RHYTHM STRIP: II
25 mm/sec; 1 cm/mV

Figure 5-25
Resting 12-Lead ECG

294

1. RATE

Atrial:

Ventricular:

2. RHYTHM

Atrial:

Ventricular:

3. WAVES

P waves present:

Appearance:

Consistent:

Relation to QRS:

Q waves present:

Leads:

Pathological:

T waves present:

Morphology:

4. INTERVALS

P-R interval:

Consistent:

QRS:

Appearance:

Consistent:

Q-T interval:

5. AXIS

Quadrant:

Degrees:

6. HYPERTROPHY

Atrial:

Ventricular:

7. MYOCARDIAL INFARCTION

Q waves:

S-T displacement:

8. ISCHEMIA

S-T displacement:

9. POSSIBLE DRUG EFFECTS

10. ECG ANALYSIS

11. INTERPRETATION

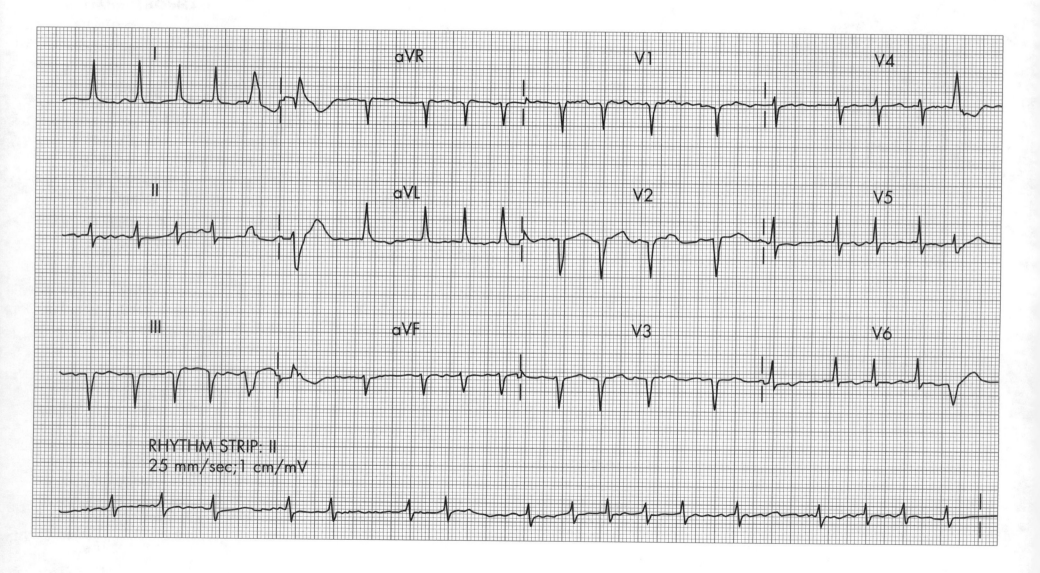

Figure 5-26
Resting 12-Lead ECG
296

1. RATE

Atrial:

Ventricular:

2. RHYTHM

Atrial:

Ventricular:

3. WAVES

P waves present:

Appearance:

Consistent:

Relation to QRS:

Q waves present:

Leads:

Pathological:

T waves present:

Morphology:

4. INTERVALS

P-R interval:

Consistent:

QRS:

Appearance:

Consistent:

Q-T interval:

5. AXIS

Quadrant:

Degrees:

6. HYPERTROPHY

Atrial:

Ventricular:

7. MYOCARDIAL INFARCTION

Q waves:

S-T displacement:

8. ISCHEMIA

S-T displacement:

9. POSSIBLE DRUG EFFECTS

10. ECG ANALYSIS

11. INTERPRETATION

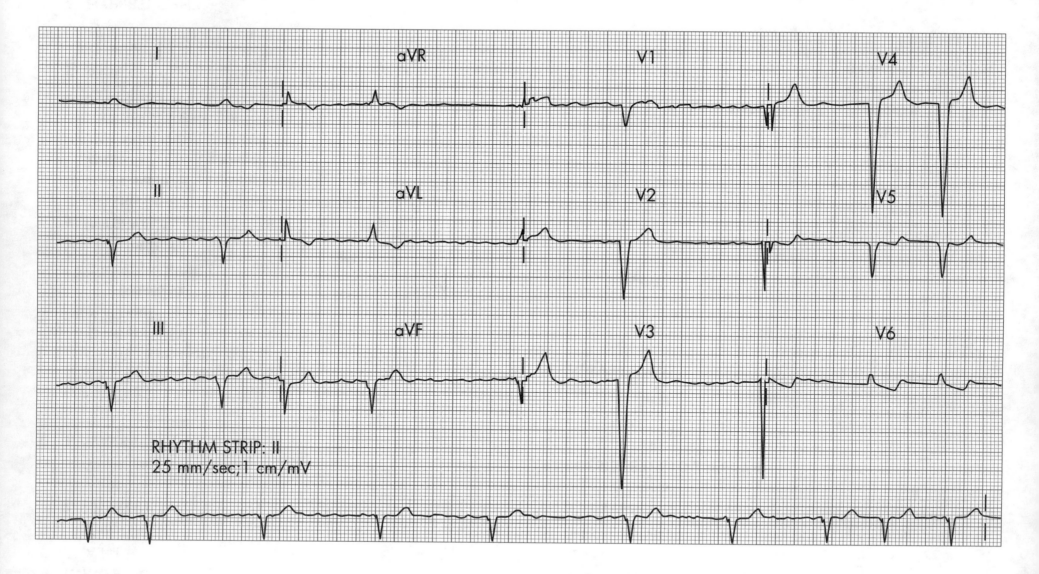

Figure 5-27
Resting 12-Lead ECG
298

I. RATE

    Atrial:

    Ventricular:

2. RHYTHM

    Atrial:

    Ventricular:

3. WAVES

    P waves present:

        Appearance:

        Consistent:

        Relation to QRS:

    Q waves present:

        Leads:

        Pathological:

    T waves present:

        Morphology:

4. INTERVALS

    P-R interval:

        Consistent:

    QRS:

        Appearance:

        Consistent:

    Q-T interval:

5. AXIS

    Quadrant:

    Degrees:

6. HYPERTROPHY

    Atrial:

    Ventricular:

7. MYOCARDIAL INFARCTION

    Q waves:

    S-T displacement:

8. ISCHEMIA

    S-T displacement:

9. POSSIBLE DRUG EFFECTS

10. ECG ANALYSIS

11. INTERPRETATION

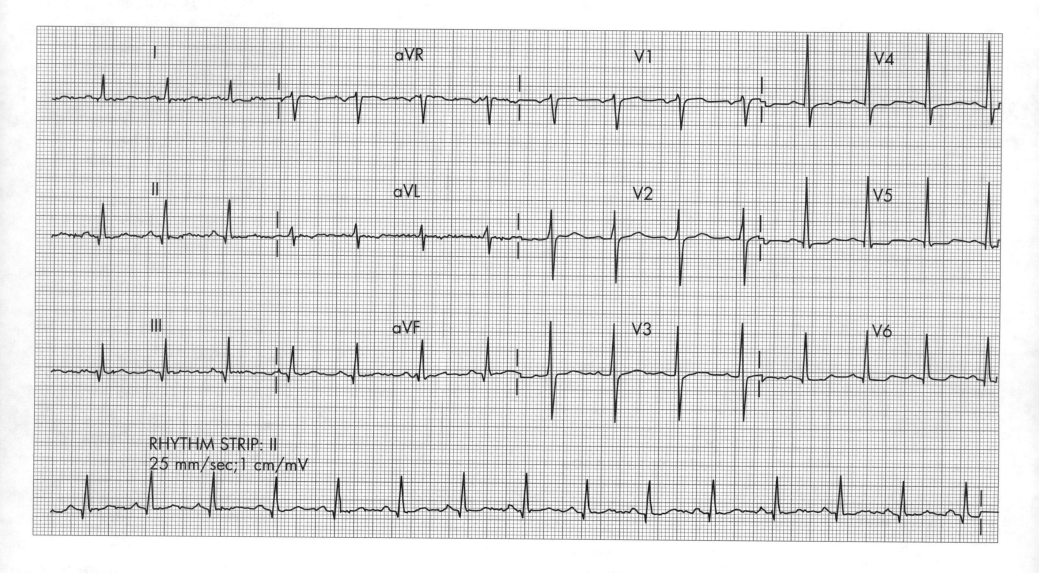

I aVR V1 V4

II aVL V2 V5

III aVF V3 V6

RHYTHM STRIP: II
25 mm/sec;1 cm/mV

Figure 5-28
Resting 12-Lead ECG

300

1. RATE

Atrial:

Ventricular:

2. RHYTHM

Atrial:

Ventricular:

3. WAVES

P waves present:

Appearance:

Consistent:

Relation to QRS:

Q waves present:

Leads:

Pathological:

T waves present:

Morphology:

4. INTERVALS

P-R interval:

Consistent:

QRS:

Appearance:

Consistent:

Q-T interval:

5. AXIS

Quadrant:

Degrees:

6. HYPERTROPHY

Atrial:

Ventricular:

7. MYOCARDIAL INFARCTION

Q waves:

S-T displacement:

8. ISCHEMIA

S-T d splacement:

9. POSSIBLE DRUG EFFECTS

10. ECG ANALYSIS

11. INTERPRETATION

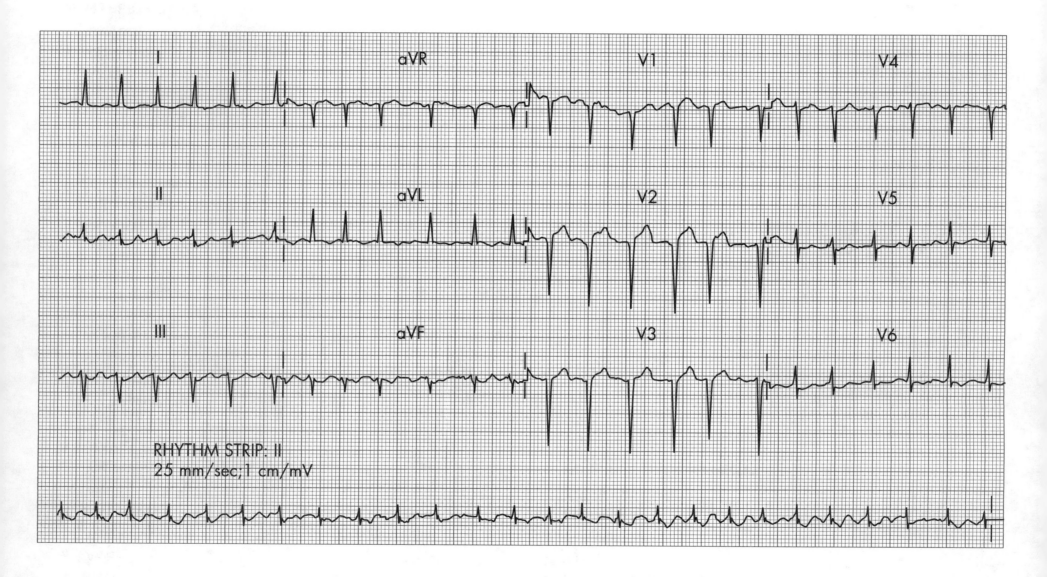

Figure 5-29
Resting 12-Lead ECG
302

1. **RATE**

   Atrial:

   Ventricular:

2. **RHYTHM**

   Atrial:

   Ventricular:

3. **WAVES**

   P waves present:

   Appearance:

   Consistent:

   Relation to QRS:

   Q waves present:

   Leads:

   Pathological:

   T waves present:

   Morphology:

4. **INTERVALS**

   P-R interval:

   Consistent:

   QRS:

   Appearance:

   Consistent:

   Q-T interval:

5. **AXIS**

   Quadrant:

   Degrees:

6. **HYPERTROPHY**

   Atrial:

   Ventricular:

7. **MYOCARDIAL INFARCTION**

   Q waves:

   S-T displacement:

8. **ISCHEMIA**

   S-T displacement:

9. **POSSIBLE DRUG EFFECTS**

10. **ECG ANALYSIS**

11. **INTERPRETATION**

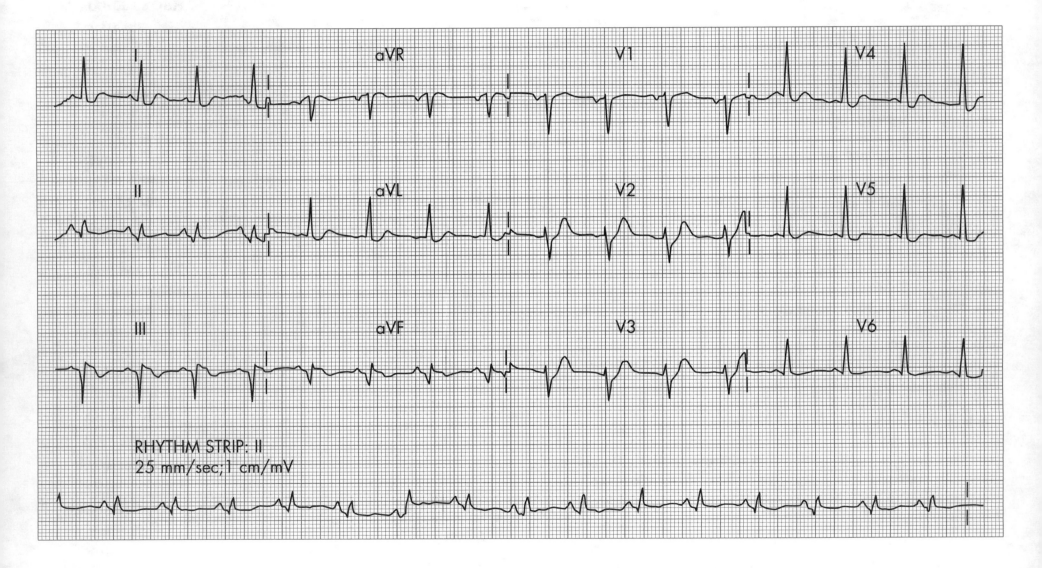

RHYTHM STRIP: II
25 mm/sec;1 cm/mV

Figure 5-30
Resting 12-Lead ECG

1. RATE

   Atrial:

   Ventricular:

2. RHYTHM

   Atrial:

   Ventricular:

3. WAVES

   P waves present:

      Appearance:

      Consistent:

      Relation to QRS:

   Q waves present:

      Leads:

      Pathological:

   T waves present:

      Morphology:

4. INTERVALS

   P-R interval:

      Consistent:

   QRS:

      Appearance:

      Consistent:

   Q-T interval:

5. AXIS

   Quadrant:

   Degrees:

6. HYPERTROPHY

   Atrial:

   Ventricular:

7. MYOCARDIAL INFARCTION

   Q waves:

   S-T displacement:

8. ISCHEMIA

   S-T displacement:

9. POSSIBLE DRUG EFFECTS

10. ECG ANALYSIS

11. INTERPRETATION

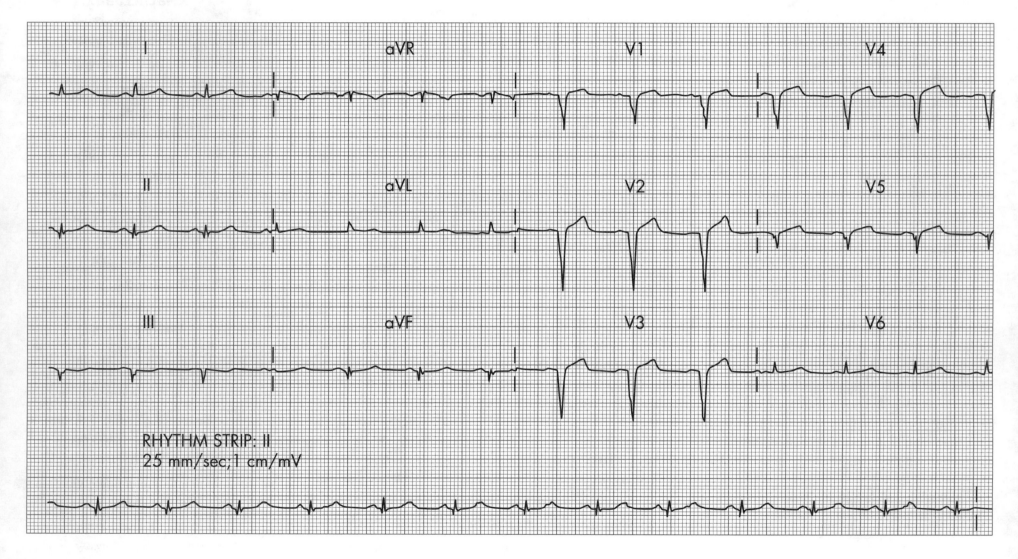

I aVR V1 V4

II aVL V2 V5

III aVF V3 V6

RHYTHM STRIP: II
25 mm/sec;1 cm/mV

Figure 5-31
Resting 12-Lead ECG
ECG #1 of 2
306

1. RATE

Atrial:

Ventricular:

2. RHYTHM

Atrial:

Ventricular:

3. WAVES

P waves present:

Appearance:

Consistent:

Relation to QRS:

Q waves present:

Leads:

Pathological:

T waves present:

Morphology:

4. INTERVALS

P-R interval:

Consistent:

QRS:

Appearance:

Consistent:

Q-T interval:

5. AXIS

Quadrant:

Degrees:

6. HYPERTROPHY

Atrial:

Ventricular:

7. MYOCARDIAL INFARCTION

Q waves:

S-T displacement:

8. ISCHEMIA

S-T displacement:

9. POSSIBLE DRUG EFFECTS

10. ECG ANALYSIS

11. INTERPRETATION

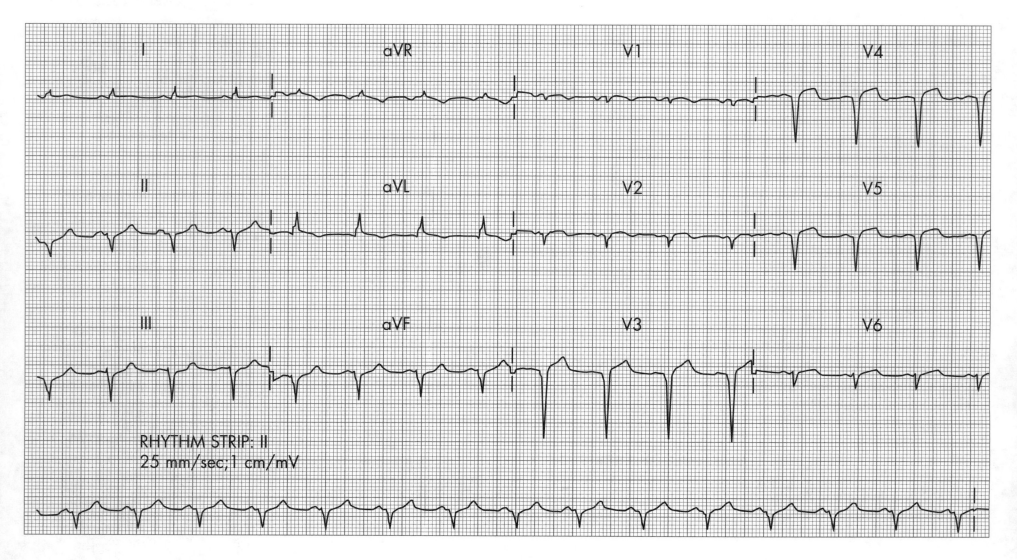

I aVR V1 V4

II aVL V2 V5

III aVF V3 V6

RHYTHM STRIP: II
25 mm/sec;1 cm/mV

Figure 5-32
Resting 12-Lead ECG
ECG #2 of 2
308

1. **RATE**

   Atrial:

   Ventricular:

2. **RHYTHM**

   Atrial:

   Ventricular:

3. **WAVES**

   P waves present:

   Appearance:

   Consistent:

   Relation to QRS:

   Q waves present:

   Leads:

   Pathological:

   T waves present:

   Morphology:

4. **INTERVALS**

   P-R interval:

   Consistent:

   QRS:

   Appearance:

   Consistent:

   Q-T interval:

5. **AXIS**

   Quadrant:

   Degrees:

6. **HYPERTROPHY**

   Atrial:

   Ventricular:

7. **MYOCARDIAL INFARCTION**

   Q waves:

   S-T displacement:

8. **ISCHEMIA**

   S-T displacement:

9. **POSSIBLE DRUG EFFECTS**

10. **ECG ANALYSIS**

11. **INTERPRETATION**

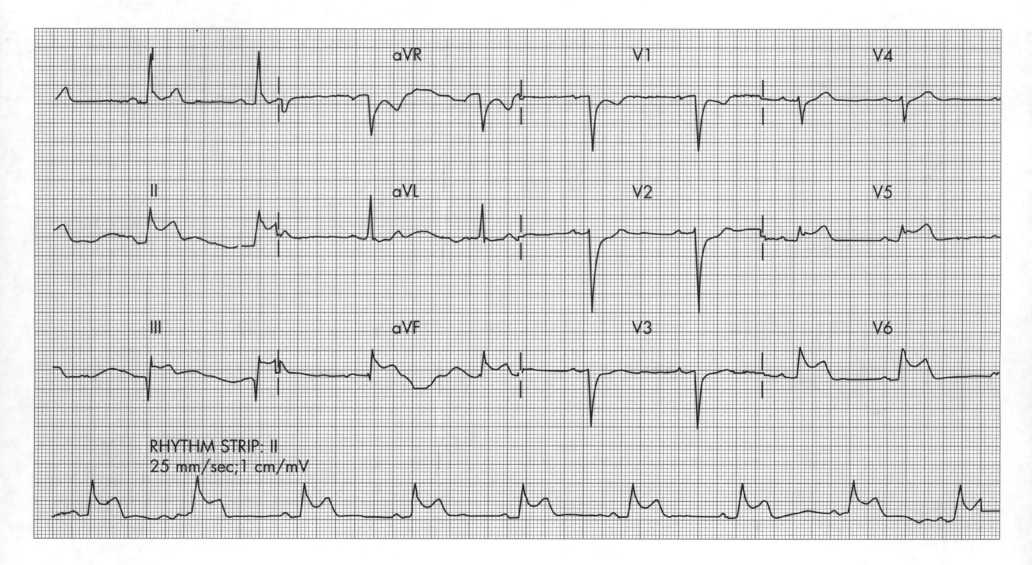

aVR V1 V4

II aVL V2 V5

III aVF V3 V6

RHYTHM STRIP: II
25 mm/sec; 1 cm/mV

Figure 5-33
Resting 12-Lead ECG
ECG #1 of 3
310

1. RATE

Atrial:

Ventricular:

2. RHYTHM

Atrial:

Ventricular:

3. WAVES

P waves present:

Appearance:

Consistent:

Relation to QRS:

Q waves present:

Leads:

Pathological:

T waves present:

Morphology:

4. INTERVALS

P-R interval:

Consistent:

QRS:

Appearance:

Consistent:

Q-T interval:

5. AXIS

Quadrant:

Degrees:

6. HYPERTROPHY

Atrial:

Ventricular:

7. MYOCARDIAL INFARCTION

Q waves:

S-T displacement:

8. ISCHEMIA

S-T displacement:

9. POSSIBLE DRUG EFFECTS

10. ECG ANALYSIS

11. INTERPRETATION

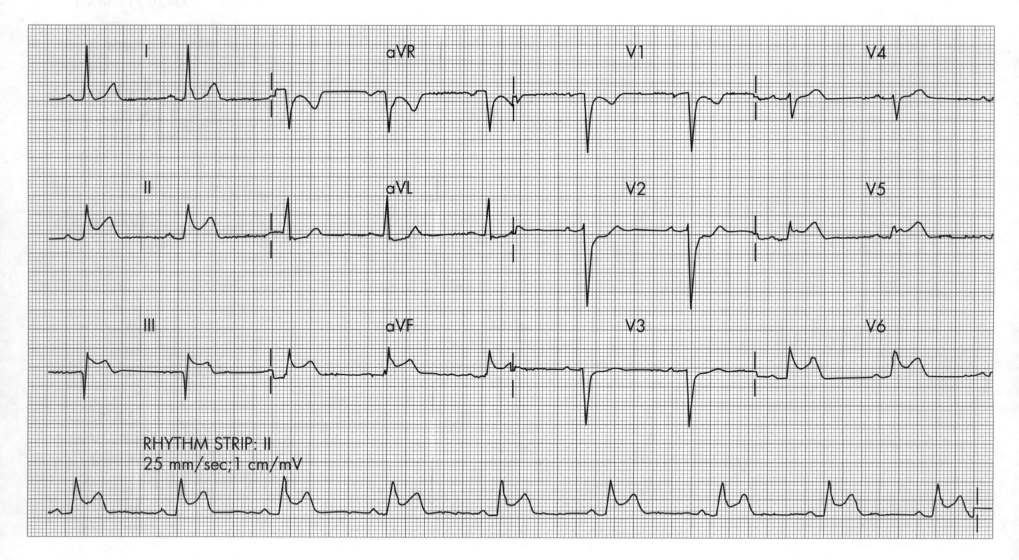

Figure 5-34
Resting 12-Lead ECG
ECG #2 of 3

312

1. RATE

Atrial:

Ventricular:

2. RHYTHM

Atrial:

Ventricular:

3. WAVES

P waves present:

    Appearance:

    Consistent:

    Relation to QRS:

Q waves present:

    Leads:

    Pathological:

T waves present:

    Morphology:

4. INTERVALS

P-R interval:

    Consistent:

QRS:

    Appearance:

    Consistent:

Q-T interval:

5. AXIS

Quadrant:

Degrees:

6. HYPERTROPHY

Atrial:

Ventricular:

7. MYOCARDIAL INFARCTION

Q waves:

S-T displacement:

8. ISCHEMIA

S-T displacement:

9. POSSIBLE DRUG EFFECTS

10. ECG ANALYSIS

11. INTERPRETATION

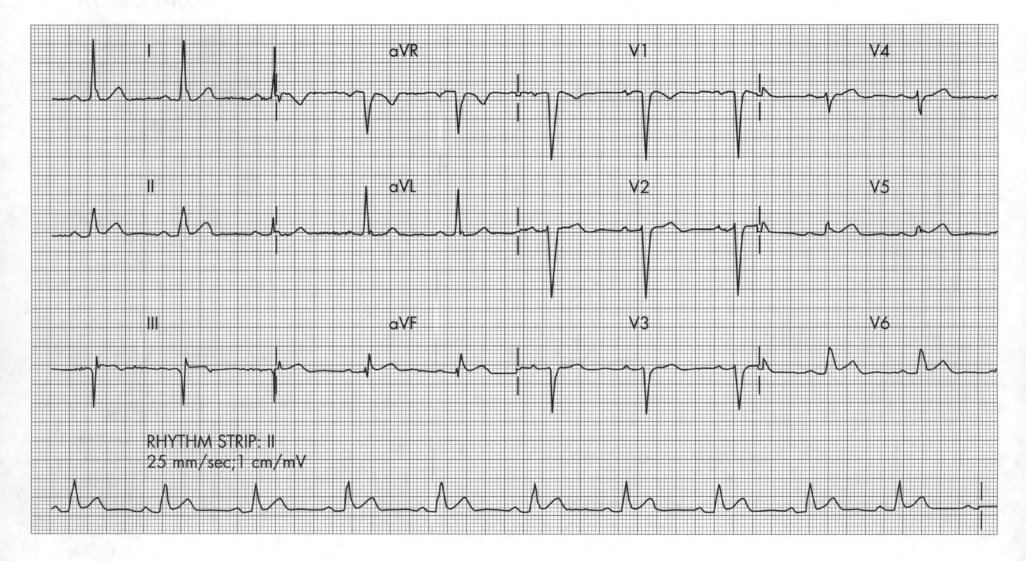

I aVR V1 V4

II aVL V2 V5

III aVF V3 V6

RHYTHM STRIP: II
25 mm/sec;1 cm/mV

Figure 5-35
Resting 12-Lead ECG
ECG #3 of 3
314

1. **RATE**

   Atrial:

   Ventricular:

2. **RHYTHM**

   Atrial:

   Ventricular:

3. **WAVES**

   P waves present:

       Appearance:

       Consistent:

       Relation to QRS:

   Q waves present:

       Leads:

       Pathological:

   T waves present:

       Morphology:

4. **INTERVALS**

   P-R interval:

       Consistent:

   QRS:

       Appearance:

       Consistent:

   Q-T interval:

5. **AXIS**

   Quadrant:

   Degrees:

6. **HYPERTROPHY**

   Atrial:

   Ventricular:

7. **MYOCARDIAL INFARCTION**

   Q waves:

   S-T displacement:

8. **ISCHEMIA**

   S-T displacement:

9. **POSSIBLE DRUG EFFECTS**

10. **ECG ANALYSIS**

11. **INTERPRETATION**

Part VI

Cardiac Pacemakers and Medication Effects

PACEMAKER—12-LEAD ECG ANALYSIS

Mechanical pacemakers can make ECG interpretations difficult. Underlying rhythms may be virtually impossible to read with a pacemaker that is functioning over 50% of the time. Ischemia and myocardial infarctions are difficult, if not impossible, to diagnose using a primarily paced 12-lead tracing. Usually the more important issues concerning practitioners examining ECGs of patients with pacemakers are whether or not the pacemaker functions and whether it functions as it was programmed.

The Intersociety Committee on Heart Disease (ICHD) has established the codes listed below to describe pacemaker operation. The first letter describes the chamber paced, the second letter describes the chamber sensed, and the third letter describes the mode of response. If a fourth letter is used in a description, it stands for the special features of the pacemaker.

The most frequently encountered single chamber pacemaker is the ventricular demand pacemaker. The ICHD code is **VVI,** meaning the ventricle is the chamber paced (V) and sensed (V), and the mode of response to a sensed QRS is inhibition (I).

Dual chamber pacemakers (**DDD**) are capable of sensing and pacing either the ventricle or the atrium at any one time. The pacemaker may be functioning in the **AAI** (atrial demand), **VVI** (ventricular demand), **VAT** or **VDD** (atrial synchronous), or **DVI** (atrial—ventricular sequential) mode. If in the **VAT** or **VDD** mode, the ventricles are triggered at a preset interval following the sensing of a P wave.

PACEMAKER IDENTIFICATION CODES INTERSOCIETY COMMITTEE ON HEART DISEASE			
Letter 1 *Chamber Paced*	**Letter 2** *Chamber Sensed*	**Letter 3** *Mode of Response*	**Letter 4** *Features*
V = Ventricle **A** = Atrium **D** = Dual chamber **S** = Single chamber	**V** = Ventricle **A** = Atrium **D** = Dual chamber **S** = Single chamber	**I** = Inhibits pacing **T** = Triggered **D** = Dual both I & T **0** = None	**P** = Programmable **M** = Multi-programmable **C** = Communicating **R** = Rate modulating

When analyzing a 12-lead ECG in which pacemaker spikes are seen, the student should use the following sequence of analysis:

Complete steps 1 through 7 (the same as nonpaced 12-lead tracings) as completely as possible and determine the underlying rhythm. Use only nonpaced beats in this analysis.

1. Rate
2. Rhythm
3. Waves
   P waves
   Q waves
   T waves
4. Intervals
   P-R
   QRS
   Q-T
5. Axis
6. Hypertrophy
7. MI

Assess pacemaker type and function:

8. Determine type of pacemaker
   Examine pacemaker spikes and their relationship to the P waves and to QRS complexes
9. Calculate pacemaker rate
10. Calculate AV delay for atrial pacemakers
11. Assess pacemaker sensing function
    Examine the ECG for any unexpected pauses
12. Assess pacemaker capture function
    Observe for any pacemaker spikes that are **not** followed by an AV delay and/or proper ventricular response

Analyze information and interpret ECG:

13. ECG analysis
    Summarize pertinent information
14. Interpretation
    List underlying rhythm, abnormalities, and pacemaker function

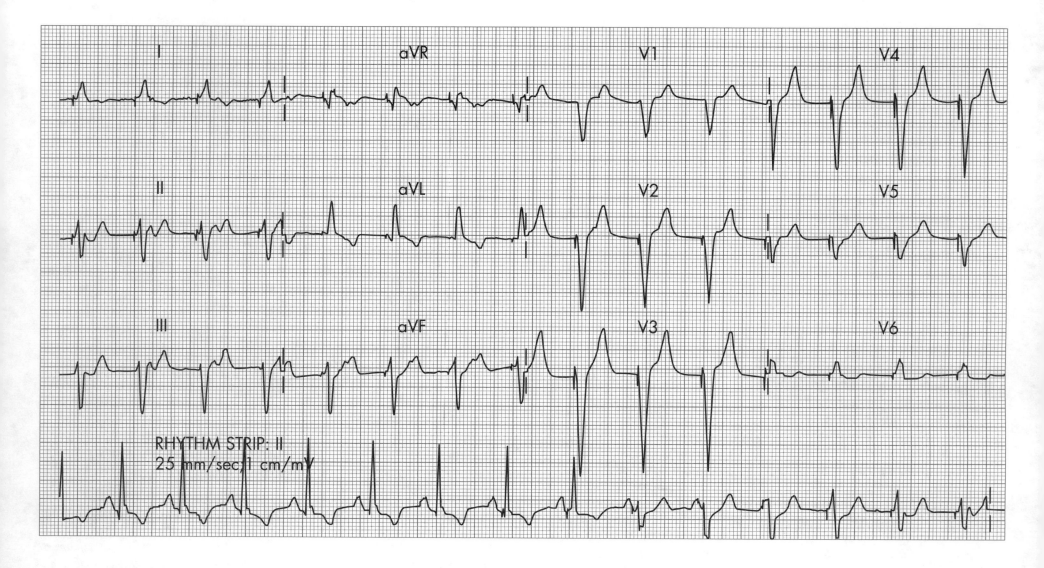

Figure 6-1
Resting 12-Lead ECG

1. **RATE**
   Atrial:
   Ventricular:

2. **RHYTHM**
   Atrial:
   Ventricular:

3. **WAVES**
   P waves present:
   　　Appearance:
   　　Consistent:
   　　Relation to QRS:
   Q waves present:
   　　Leads:
   　　Pathological:
   T waves present:
   　　Morphology:

4. **INTERVALS**
   P-R interval:
   　　Consistent:
   QRS:
   　　Appearance:
   　　Consistent:
   Q-T interval:

5. **AXIS**
   Quadrant:
   Degrees:

6. **HYPERTROPHY**
   Atrial:
   Ventricular:

7. **MYOCARDIAL INFARCTION**
   Q waves:
   S-T displacement:

8. **PACEMAKER TYPE**
   Spikes present:
   Relationship to P wave:
   AV delay:
   Relationship to QRS:

9. **PACEMAKER RATE**
   Atria:
   Ventricular:

10. **PACEMAKER SENSING**
    Unexpected pauses:

11. **PACEMAKER CAPTURE**
    Spikes without depolarization:

12. **POSSIBLE DRUG EFFECTS**

13. **ECG ANALYSIS**

14. **INTERPRETATION**
    Underlying rhythm:

    Mechanical pacemaker:

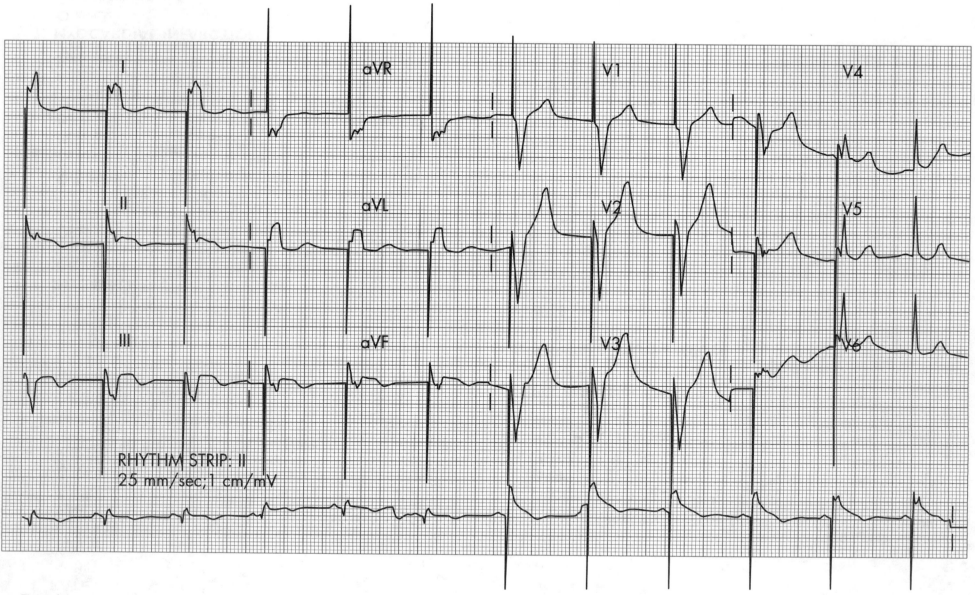

I   aVR   V1   V4

II   aVL   V2   V5

III   aVF   V3   V6

RHYTHM STRIP: II
25 mm/sec; 1 cm/mV

Figure 6-2
Resting 12-Lead ECG

322

1. RATE
Atrial:
Ventricular:

2. RHYTHM
Atrial:
Ventricular:

3. WAVES
P waves present:
    Appearance:
    Consistent:
    Relation to QRS:
Q waves present:
    Leads:
    Pathological:
T waves present:
    Morphology:

4. INTERVALS
P-R interval:
    Consistent:
QRS:
    Appearance:
    Consistent:
Q-T interval:

5. AXIS
Quadrant:
Degrees:

6. HYPERTROPHY
Atrial:
Ventricular:

7. MYOCARDIAL INFARCTION
Q waves:
S-T displacement:

8. PACEMAKER TYPE
Spikes present:
Relationship to P wave:
AV delay:
Relationship to QRS:

9. PACEMAKER RATE
Atrial:
Ventricular:

10. PACEMAKER SENSING
Unexpected pauses:

11. PACEMAKER CAPTURE
Spikes without depolarization:

12. POSSIBLE DRUG EFFECTS

13. ECG ANALYSIS

14. INTERPRETATION
Underlying rhythm:

Mechanical pacemaker:

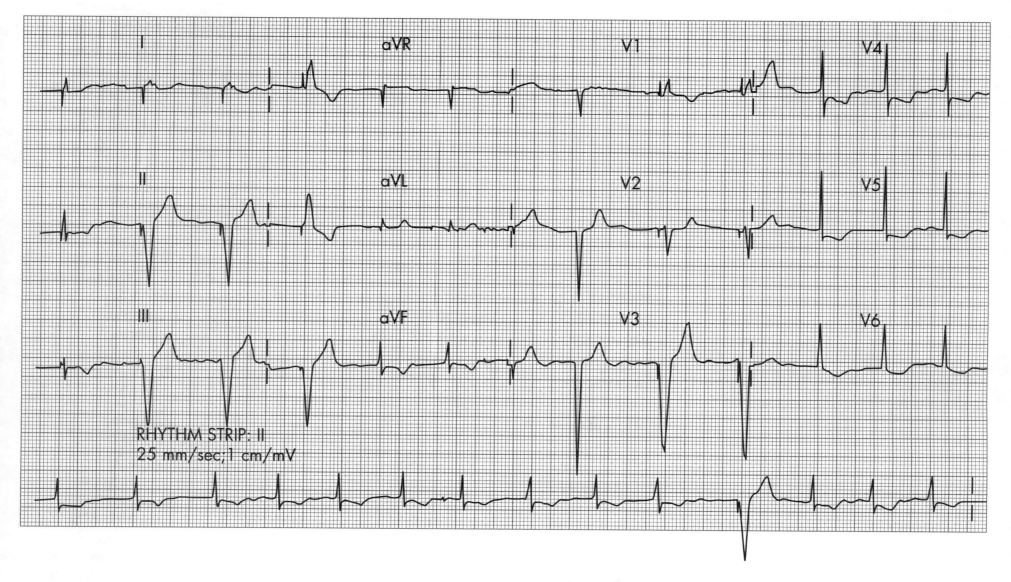

Figure 6-3
Resting 12-Lead ECG

324

1. **RATE**
   Atrial:
   Ventricular:

2. **RHYTHM**
   Atrial:
   Ventricular:

3. **WAVES**
   P waves present:
      Appearance:
      Consistent:
      Relation to QRS:
   Q waves present:
      Leads:
      Pathological:
   T waves present:
      Morphology:

4. **INTERVALS**
   P-R interval:
      Consistent:
   QRS:
      Appearance:
      Consistent:
   Q-T interval:

5. **AXIS**
   Quadrant:
   Degrees:

6. **HYPERTROPHY**
   Atrial:
   Ventricular:

7. **MYOCARDIAL INFARCTION**
   Q waves:
   S-T displacement:

8. **PACEMAKER TYPE**
   Spikes present:
   Relationship to P wave:
   AV delay:
   Relationship to QRS:

9. **PACEMAKER RATE**
   Atrial:
   Ventricular:

10. **PACEMAKER SENSING**
    Unexpected pauses:

11. **PACEMAKER CAPTURE**
    Spikes without depolarization:

12. **POSSIBLE DRUG EFFECTS**

13. **ECG ANALYSIS**

14. **INTERPRETATION**
    Underlying rhythm:

    Mechanical pacemaker:

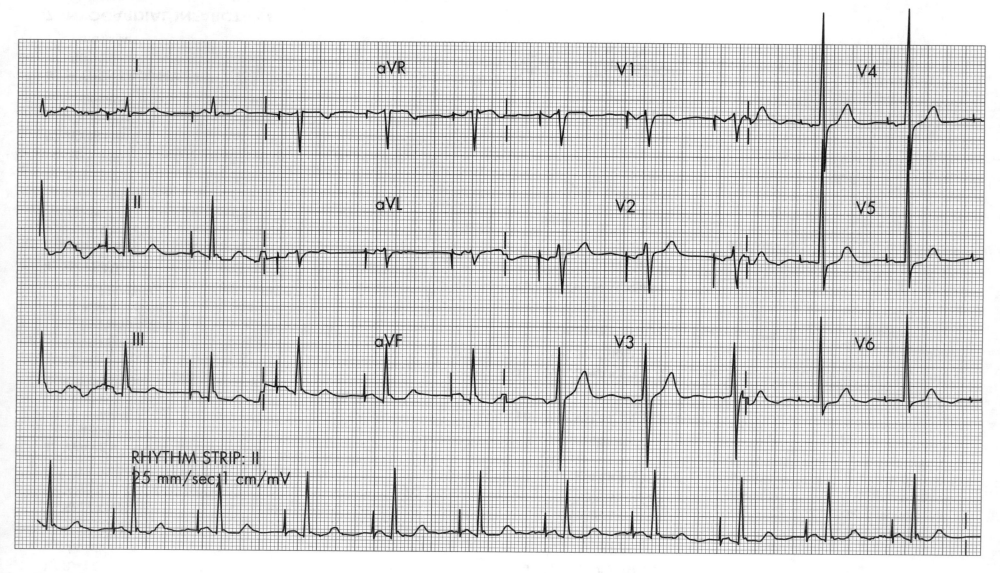

Figure 6-4
Resting 12-Lead ECG

1. **RATE**
   Atrial:
   Ventricular:

2. **RHYTHM**
   Atrial:
   Ventricular:

3. **WAVES**
   P waves present:
       Appearance:
       Consistent:
       Relation to QRS:
   Q waves present:
       Leads:
       Pathological:
   T waves present:
       Morphology:

4. **INTERVALS**
   P-R interval:
       Consistent:
   QRS:
       Appearance:
       Consistent:
   Q-T interval:

5. **AXIS**
   Quadrant:
   Degrees:

6. **HYPERTROPHY**
   Atrial:
   Ventricular:

7. **MYOCARDIAL INFARCTION**
   Q waves:
   S-T displacement:

8. **PACEMAKER TYPE**
   Spikes present:
   Relationship to P wave:
   AV delay:
   Relationship to QRS:

9. **PACEMAKER RATE**
   Atrial:
   Ventricular:

10. **PACEMAKER SENSING**
    Unexpected pauses:

11. **PACEMAKER CAPTURE**
    Spikes without depolarization:

12. **POSSIBLE DRUG EFFECTS**

13. **ECG ANALYSIS**

14. **INTERPRETATION**
    Underlying rhythm:

    Mechanical pacemaker:

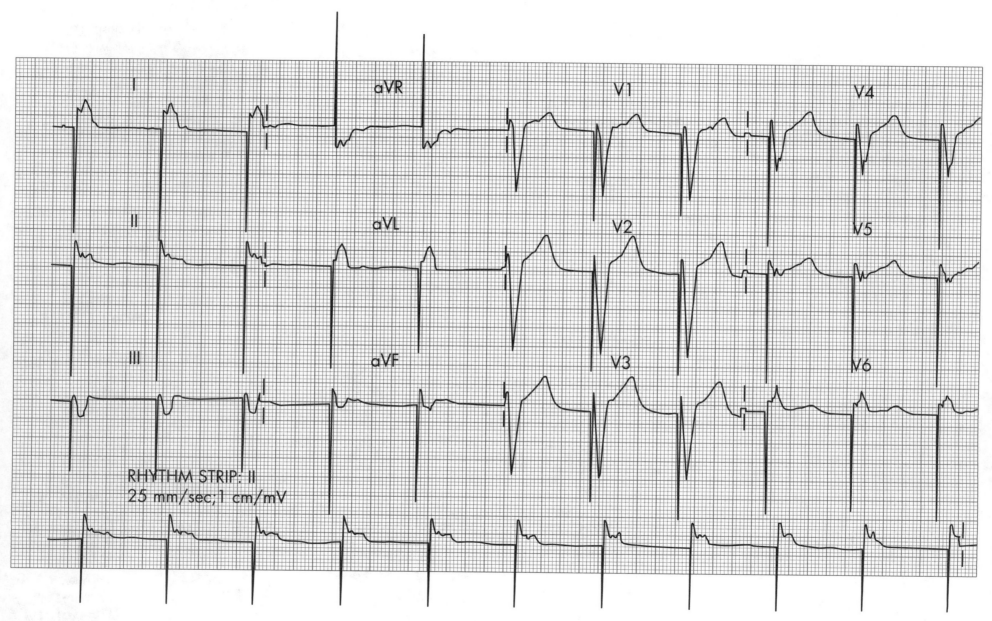

I aVR V1 V4

II aVL V2 V5

III aVF V3 V6

RHYTHM STRIP: II
25 mm/sec; 1 cm/mV

Figure 6-5
Resting 12-Lead ECG

328

1. **RATE**
   Atrial:
   Ventricular:

2. **RHYTHM**
   Atrial:
   Ventricular:

3. **WAVES**
   P waves present:
      Appearance:
      Consistent:
      Relation to QRS:
   Q waves present:
      Leads:
      Pathological:
   T waves present:
      Morphology:

4. **INTERVALS**
   P-R interval:
      Consistent:
   QRS:
      Appearance:
      Consistent:
   Q-T interval:

5. **AXIS**
   Quadrant:
   Degrees:

6. **HYPERTROPHY**
   Atrial:
   Ventricular:

7. **MYOCARDIAL INFARCTION**
   Q waves:
   S-T displacement:

8. **PACEMAKER TYPE**
   Spikes present:
   Relationship to P wave:
   AV delay:
   Relationship to QRS:

9. **PACEMAKER RATE**
   Atrial:
   Ventricular:

10. **PACEMAKER SENSING**
   Unexpected pauses:

11. **PACEMAKER CAPTURE**
   Spikes without depolarization:

12. **POSSIBLE DRUG EFFECTS**

13. **ECG ANALYSIS**

14. **INTERPRETATION**
   Underlying rhythm:

   Mechanical pacemaker:

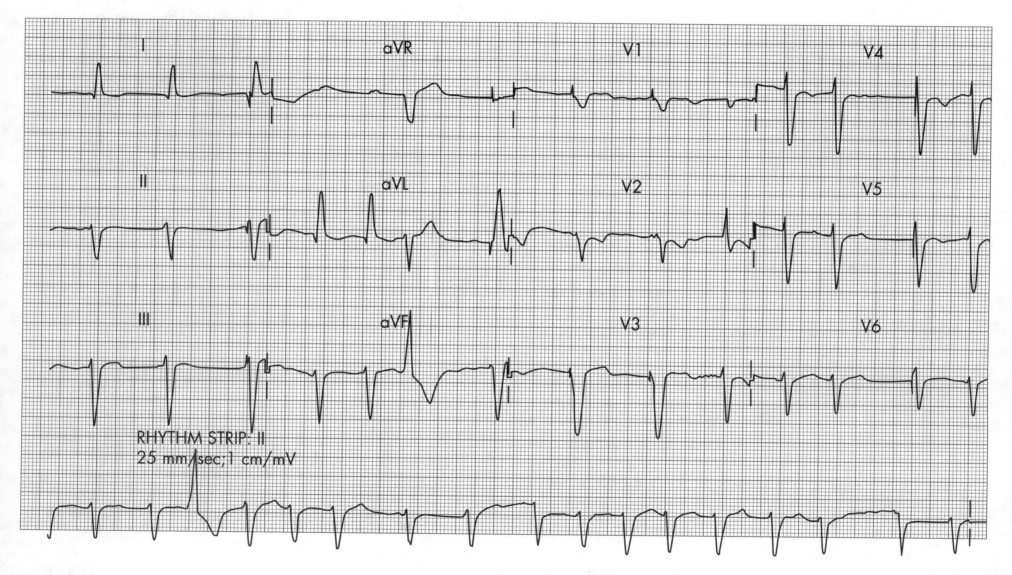

Figure 6-6
Resting 12-Lead ECG

1. RATE
  Atrial:
  Ventricular:

2. RHYTHM
  Atrial:
  Ventricular:

3. WAVES
  P waves present:
    Appearance:
    Consistent:
    Relation to QRS:
  Q waves present:
    Leads:
    Pathological:
  T waves present:
    Morphology:

4. INTERVALS
  P-R interval:
    Consistent:
  QRS:
    Appearance:
    Consistent:
  Q-T interval:

5. AXIS
  Quadrant:
  Degrees:

6. HYPERTROPHY
  Atrial:
  Ventricular:

7. MYOCARDIAL INFARCTION
  Q waves:
  S-T displacement:

8. PACEMAKER TYPE
  Spikes present:
  Relationship to P wave:
  AV delay:
  Relationship to QRS:

9. PACEMAKER RATE
  Atrial:
  Ventricular:

10. PACEMAKER SENSING
  Unexpected pauses:

11. PACEMAKER CAPTURE
  Spikes without depolarization:

12. POSSIBLE DRUG EFFECTS

13. ECG ANALYSIS

14. INTERPRETATION
  Underlying rhythm:

  Mechanical pacemaker:

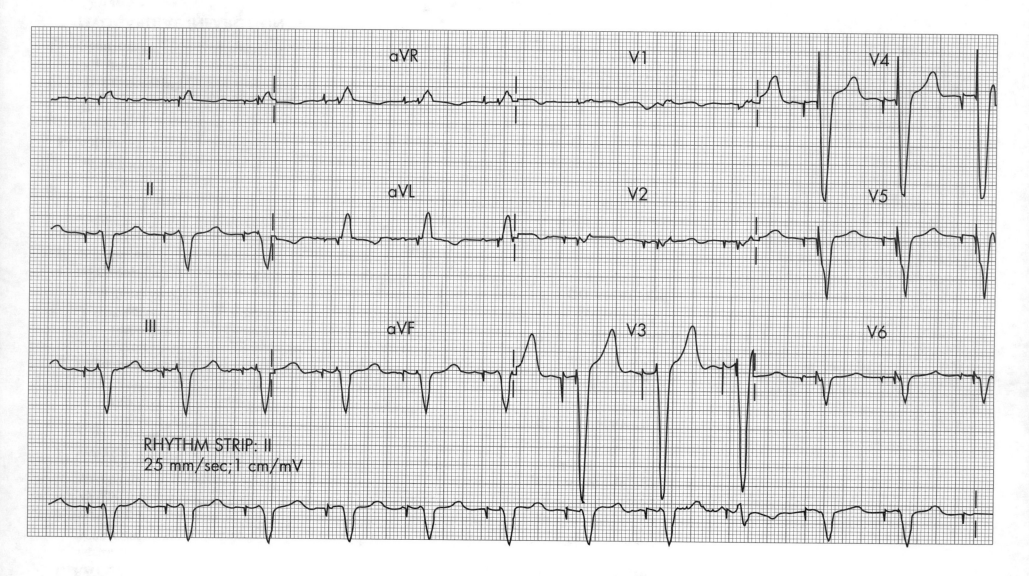

I aVR V1 V4

II aVL V2 V5

III aVF V3 V6

RHYTHM STRIP: II
25 mm/sec; 1 cm/mV

Figure 6-7
Resting 12-Lead ECG

332

I. RATE
Atrial:
Ventricular:

2. RHYTHM
Atrial:
Ventricular:

3. WAVES
P waves present:
    Appearance:
    Consistent:
    Relation to QRS:
Q waves present:
    Leads:
    Pathological:
T waves present:
    Morphology:

4. INTERVALS
P-R interval:
    Consistent:
QRS:
    Appearance:
    Consistent:
Q-T interval:

5. AXIS
Quadrant:
Degrees:

6. HYPERTROPHY
Atrial:
Ventricular:

7. MYOCARDIAL INFARCTION
Q waves:
S-T displacement:

8. PACEMAKER TYPE
Spikes present:
Relationship to P wave:
AV delay:
Relationship to QRS:

9. PACEMAKER RATE
Atrial:
Ventricular:

10. PACEMAKER SENSING
Unexpected pauses:

11. PACEMAKER CAPTURE
Spikes without depolarization:

12. POSSIBLE DRUG EFFECTS

13. ECG ANALYSIS

14. INTERPRETATION
Underlying rhythm:

Mechanical pacemaker:

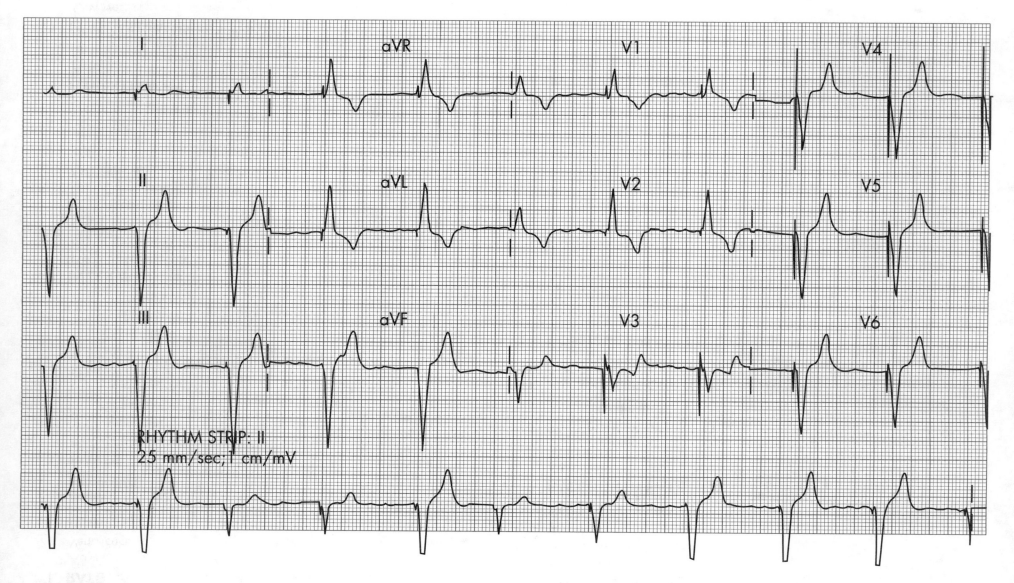

Figure 6-8
Resting 12-Lead ECG

1. RATE
Atrial:
Ventricular:

2. RHYTHM
Atrial:
Ventricular:

3. WAVES
P waves present:
    Appearance:
    Consistent:
    Relation to QRS:
Q waves present:
    Leads:
    Pathological:
T waves present:
    Morphology:

4. INTERVALS
P-R interval:
    Consistent:
QRS:
    Appearance:
    Consistent:
Q-T interval:

5. AXIS
Quadrant:
Degrees:

6. HYPERTROPHY
Atrial:
Ventricular:

7. MYOCARDIAL INFARCTION
Q waves:
S-T displacement:

8. PACEMAKER TYPE
Spikes present:
Relationship to P wave:
AV delay:
Relationship to QRS:

9. PACEMAKER RATE
Atrial:
Ventricular:

10. PACEMAKER SENSING
Unexpected pauses:

11. PACEMAKER CAPTURE
Spikes without depolarization:

12. POSSIBLE DRUG EFFECTS

13. ECG ANALYSIS

14. INTERPRETATION
Underlying rhythm:

Mechanical pacemaker:

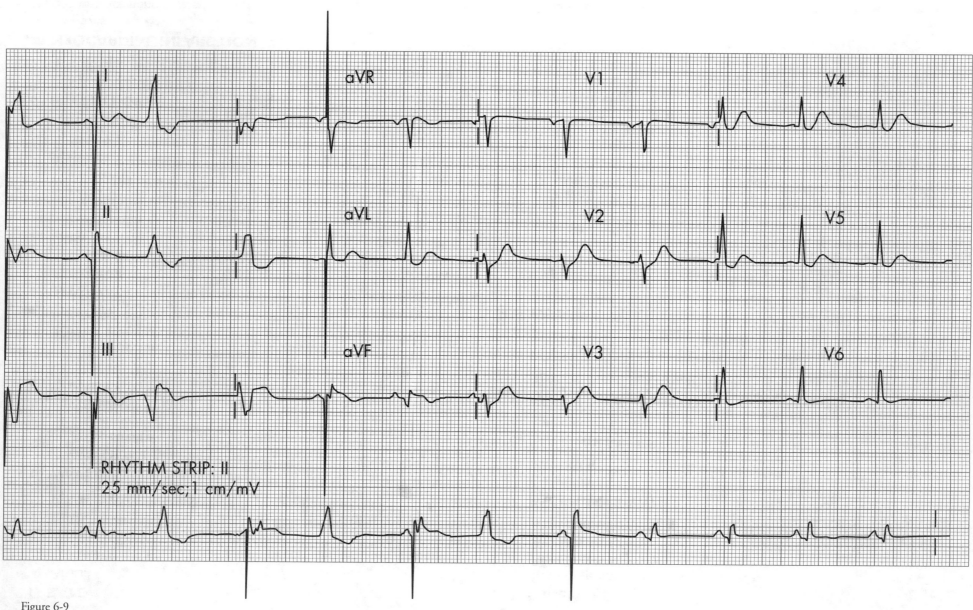

I   aVR   V1   V4

II   aVL   V2   V5

III   aVF   V3   V6

RHYTHM STRIP: II
25 mm/sec; 1 cm/mV

Figure 6-9
Resting 12-Lead ECG

336

1. RATE
   Atrial:
   Ventricular:

2. RHYTHM
   Atrial:
   Ventricular:

3. WAVES
   P waves present:
      Appearance:
      Consistent:
      Relation to QRS:
   Q waves present:
      Leads:
      Pathological:
   T waves present:
      Morphology:

4. INTERVALS
   P-R interval:
      Consistent:
   QRS:
      Appearance:
      Consistent:
   Q-T interval:

5. AXIS
   Quadrant:
   Degrees:

6. HYPERTROPHY
   Atrial:
   Ventricular:

7. MYOCARDIAL INFARCTION
   Q waves:
   S-T displacement:

8. PACEMAKER TYPE
   Spikes present:
   Relationship to P wave:
   AV delay:
   Relationship to QRS:

9. PACEMAKER RATE
   Atrial:
   Ventricular:

10. PACEMAKER SENSING
   Unexpected pauses:

11. PACEMAKER CAPTURE
   Spikes without depolarization:

12. POSSIBLE DRUG EFFECTS

13. ECG ANALYSIS

14. INTERPRETATION
   Underlying rhythm:

   Mechanical pacemaker:

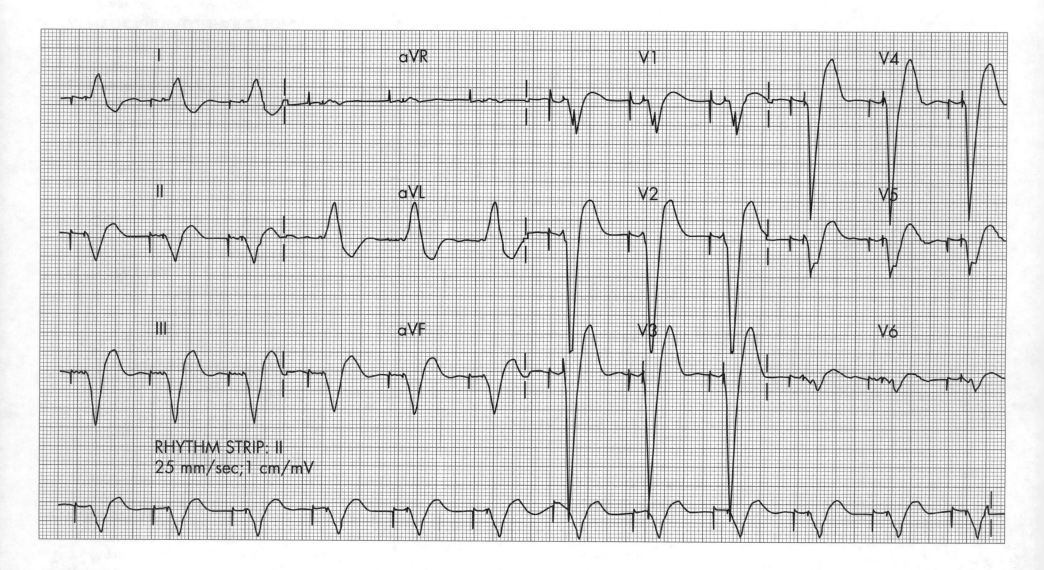

RHYTHM STRIP: II
25 mm/sec;1 cm/mV

Figure 6-10
Resting 12-Lead ECG

338

1. RATE
Atrial:
Ventricular:

2. RHYTHM
Atrial:
Ventricular:

3. WAVES
P waves present:
Appearance:
Consistent:
Relation to QRS:
Q waves present:
Leads:
Pathological:
T waves present:
Morphology:

4. INTERVALS
P-R interval:
Consistent:
QRS:
Appearance:
Consistent:
Q-T interval:

5. AXIS
Quadrant:
Degrees:

6. HYPERTROPHY
Atrial:
Ventricular:

7. MYOCARDIAL INFARCTION
Q waves:
S-T displacement:

8. PACEMAKER TYPE
Spikes present:
Relationship to P wave:
AV delay:
Relationship to QRS:

9. PACEMAKER RATE
Atrial:
Ventricular:

10. PACEMAKER SENSING
Unexpected pauses:

11. PACEMAKER CAPTURE
Spikes without depolarization:

12. POSSIBLE DRUG EFFECTS

13. ECG ANALYSIS

14. INTERPRETATION
Underlying rhythm:

Mechanical pacemaker:

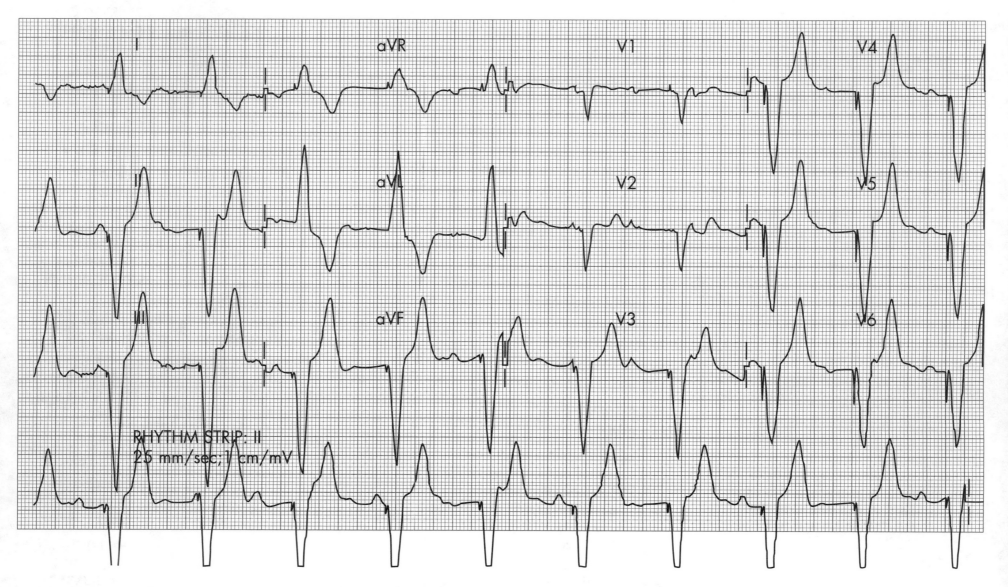

I aVR V1 V4

II aVL V2 V5

III aVF V3 V6

RHYTHM STRIP: II
25 mm/sec; 1 cm/mV

Figure 6-11
Resting 12-Lead ECG
340

1. **RATE**
   Atrial:
   Ventricular:

2. **RHYTHM**
   Atrial:
   Ventricular:

3. **WAVES**
   P waves present:
       Appearance:
       Consistent:
       Relation to QRS:
   Q waves present:
       Leads:
       Pathological:
   T waves present:
       Morphology:

4. **INTERVALS**
   P-R interval:
       Consistent:
   QRS:
       Appearance:
       Consistent:
   Q-T interval:

5. **AXIS**
   Quadrant:
   Degrees:

6. **HYPERTROPHY**
   Atrial:
   Ventricular:

7. **MYOCARDIAL INFARCTION**
   Q waves:
   S-T displacement:

8. **PACEMAKER TYPE**
   Spikes present:
   Relationship to P wave:
   AV delay:
   Relationship to QRS:

9. **PACEMAKER RATE**
   Atrial:
   Ventricular:

10. **PACEMAKER SENSING**
    Unexpected pauses:

11. **PACEMAKER CAPTURE**
    Spikes without depolarization:

12. **POSSIBLE DRUG EFFECTS**

13. **ECG ANALYSIS**

14. **INTERPRETATION**
    Underlying rhythm:

    Mechanical pacemaker:

MEDICATIONS

Almost any medication, if taken in high doses, can cause a cardiac dysrhythmia. The following are commonly used medications that may alter the electrocardiogram:

Digitalis preparations

Possible ECG effect:
- Bradyarrhythmias or tachyarrhythmias
- Blocks
- S-T segment depression (characteristic "scooped" appearance)

Tricyclic antidepressants

- Prolonged Q-T interval

Phenothiazines

- Prolonged Q-T interval
- Prominent U wave

Quinidine and other type I antiarrhythmic medications

- Prolonged Q-T interval
- S-T segment depression
- Flat T waves
- Possible U waves

METABOLIC CONDITIONS

Hyperkalemia

- Typically tall peaked T waves

Hypokalemia

- Flat T waves merge with prominent U waves
- Prolonged Q-T interval

Hypercalcemia

- Short Q-T interval

Hypocalcemia

- Prolonged Q-T interval

Hypomagnesemia

- Flat T waves merge with prominent U waves
- Prolonged Q-T interval
- Mimics hypokalemia

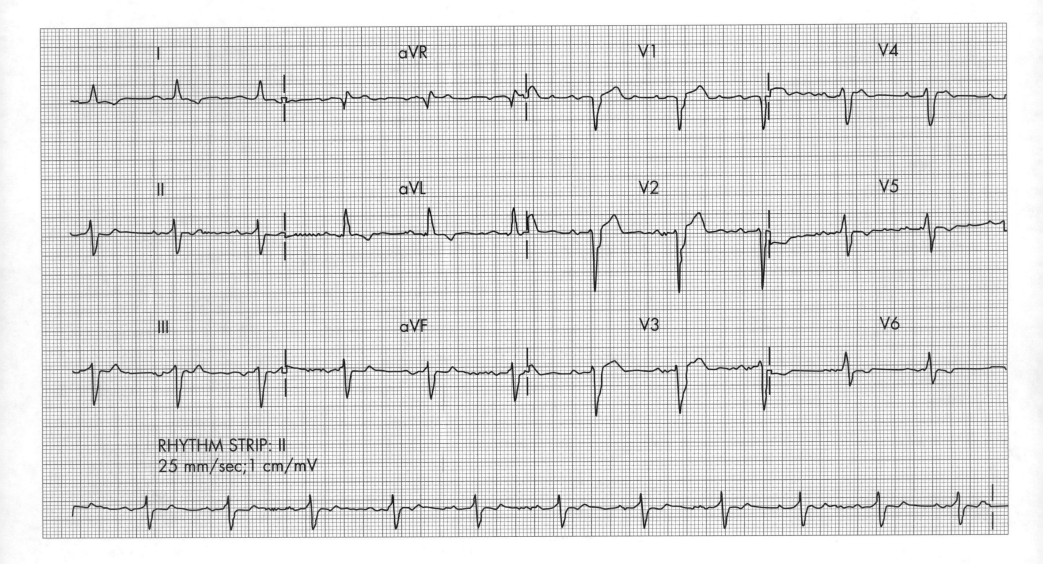

I   aVR   V1   V4

II   aVL   V2   V5

III   aVF   V3   V6

RHYTHM STRIP: II
25 mm/sec;1 cm/mV

Figure 6-12
Resting 12-Lead ECG
344

1. RATE

Atrial:

Ventricular:

2. RHYTHM

Atrial:

Ventricular:

3. WAVES

P waves present:

Appearance:

Consistent:

Relation to QRS:

Q waves present:

Leads:

Pathological:

T waves present:

Morphology:

4. INTERVALS

P-R interval:

Consistent:

QRS:

Appearance:

Consistent:

Q-T interval:

5. AXIS

Quadrant:

Degrees:

6. HYPERTROPHY

Atrial:

Ventricular:

7. MYOCARDIAL INFARCTION

Q waves:

S-T displacement:

8. ISCHEMIA

S-T displacement:

9. POSSIBLE DRUG EFFECTS

10. ECG ANALYSIS

11. INTERPRETATION

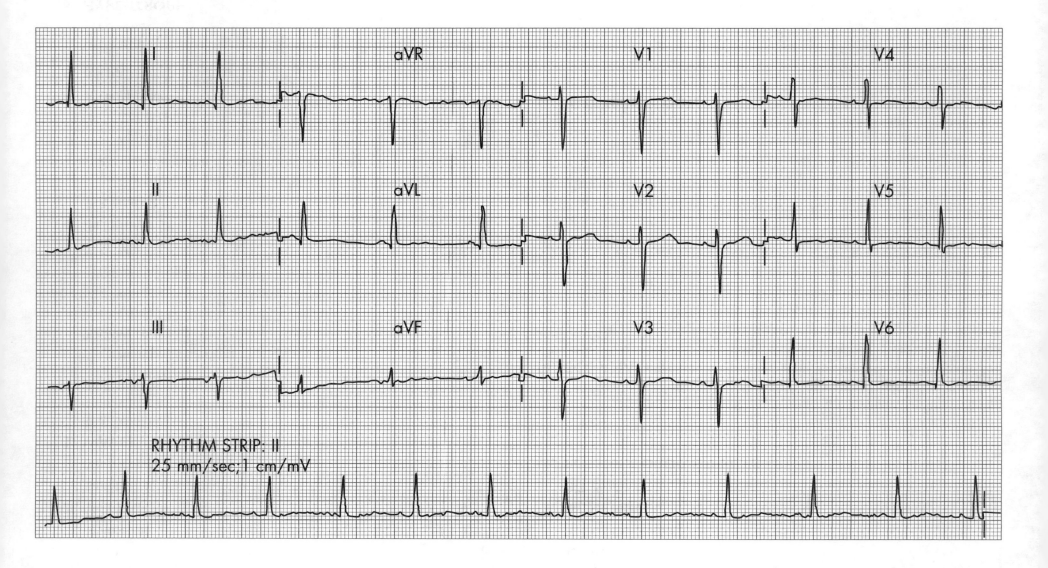

RHYTHM STRIP: II
25 mm/sec;1 cm/mV

Figure 6-13
Resting 12-Lead ECG
346

1. **RATE**

   Atrial:

   Ventricular:

2. **RHYTHM**

   Atrial:

   Ventricular:

3. **WAVES**

   P waves present:

       Appearance:

       Consistent:

       Relation to QRS:

   Q waves present:

       Leads:

       Pathological:

   T waves present:

       Morphology:

4. **INTERVALS**

   P-R interval:

       Consistent:

   QRS:

       Appearance:

       Consistent:

   Q-T interval:

5. **AXIS**

   Quadrant:

   Degrees:

6. **HYPERTROPHY**

   Atrial:

   Ventricular:

7. **MYOCARDIAL INFARCTION**

   Q waves:

   S-T displacement:

8. **ISCHEMIA**

   S-T displacement:

9. **POSSIBLE DRUG EFFECTS**

10. **ECG ANALYSIS**

11. **INTERPRETATION**

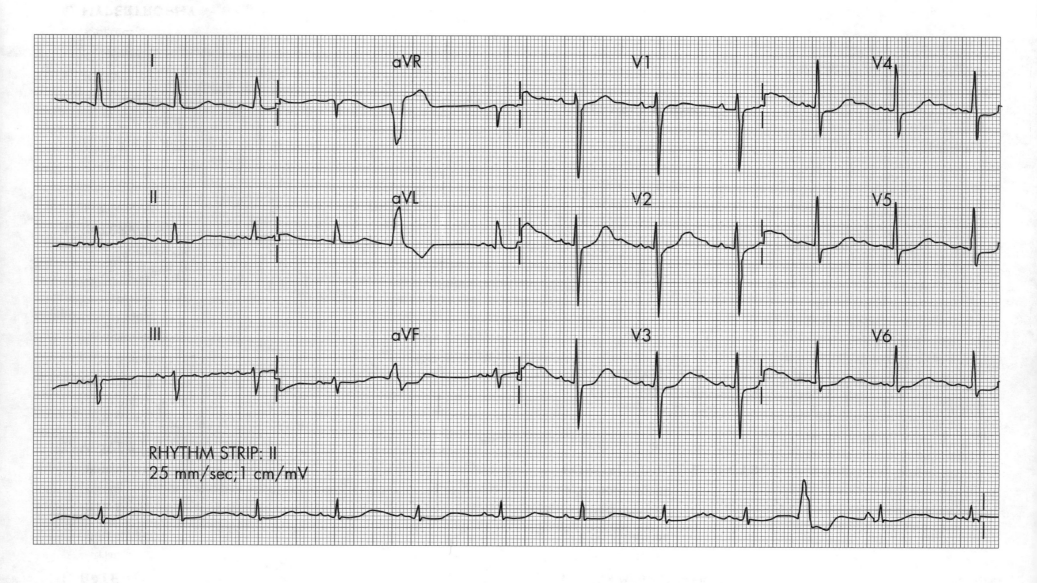

Figure 6-14
Resting 12-Lead ECG

348

1. RATE

    Atrial:

    Ventricular:

2. RHYTHM

    Atrial:

    Ventricular:

3. WAVES

    P waves present:

        Appearance:

        Consistent:

        Relation to QRS:

    Q waves present:

        Leads:

        Pathological:

    T waves present:

        Morphology:

4. INTERVALS

    P-R interval:

        Consistent:

    QRS:

        Appearance:

        Consistent:

    Q-T interval:

5. AXIS

    Quadrant:

    Degrees:

6. HYPERTROPHY

    Atrial:

    Ventricular:

7. MYOCARDIAL INFARCTION

    Q waves:

    S-T displacement:

8. ISCHEMIA

    S-T displacement:

9. POSSIBLE DRUG EFFECTS

10. ECG ANALYSIS

11. INTERPRETATION

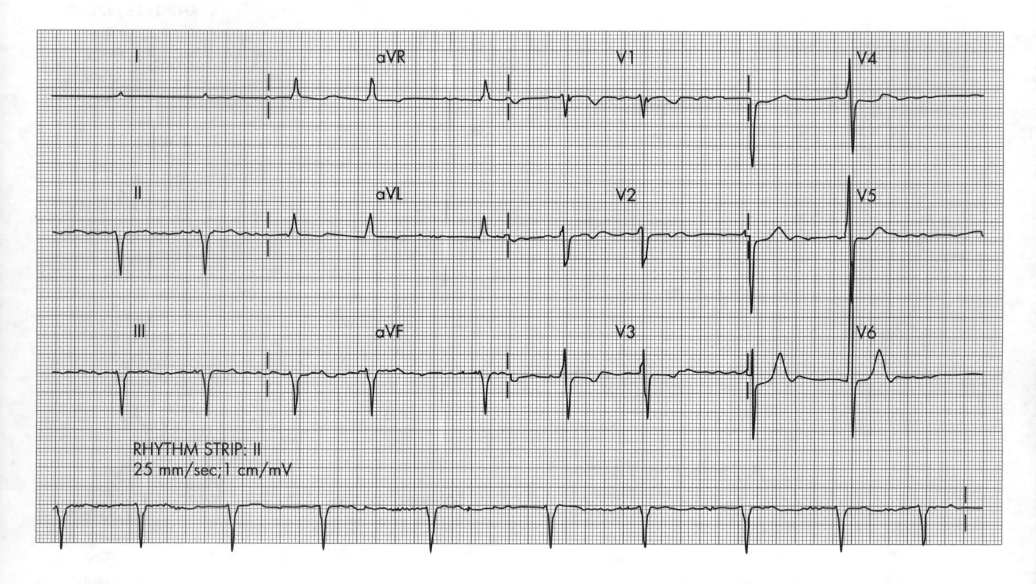

RHYTHM STRIP: II
25 mm/sec; 1 cm/mV

Figure 6-15
Resting 12-Lead ECG

350

1. RATE

Atrial:

Ventricular:

2. RHYTHM

Atrial:

Ventricular:

3. WAVES

P waves present:

Appearance:

Consistent:

Relation to QRS:

Q waves present:

Leads:

Pathological:

T waves present:

Morphology:

4. INTERVALS

P-R interval:

Consistent:

QRS:

Appearance:

Consistent:

Q-T interval:

5. AXIS

Quadrant:

Degrees:

6. HYPERTROPHY

Atrial:

Ventricular:

7. MYOCARDIAL INFARCTION

Q waves:

S-T displacement:

8. ISCHEMIA

S-T displacement:

9. POSSIBLE DRUG EFFECTS

10. ECG ANALYSIS

11. INTERPRETATION

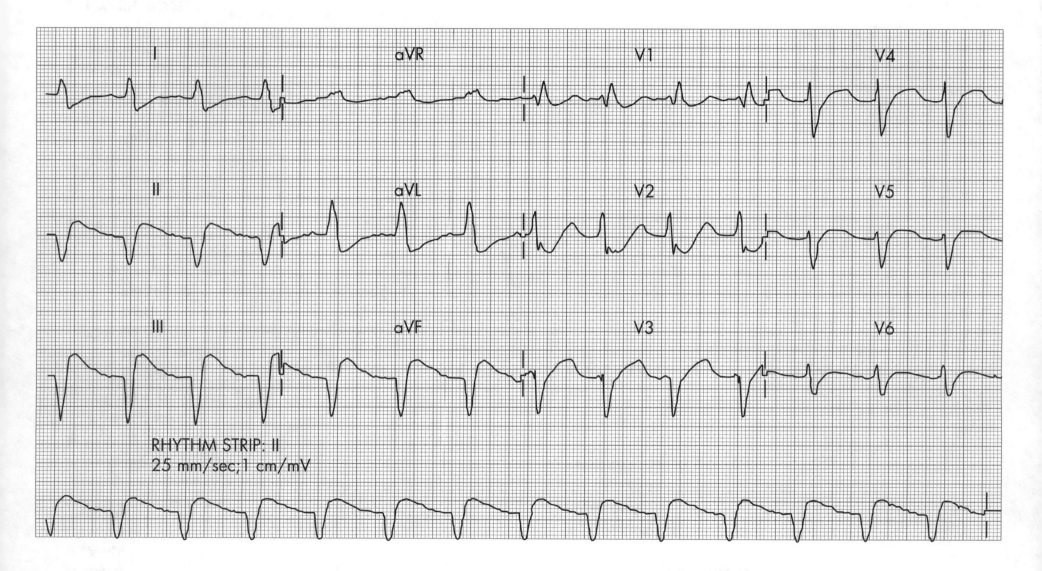

RHYTHM STRIP: II
25 mm/sec;1 cm/mV

Figure 6-16
Resting 12-Lead ECG
352

1. RATE

Atrial:

Ventricular:

2. RHYTHM

Atrial:

Ventricular:

3. WAVES

P waves present:

Appearance:

Consistent:

Relation to QRS:

Q waves present:

Leads:

Pathological:

T waves present:

Morphology:

4. INTERVALS

P-R interval:

Consistent:

QRS:

Appearance:

Consistent:

Q-T interval:

5. AXIS

Quadrant:

Degrees:

6. HYPERTROPHY

Atrial:

Ventricular:

7. MYOCARDIAL INFARCTION

Q waves:

S-T displacement:

8. ISCHEMIA

S-T displacement:

9. POSSIBLE DRUG EFFECTS

10. ECG ANALYSIS

11. INTERPRETATION

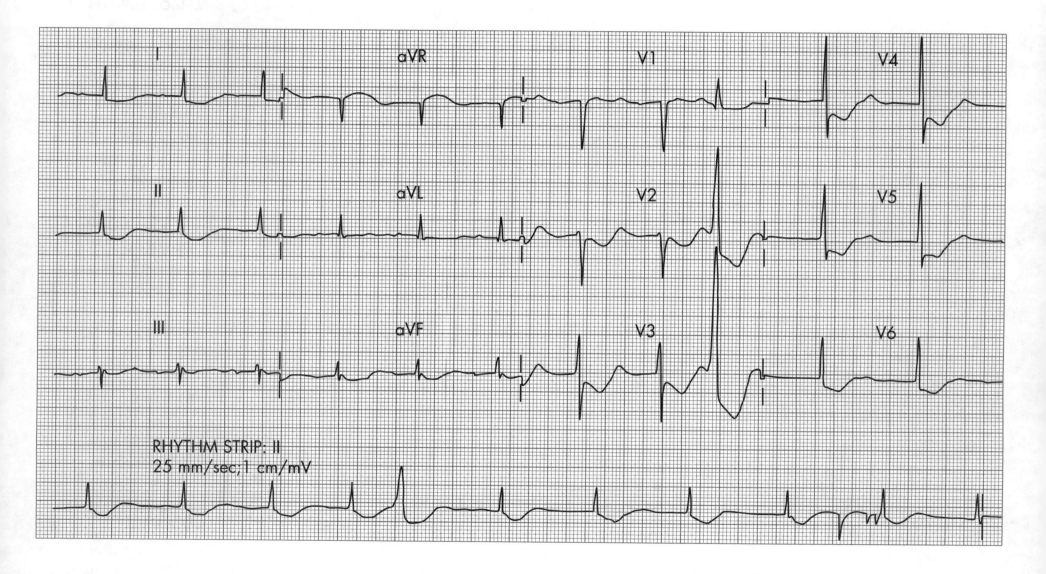

I   aVR   V1   V4

II   aVL   V2   V5

III   aVF   V3   V6

RHYTHM STRIP: II
25 mm/sec; 1 cm/mV

Figure 6-17
Resting 12-Lead ECG
354

1. RATE

Atrial:

Ventricular:

2. RHYTHM

Atrial:

Ventricular:

3. WAVES

P waves present:

Appearance:

Consistent:

Relation to QRS:

Q waves present:

Leads:

Pathological:

T waves present:

Morphology:

4. INTERVALS

P-R interval:

Consistent:

QRS:

Appearance:

Consistent:

Q-T interval:

5. AXIS

Quadrant:

Degrees:

6. HYPERTROPHY

Atrial:

Ventricular:

7. MYOCARDIAL INFARCTION

Q waves:

S-T displacement:

8. ISCHEMIA

S-T displacement:

9. POSSIBLE DRUG EFFECTS

10. ECG ANALYSIS

11. INTERPRETATION

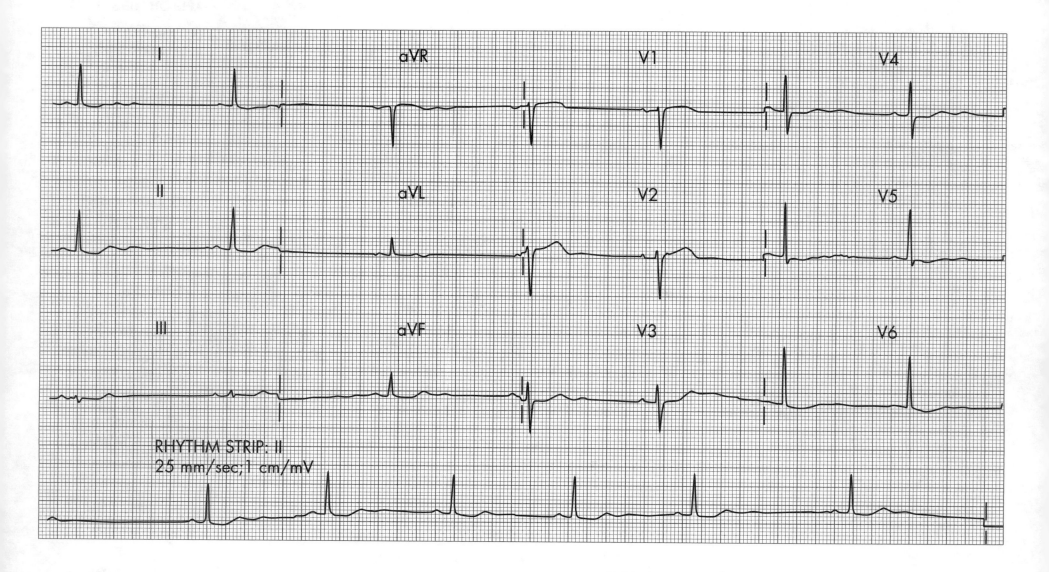

Figure 6-18
Resting 12-Lead ECG
356

1. RATE

    Atrial:

    Ventricular:

2. RHYTHM

    Atrial:

    Ventricular:

3. WAVES

    P waves present:

        Appearance:

        Consistent:

        Relation to QRS:

    Q waves present:

        Leads:

        Pathological:

    T waves present:

        Morphology:

4. INTERVALS

    P-R interval:

        Consistent:

    QRS:

        Appearance:

        Consistent:

    Q-T interval:

5. AXIS

    Quadrant:

    Degrees:

6. HYPERTROPHY

    Atrial:

    Ventricular:

7. MYOCARDIAL INFARCTION

    Q waves:

    S-T displacement:

8. ISCHEMIA

    S-T displacement:

9. POSSIBLE DRUG EFFECTS

10. ECG ANALYSIS

11. INTERPRETATION

Part VII

Analysis

ANALYSIS 2-1

1. RATE
Atrial: 78 bpm

Ventricular: 78 bpm

2. RHYTHM
Atrial: Regular

Ventricular: Regular

3. WAVES
P waves present: Yes

Appearance: Normal

Consistent: Yes

Relation to QRS: 1:1

Q waves present: No

Leads:

Pathological:

T waves present: Yes

Morphology: Normal

4. INTERVALS
P-R interval: 0.16 seconds

Consistent: Yes

QRS: 0.08 seconds

Appearance: Normal

Consistent: Yes

Q-T interval: 0.36 seconds

5. AXIS
Quadrant: Normal

Degrees: +60° (aVL most isoelectric)

6. HYPERTROPHY
Atrial: None

Ventricular: None

7. MYOCARDIAL INFARCTION
Q waves: None significant

S-T displacement: No significant elevation

8. ISCHEMIA
S-T displacement: No significant depression

9. POSSIBLE DRUG EFFECTS
None noted

10. ECG ANALYSIS
All variables are within normal limits (WNL).

11. INTERPRETATION
Normal sinus rhythm

1. RATE

Atrial: 67 bpm

Ventricular: 67 bpm

2. RHYTHM

Atrial: Regular

Ventricular: Regular

3. WAVES

P waves present: Yes

Appearance: Normal

Consistent: Yes

Relation to QRS: 1:1

Q waves present: No

Leads:

Pathological:

T waves present: Yes

Morphology: Normal

4. INTERVALS

P-R interval: 0.16 seconds

Consistent: Yes

QRS: 0.08 seconds

Appearance: Normal

Consistent: Yes

Q-T interval: 0.36 seconds

5. AXIS

Quadrant: Normal

Degrees: +60° (aVL most isoelectric)

6. HYPERTROPHY

Atrial: None

Ventricular: None

7. MYOCARDIAL INFARCTION

Q waves: None significant

S-T displacement: 1 mm diffuse S-T elevation

8. ISCHEMIA

S-T displacement: No significant depression

9. POSSIBLE DRUG EFFECTS

None noted

10. ECG ANALYSIS

The rate is 67 bpm, rhythm is regular, and intervals and axis are WNL. Although there is slight (1 mm) S-T elevation noted throughout, it is not a significant finding. The reason for this elevation may be early repolarization and may be a normal variant.

11. INTERPRETATION

Normal sinus rhythm

1. RATE

Atrial: 67 bpm

Ventricular: 67 bpm

2. RHYTHM

Atrial: Regular

Ventricular: Regular

3. WAVES

P waves present: Yes

Appearance: Normal

Consistent: Yes

Relation to QRS: 1:1

Q waves present: Small

Leads: aVL

Pathological: No

T waves present: Yes

Morphology: Normal

4. INTERVALS

P-R interval: 0.16 seconds

Consistent: Yes

QRS: 0.08 seconds

Appearance: Normal

Consistent: Yes

Q-T interval: 0.40 seconds

5. AXIS

Quadrant: Normal

Degrees: +35° (III most isoelectric, slightly positive)

6. HYPERTROPHY

Atrial: None

Ventricular: None

7. MYOCARDIAL INFARCTION

Q waves: None significant

S-T displacement: No significant elevation

8. ISCHEMIA

S-T displacement: No significant depression

9. POSSIBLE DRUG EFFECTS

None noted

10. ECG ANALYSIS

All variables are WNL.

11. INTERPRETATION

Normal sinus rhythm

I. RATE

Atrial: 67 to 88 bpm

Ventricular: 67 to 88 bpm

2. RHYTHM

Atrial: Regular, variable

Ventricular: Regular, variable

3. WAVES

P waves present: Yes

    Appearance: Normal

    Consistent: Yes

    Relation to QRS: 1:1

Q waves present: Small

    Leads: II, III

    Pathological: No

T waves present: Yes

    Morphology: Flat I, aVL, V_{5-6}

4. INTERVALS

P-R interval: 0.18 seconds

    Consistent: Yes

QRS: 0.08 seconds

    Appearance: Normal

    Consistent: Yes

Q-T interval: 0.36 seconds

5. AXIS

Quadrant: Normal

Degrees: +30° (III most isoelectric)

6. HYPERTROPHY

Atrial: None

Ventricular: None

7. MYOCARDIAL INFARCTION

Q waves: None significant

S-T displacement: No significant elevation

8. ISCHEMIA

S-T displacement: No significant depression

9. POSSIBLE DRUG EFFECTS

None noted

10. ECG ANALYSIS

The rate is from 67 to 88 bpm and the rhythm varies slightly, probably with breathing. Intervals and axis are WNL. Nonspecific T wave flattening is noted in the lateral leads (I, aVL, V_{5-6}) as well as baseline artifact in V_1.

11. INTERPRETATION

Sinus arrhythmia

- Nonspecific lateral T wave changes

ANALYSIS 2-5

1. RATE

Atrial: 84 bpm

Ventricular: 84 bpm

2. RHYTHM

Atrial: Regular

Ventricular: Regular

3. WAVES

P waves present: Yes

   Appearance: Normal

   Consistent: Yes

   Relation to QRS: 1:1

Q waves present: No

   Leads:

   Pathological:

T waves present: Yes

   Morphology: Normal

4. INTERVALS

P-R interval: 0.18 seconds

   Consistent: Yes

QRS: 0.08 seconds

   Appearance: Normal

   Consistent: Yes

Q-T interval: 0.38 seconds

5. AXIS

Quadrant: Normal

Degrees: +75° (I and aVL most isoelectric)

6. HYPERTROPHY

Atrial: None

Ventricular: None

7. MYOCARDIAL INFARCTION

Q waves: None pathological

S-T displacement: No significant elevation

8. ISCHEMIA

S-T displacement: No significant depression

9. POSSIBLE DRUG EFFECTS

None noted

10. ECG ANALYSIS

All variables are WNL.

11. INTERPRETATION

Normal sinus rhythm

1. RATE

Atrial: 58 to 70 bpm

Ventricular: 58 to 70 bpm

2. RHYTHM

Atrial: Regular, variable

Ventricular: Regular, variable

3. WAVES

P waves present: Yes

    Appearance: Normal

    Consistent: Yes

    Relation to QRS: 1:1

Q waves present: No

    Leads:

    Pathological:

T waves present: Yes

    Morphology: Normal

4. INTERVALS

P-R interval: 0.16 seconds

    Consistent: Yes

QRS: 0.08 seconds

    Appearance: Normal

    Consistent: Yes

Q-T interval: 0.36 seconds

5. AXIS

Quadrant: Normal

Degrees: +50° (aVL most isoelectric, slightly positive)

6. HYPERTROPHY

Atrial: None

Ventricular: None

7. MYOCARDIAL INFARCTION

Q waves: None significant

S-T displacement: No significant elevation

8. ISCHEMIA

S-T displacement: No significant depression

9. POSSIBLE DRUG EFFECTS

None noted

10. ECG ANALYSIS

The rate is from 58 to 70 bpm, and the rhythm varies slightly, probably in sequence with breathing. Intervals and axis are WNL.

11. INTERPRETATION

Sinus arrhythmia

1. RATE

Atrial: 93 bpm

Ventricular: 93 bpm

2. RHYTHM

Atrial: Regular

Ventricular: Regular

3. WAVES

P waves present: Yes

Appearance: Normal

Consistent: Yes

Relation to QRS: 1:1

Q waves present: No

Leads:

Pathological:

T waves present: Yes

Morphology: Normal

4. INTERVALS

P-R interval: 0.16 seconds

Consistent: Yes

QRS: 0.08 seconds

Appearance: Normal

Consistent: Yes

Q-T interval: 0.32 seconds

5. AXIS

Quadrant: Normal

Degrees: +45° (III and aVL most isoelectric)

6. HYPERTROPHY

Atrial: None

Ventricular: None

7. MYOCARDIAL INFARCTION

Q waves: None significant

S-T displacement: No significant elevation

8. ISCHEMIA

S-T displacement: No significant depression

9. POSSIBLE DRUG EFFECTS

None noted

10. ECG ANALYSIS

All variables are WNL.

11. INTERPRETATION

Normal sinus rhythm

1. RATE

Atrial: 68 bpm

Ventricular: 68 bpm

2. RHYTHM

Atrial: Regular

Ventricular: Regular

3. WAVES

P waves present: Yes

Appearance: Normal

Consistent: Yes

Relation to QRS: 1:1

Q waves present: No

Leads:

Pathological:

T waves present: Yes

Morphology: Normal

4. INTERVALS

P-R interval: 0.18 seconds

Consistent: Yes

QRS: 0.08 seconds

Appearance: Normal

Consistent: Yes

Q-T interval: 0.40 seconds

5. AXIS

Quadrant: Normal

Degrees: +15° (III and aVF most isoelectric)

6. HYPERTROPHY

Atrial: None

Ventricular: None

7. MYOCARDIAL INFARCTION

Q waves: None significant

S-T displacement: No significant elevation

8. ISCHEMIA

S-T displacement: No significant depression

9. POSSIBLE DRUG EFFECTS

None noted

10. ECG ANALYSIS

All variables are WNL. Baseline artifact is seen in I, II, and III.

11. INTERPRETATION

Normal sinus rhythm

1. RATE

Atrial: 65 to 75 bpm

Ventricular: 65 to 75 bpm

2. RHYTHM

Atrial: Regular, variable

Ventricular: Regular, variable

3. WAVES

P waves present: Yes

    Appearance: Normal

    Consistent: Yes

    Relation to QRS: 1:1

Q waves present: Yes

    Leads: III, aVF

    Pathological: No

T waves present: Yes

    Morphology: Normal

4. INTERVALS

P-R interval: 0.16 seconds

    Consistent: Yes

QRS: 0.08 seconds

    Appearance: Normal

    Consistent: Yes

Q-T interval: 0.38 seconds

5. AXIS

Quadrant: Normal

Degrees: +15° (aVF most isoelectric, slightly positive)

6. HYPERTROPHY

Atrial: None

Ventricular: None

7. MYOCARDIAL INFARCTION

Q waves: None significant

S-T displacement: No significant elevation

8. ISCHEMIA

S-T displacement: No significant depression

9. POSSIBLE DRUG EFFECTS

None noted

10. ECG ANALYSIS

The rate is from 65 to 75 bpm and the rhythm varies slightly, probably with breathing. Intervals and axis are WNL. Q waves noted in III and aVF are a nonpathological finding because they are not one-third the height of the QRS or greater than 1 mm wide.

11. INTERPRETATION

Sinus arrhythmia

1. RATE

Atrial: 70 bpm

Ventricular: 70 bpm

2. RHYTHM

Atrial: Regular

Ventricular: Regular

3. WAVES

P waves present: Yes

    Appearance: Normal

    Consistent: Yes

    Relation to QRS: 1:1

Q waves present: Small Q

    Leads: III

    Pathological: No

T waves present: Yes

    Upright in I, II, V_{3-6}: Yes

4. INTERVALS

P-R interval: 0.16 seconds

    Consistent: Yes

QRS: 0.08 seconds

    Appearance: Normal

    Consistent: Yes

Q-T interval: 0.42 seconds

5. AXIS

Quadrant: Normal

Degrees: +45° (III most isoelectric, slightly positive)

6. HYPERTROPHY

Atrial: None

Ventricular: None

7. MYOCARDIAL INFARCTION

Q waves: None significant

S-T displacement: No significant elevation

8. ISCHEMIA

S-T displacement: No significant depression

9. POSSIBLE DRUG EFFECTS

None noted

10. ECG ANALYSIS

All variables are WNL. It should be noted that the S-T segment and T waves are flat in V_{2-5}, which is a nonspecific finding. Also the T in V_2 is inverted, which can be a normal occurrence.

11. INTERPRETATION

Normal sinus rhythm

- Nonspecific anterior S-T and T wave changes

ANALYSIS 2-11

1. RATE

Atrial: 60 bpm

Ventricular: 60 bpm

2. RHYTHM

Atrial: Regular

Ventricular: Regular

3. WAVES

P waves present: Yes

    Appearance: Normal

    Consistent: Yes

    Relation to QRS: 1:1

Q waves present: Small

    Leads: III, aVF

    Pathological: No

T waves present: Yes

    Morphology: Normal

4. INTERVALS

P-R interval: 0.16 seconds

    Consistent: Yes

QRS: 0.08 seconds

    Appearance: Normal

    Consistent: Yes

Q-T interval: 0.40 seconds

5. AXIS

Quadrant: Normal

Degrees: +30° (III most isoelectric)

6. HYPERTROPHY

Atrial: None

Ventricular: None

7. MYOCARDIAL INFARCTION

Q waves: None significant

S-T displacement: No significant elevation

8. ISCHEMIA

S-T displacement: No significant depression

9. POSSIBLE DRUG EFFECTS

None noted

10. ECG ANALYSIS

All variables are WNL.

11. INTERPRETATION

Normal sinus rhythm

1. RATE

Atrial: 86 bpm

Ventricular: 86 bpm

2. RHYTHM

Atrial: Regular

Ventricular: Regular

3. WAVES

P waves present: Yes

  Appearance: Normal

  Consistent: Yes

  Relation to QRS: 1:1

Q waves present: Yes

  Leads: III

  Pathological: No

T waves present: Yes

  Morphology: Normal

4. INTERVALS

P-R interval: 0.18 seconds

  Consistent: Yes

QRS: 0.08 seconds

  Appearance: Normal

  Consistent: Yes

Q-T interval: 0.38 seconds

5. AXIS

Quadrant: Normal

Degrees: +15° (aVF most isoelectric, slightly positive)

6. HYPERTROPHY

Atrial: None

Ventricular: None

7. MYOCARDIAL INFARCTION

Q waves: None significant

S-T displacement: No significant elevation

8. ISCHEMIA

S-T displacement: No significant depression

9. POSSIBLE DRUG EFFECTS

None noted

10. ECG ANALYSIS

All variables are WNL. The Q wave in III is an isolated finding and is not significant.

11. INTERPRETATION

Normal sinus rhythm

ANALYSIS 2-13

1. RATE

Atrial: 78 to 84 bpm

Ventricular: 78 to 84 bpm

2. RHYTHM

Atrial: Regular, variable

Ventricular: Regular, variable

3. WAVES

P waves present: Yes

    Appearance: Normal

    Consistent: Yes

    Relation to QRS: 1:1

Q waves present: No

    Leads:

    Pathological:

T waves present: Yes

    Morphology: Normal

4. INTERVALS

P-R interval: 0.16 seconds

    Consistent: Yes

QRS: 0.08 seconds

    Appearance: Normal

    Consistent: Yes

Q-T interval: 0.32 seconds

5. AXIS

Quadrant: Normal

Degrees: +60° (aVL most isoelectric)

6. HYPERTROPHY

Atrial: None

Ventricular: None

7. MYOCARDIAL INFARCTION

Q waves: None significant

S-T displacement: No significant elevation

8. ISCHEMIA

S-T displacement: No significant depression

9. POSSIBLE DRUG EFFECTS

None noted

10. ECG ANALYSIS

The rate is 78 to 84 bpm and the rhythm is slightly variable, probably with breathing. Intervals and axis are WNL. The R wave does not progress in amplitude in V_1 through V_2. This finding may indicate an old anterior MI, however, without patient history this is not conclusive. Slight diffuse S-T elevation, which is nonconclusive, is noted.

11. INTERPRETATION

Sinus arrhythmia

- Poor R wave progression

1. RATE

Atrial: 66 bpm

Ventricular: 66 bpm

2. RHYTHM

Atrial: Regular

Ventricular: Regular

3. WAVES

P waves present: Yes

Appearance: Normal

Consistent: Yes

Relation to QRS: 1:1

Q waves present: Yes

Leads: III

Pathological: No

T waves present: Yes

Morphology: Normal

4. INTERVALS

P-R interval: 0.16 seconds

Consistent: Yes

QRS: 0.10 seconds

Appearance: Normal

Consistent: Yes

Q-T interval: 0.38 seconds

5. AXIS

Quadrant: Normal

Degrees: +15° (III and aVF most isoelectric)

6. HYPERTROPHY

Atrial: None

Ventricular: None

7. MYOCARDIAL INFARCTION

Q waves: None significant

S-T displacement: No significant elevation

8. ISCHEMIA

S-T displacement: No significant depression

9. POSSIBLE DRUG EFFECTS

None noted

10. ECG ANALYSIS

All variables are WNL. The Q wave in II is an isolated finding and is not significant.

11. INTERPRETATION

Normal sinus rhythm

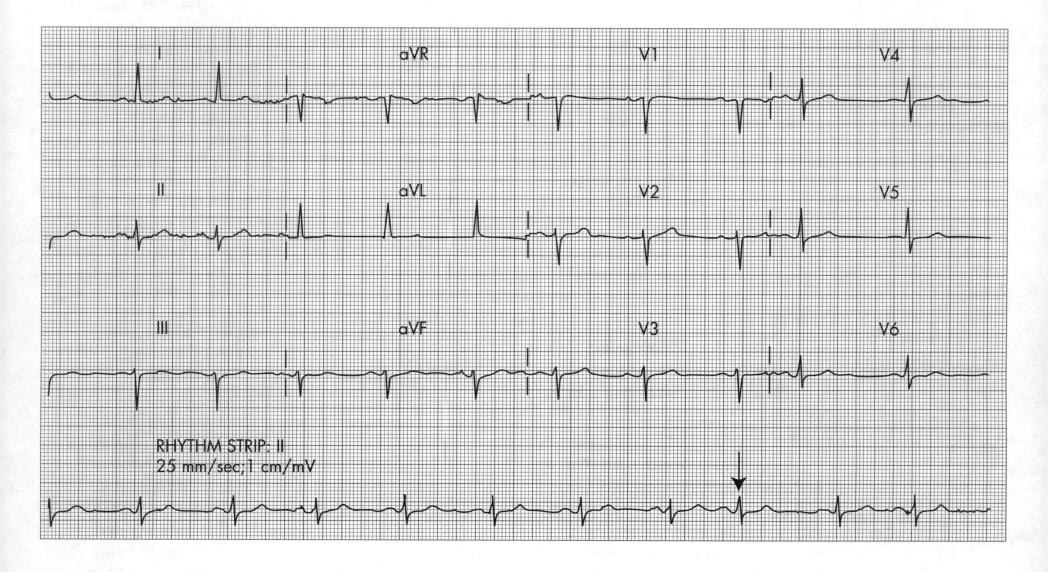

Figure 2-15
Resting 12-Lead ECG
374

1. RATE

Atrial: 56 to 67 bpm

Ventricular: 56 to 67 bpm

2. RHYTHM

Atrial: Regular, rhythmic variation

Ventricular: Regular, rhythmic variation

3. WAVES

P waves present: Yes

    Appearance: Normal

    Consistent: Yes

    Relation to QRS: 1:1

Q waves present: No

    Leads:

    Pathological:

T waves present: Yes

    Morphology: Normal

4. INTERVALS

P-R interval: 0.18 seconds

    Consistent: Yes

QRS: 0.08 seconds

    Appearance: Normal

    Consistent: Yes

Q-T interval: 0.40 seconds

5. AXIS

Quadrant: Left

Degrees: −30° (II most isoelectric)

6. HYPERTROPHY

Atrial: None

Ventricular: None

7. MYOCARDIAL INFARCTION

Q waves: None significant

S-T displacement: No significant elevation

8. ISCHEMIA

S-T displacement: No significant depression

9. POSSIBLE DRUG EFFECTS

None noted

10. ECG ANALYSIS

The rate is 56 to 67 bpm; intervals are WNL. The rhythm is variable but rhythmic and likely timed with respiration. The axis is in the left quadrant. The eighth and tenth beats on the rhythm strip are slightly early, however because they are only slightly early, they are likely timed with respiration.

11. INTERPRETATION

Sinus arrhythmia

    • Left axis deviation

1. RATE

Atrial: 56 bpm

Ventricular: 56 bpm

2. RHYTHM

Atrial: Regular

Ventricular: Regular

3. WAVES

P waves present: Yes

Appearance: Normal

Consistent: Yes

Relation to QRS: 1:1

Q waves present: No

Leads:

Pathological:

T waves present: Yes

Morphology: Normal

4. INTERVALS

P-R interval: 0.18 seconds

Consistent: Yes

QRS: 0.08 seconds

Appearance: Normal

Consistent: Yes

Q-T interval: 0.40 seconds

5. AXIS

Quadrant: Normal

Degrees: +60° (aVL most isoelectric)

6. HYPERTROPHY

Atrial: None

Ventricular: None

7. MYOCARDIAL INFARCTION

Q waves: None significant

S-T displacement: No significant elevation

8. ISCHEMIA

S-T displacement: No significant depression

9. POSSIBLE DRUG EFFECTS

None noted

10. ECG ANALYSIS

All variables are WNL.

11. INTERPRETATION

Normal sinus rhythm

1. RATE

Atrial: 66 bpm

Ventricular: 66 bpm

2. RHYTHM

Atrial: Regular

Ventricular: Regular

3. WAVES

P waves present: Yes

    Appearance: Normal

    Consistent: Yes

    Relation to QRS: 1:1

Q waves present: No

    Leads:

    Pathological:

T waves present: Yes

    Morphology: Normal

4. INTERVALS

P-R interval: 0.14 seconds

    Consistent: Yes

QRS: 0.08 seconds

    Appearance: Normal

    Consistent: 0.08 seconds

Q-T interval: 0.38 seconds

5. AXIS

Quadrant: Normal

Degrees: +90° (I most isoelectric)

6. HYPERTROPHY

Atrial: None

Ventricular: None

7. MYOCARDIAL INFARCTION

Q waves: None significant

S-T displacement: No significant elevation

8. ISCHEMIA

S-T displacement: No significant depression

9. POSSIBLE DRUG EFFECTS

None noted

10. ECG ANALYSIS

All variables are WNL.

11. INTERPRETATION

Normal sinus rhythm

ANALYSIS 2-18

1. RATE
Atrial: 95 bpm

Ventricular: 95 bpm

2. RHYTHM
Atrial: Regular

Ventricular: Regular

3. WAVES
P waves present: Yes

    Appearance: Normal

    Consistent: Yes

    Relation to QRS: 1:1

Q waves present: Yes

    Leads: III

    Pathological: No

T waves present: Yes

    Morphology: Normal

4. INTERVALS
P-R interval: 0.16 seconds

    Consistent: Yes

QRS: 0.06 seconds

    Appearance: Normal

    Consistent: Yes

Q-T interval: 0.36 seconds

5. AXIS
Quadrant: Normal

Degrees: +45° (aVL and III most isoelectric)

6. HYPERTROPHY
Atrial: None noted

Ventricular: None noted

7. MYOCARDIAL INFARCTION
Q waves: None significant

S-T displacement: No significant elevation

8. ISCHEMIA
S-T displacement: No significant depression

9. POSSIBLE DRUG EFFECTS
None noted

10. ECG ANALYSIS
All variables are WNL.

11. INTERPRETATION
Normal sinus rhythm

1. RATE

Atrial: 96 bpm

Ventricular: 96 bpm

2. RHYTHM

Atrial: Regular

Ventricular: Regular

3. WAVES

P waves present: Yes

    Appearance: Normal

    Consistent: Yes

    Relation to QRS: 1:1

Q waves present: Yes

    Leads: III

    Pathological: No

T waves present: Yes

    Morphology: Normal

4. INTERVALS

P-R interval: 0.18 seconds

    Consistent: Yes

QRS: 0.08 seconds

    Appearance: Normal

    Consistent: Yes

Q-T interval: 0.36 seconds

5. AXIS

Quadrant: Normal

Degrees: +45° (III and aVL most isoelectric)

6. HYPERTROPHY

Atrial: None noted

Ventricular: None noted

7. MYOCARDIAL INFARCTION

Q waves: None significant

S-T displacement: No significant elevation

8. ISCHEMIA

S-T displacement: No significant depression

9. POSSIBLE DRUG EFFECTS

None noted

10. ECG ANALYSIS

All variables are WNL.

11. INTERPRETATION

Normal sinus rhythm

1. RATE

Atrial: 68 to 86 bpm

Ventricular: 68 to 86 bpm

2. RHYTHM

Atrial: Regular, variable

Ventricular: Regular, variable

3. WAVES

P waves present: Yes

    Appearance: Normal

    Consistent: Yes

    Relation to QRS: 1:1

Q waves present: Yes

    Leads: III, aVF

    Pathological: No

T waves present: Yes

    Morphology: Normal

4. INTERVALS

P-R interval: 0.16 seconds

    Consistent: Yes

QRS: 0.08 seconds

    Appearance: Normal

    Consistent: Yes

Q-T interval: 0.36 seconds

5. AXIS

Quadrant: Normal

Degrees: +40° (III most isoelectric, slightly positive)

6. HYPERTROPHY

Atrial: None

Ventricular: None

7. MYOCARDIAL INFARCTION

Q waves: None significant

S-T displacement: No significant elevation

8. ISCHEMIA

S-T displacement: No significant depression

9. POSSIBLE DRUG EFFECTS

None noted

10. ECG ANALYSIS

The rate is from 68 to 86 bpm, and the rhythm varies slightly, probably in sequence with breathing. Intervals and axis are WNL. The Q waves in III and aVF are not classified as pathological because they are not one-third the height of the QRS or 1 mm wide.

11. INTERPRETATION

Sinus arrhythmia

1. RATE
Atrial: 70 bpm

Ventricular: 70 bpm

2. RHYTHM
Atrial: Regular

Ventricular: Regular

3. WAVES
P waves present: Yes

    Appearance: Normal

    Consistent: Yes

    Relation to QRS: 1:1

Q waves present: No

    Leads:

    Pathological:

T waves present: Yes

    Morphology: Normal

4. INTERVALS
P-R interval: 0.16 seconds

    Consistent: Yes

QRS: 0.08 seconds

    Appearance: Normal

    Consistent: Yes

Q-T interval: 0.36 seconds

5. AXIS
Quadrant: Normal

Degrees: +45° (aVL and III most isoelectric)

6. HYPERTROPHY
Atrial: None

Ventricular: None

7. MYOCARDIAL INFARCTION
Q waves: None significant

S-T displacement: No significant elevation

8. ISCHEMIA
S-T displacement: No significant depression

9. POSSIBLE DRUG EFFECTS
None noted

10. ECG ANALYSIS
All variables are WNL.

11. INTERPRETATION
Normal sinus rhythm

1. RATE
Atrial: 70 bpm

Ventricular: 70 bpm

2. RHYTHM
Atrial: Regular

Ventricular: Regular

3. WAVES
P waves present: Yes

    Appearance: Normal

    Consistent: Yes

    Relation to QRS: 1:1

Q waves present: Yes

    Leads: aVL

    Pathological: No

T waves present: Yes

    Morphology: Flat

4. INTERVALS
P-R interval: 0.14 seconds

    Consistent: Yes

QRS: 0.08 seconds

    Appearance: Normal

    Consistent: Yes

Q-T interval: 0.40 seconds

5. AXIS
Quadrant: Normal

Degrees: +30° (III most isoelectric)

6. HYPERTROPHY
Atrial: None

Ventricular: None

7. MYOCARDIAL INFARCTION
Q waves: None significant

S-T displacement: No significant elevation

8. ISCHEMIA
S-T displacement: No significant depression

9. POSSIBLE DRUG EFFECTS
None noted

10. ECG ANALYSIS
The rate, rhythm, intervals, and axis are all WNL, however, it should be noted that the T waves in the inferior and low lateral leads are flat. This is of little significance unless the patient has a history of ischemia or if these findings were a change from a previous ECG. The beginning of the QRS in lead II is somewhat "sweeping." This is often called a delta wave and if found in conjunction with a short P-R interval would be indicative of Wolff-Parkinson-White syndrome.

11. INTERPRETATION
Normal sinus rhythm

- Diffuse nonspecific T wave flattening

1. RATE

Atrial: 68 bpm

Ventricular: 68 bpm

2. RHYTHM

Atrial: Regular

Ventricular: Regular

3. WAVES

P waves present: Yes

    Appearance: Normal

    Consistent: Yes

    Relation to QRS: 1:1

Q waves present: Yes

    Leads: III

    Pathological: No

T waves present: Yes

    Morphology: Normal

4. INTERVALS

P-R interval: 0.18 seconds

    Consistent: Yes

QRS: 0.08 seconds

    Appearance: Normal

    Consistent: Yes

Q-T interval: 0.38 seconds

5. AXIS

Quadrant: Normal

Degrees: +45° (III and aVL most isoelectric)

6. HYPERTROPHY

Atrial: None

Ventricular: None

7. MYOCARDIAL INFARCTION

Q waves: None significant

S-T displacement: No significant elevation

8. ISCHEMIA

S-T displacement: No significant depression

9. POSSIBLE DRUG EFFECTS

None noted

10. ECG ANALYSIS

The rate, rhythm, intervals, and axis are all WNL. Nonspecific S-T depression in V_{5-6} should be noted. This finding needs clinical correlation to be significant, therefore patient history is essential. The rhythm strip loses signal toward the end of the strip. It appears that this is a mechanical problem.

11. INTERPRETATION

Normal sinus rhythm

- Nonspecific 1 mm S-T depression V_{5-6}

ANALYSIS 2-24

1. RATE
Atrial: 70 bpm

Ventricular: 70 bpm

2. RHYTHM
Atrial: Regular

Ventricular: Regular

3. WAVES
P waves present: Yes

    Appearance: Normal

    Consistent: Yes

    Relation to QRS: 1:1

Q waves present: No

    Leads:

    Pathological:

T waves present: Yes

    Morphology: Normal

4. INTERVALS
P-R interval: 0.18 seconds

    Consistent: Yes

QRS: 0.08 seconds

    Appearance: Normal

    Consistent: Yes

Q-T interval: 0.40 seconds

5. AXIS
Quadrant: Normal

Degrees: +15° (III, aVF most isoelectric)

6. HYPERTROPHY
Atrial: None

Ventricular: None

7. MYOCARDIAL INFARCTION
Q waves: None significant

S-T displacement: No significant elevation

8. ISCHEMIA
S-T displacement: No significant depression

9. POSSIBLE DRUG EFFECTS
None noted

10. ECG ANALYSIS
All variables are WNL. Artifact is noted in limb leads.

11. INTERPRETATION
Normal sinus rhythm

1. RATE

Atrial: 75 bpm

Ventricular: 75 bpm

2. RHYTHM

Atrial: Regular

Ventricular: Regular

3. WAVES

P waves present: Yes

    Appearance: Normal

    Consistent: Yes

    Relation to QRS: 1:1

Q waves present: No

    Leads:

    Pathological:

T waves present: Yes

    Morphology: Normal

4. INTERVALS

P-R interval: 0.16 seconds

    Consistent: Yes

QRS: 0.06 seconds

    Appearance: Normal

    Consistent: Yes

Q-T interval: 0.36 seconds

5. AXIS

Quadrant: Normal

Degrees: +80° (I most isoelectric, slightly positive)

6. HYPERTROPHY

Atrial: None

Ventricular: None

7. MYOCARDIAL INFARCTION

Q waves: None significant

S-T displacement: No significant elevation

8. ISCHEMIA

S-T displacement: No significant depression

9. POSSIBLE DRUG EFFECTS

None noted

10. ECG ANALYSIS

All variables are WNL.

11. INTERPRETATION

Normal sinus rhythm

1. RATE

Atrial: 98 bpm

Ventricular: 98 bpm

2. RHYTHM

Atrial: Regular

Ventricular: Regular

3. WAVES

P waves present: Yes

    Appearance: Normal

    Consistent: Yes

    Relation to QRS: 1:1

Q waves present: No

    Leads:

    Pathological:

T waves present: Yes

    Morphology: Normal

4. INTERVALS

P-R interval: 0.18 seconds

    Consistent: Yes

QRS: 0.08 seconds

    Appearance: Normal

    Consistent: Yes

Q-T interval: 0.30 seconds

5. AXIS

Quadrant: Normal

Degrees: +85° (I most isoelectric, slightly positive)

6. HYPERTROPHY

Atrial: None

Ventricular: None

7. MYOCARDIAL INFARCTION

Q waves: None significant

S-T displacement: No significant elevation

8. ISCHEMIA

S-T displacement: No significant depression

9. POSSIBLE DRUG EFFECTS

None noted

10. ECG ANALYSIS

All variables are WNL.

11. INTERPRETATION

Normal sinus rhythm

1. RATE

Atrial: 70 bpm

Ventricular: 70 bpm

2. RHYTHM

Atrial: Regular

Ventricular: Regular

3. WAVES

P waves present: Yes

Appearance: Normal

Consistent: Yes

Relation to QRS: 1:1

Q waves present: Yes

Leads: II

Pathological: No

T waves present: Yes

Morphology: Normal

4. INTERVALS

P-R interval: 0.18 seconds

Consistent: Yes

QRS: 0.06 seconds

Appearance: Normal

Consistent: Yes

Q-T interval: 0.40 seconds

5. AXIS

Quadrant: Normal

Degrees: +30° (III most isoelectric)

6. HYPERTROPHY

Atrial: None

Ventricular: None

7. MYOCARDIAL INFARCTION

Q waves: None significant

S-T displacement: No significant elevation

8. ISCHEMIA

S-T displacement: No significant depression

9. POSSIBLE DRUG EFFECTS

None noted

10. ECG ANALYSIS

All variables are WNL.

11. INTERPRETATION

Normal sinus rhythm

ANALYSIS 2-28

I. RATE

Atrial: 80 bpm

Ventricular: 80 bpm

2. RHYTHM

Atrial: Regular

Ventricular: Regular

3. WAVES

P waves present: Yes

   Appearance: Normal

   Consistent: Yes

   Relation to QRS: 1:1

Q waves present: No

   Leads:

   Pathological:

T waves present: Yes

   Morphology: Normal

4. INTERVALS

P-R interval: 0.16 seconds

   Consistent: Yes

QRS: 0.08 seconds

   Appearance: Normal

   Consistent: Yes

Q-T interval: 0.36 seconds

5. AXIS

Quadrant: Normal

Degrees: +0° (aVF most isoelectric)

6. HYPERTROPHY

Atrial: None

Ventricular: None

7. MYOCARDIAL INFARCTION

Q waves: None significant

S-T displacement: No significant elevation

8. ISCHEMIA

S-T displacement: No significant depression

9. POSSIBLE DRUG EFFECTS

None noted

10. ECG ANALYSIS

All variables are WNL.

11. INTERPRETATION

Normal sinus rhythm

I. RATE

Atrial: 60 bpm

Ventricular: 60 bpm

2. RHYTHM

Atrial: Regular

Ventricular: Regular

3. WAVES

P waves present: Yes

    Appearance: Normal

    Consistent: Yes

    Relation to QRS: 1:1

Q waves present: No

    Leads:

    Pathological:

T waves present: Yes

    Morphology: Normal

4. INTERVALS

P-R interval: 0.16 seconds

    Consistent: Yes

QRS: 0.08 seconds

    Appearance: Low voltage limb leads

    Consistent: Yes

Q-T interval: 0.40 seconds

5. AXIS

Quadrant: Normal

Degrees: +60° (aVL most isoelectric)

6. HYPERTROPHY

Atrial: None

Ventricular: None

7. MYOCARDIAL INFARCTION

Q waves: None significant

S-T displacement: No significant elevation

8. ISCHEMIA

S-T displacement: No significant depression

9. POSSIBLE DRUG EFFECTS

None noted

10. ECG ANALYSIS

The rate is 60 bpm, rhythm is regular, and the intervals and axis are WNL. The QRS voltage (amplitude) is low in the limb leads. This, along with a rightward shift of the axis, could be consistent with chronic pulmonary disease. Again, patient history is essential.

11. INTERPRETATION

Normal sinus rhythm

- Low limb lead voltage

1. RATE

Atrial: 80 bpm

Ventricular: 80 bpm

2. RHYTHM

Atrial: Regular

Ventricular: Regular

3. WAVES

P waves present: Yes

Appearance: Normal

Consistent: Yes

Relation to QRS: 1:1

Q waves present: No

Leads:

Pathological:

T waves present: Yes

Morphology: Normal

4. INTERVALS

P-R interval: 0.16 seconds

Consistent: Yes

QRS: 0.08 seconds

Appearance: Normal

Consistent: Yes

Q-T interval: 0.40 seconds

5. AXIS

Quadrant: Normal

Degrees: +15° (III and aVF most isoelectric)

6. HYPERTROPHY

Atrial: None

Ventricular: None

7. MYOCARDIAL INFARCTION

Q waves: None significant

S-T displacement: No significant elevation

8. ISCHEMIA

S-T displacement: No significant depression

9. POSSIBLE DRUG EFFECTS

None noted

10. ECG ANALYSIS

All variables are WNL.

11. INTERPRETATION

Normal sinus rhythm

1. RATE

Atrial: 92 bpm

Ventricular: 92 bpm

2. RHYTHM

Atrial: Regular

Ventricular: Regular

3. WAVES

P waves present: Yes

    Appearance: Normal

    Consistent: Yes

    Relation to QRS: 1:1

Q waves present: Yes

    Leads: II, III, aVF

    Pathological: No

T waves present: Yes

    Morphology: Normal

4. INTERVALS

P-R interval: 0.14 seconds

    Consistent: Yes

QRS: 0.08 seconds

    Appearance: Normal

    Consistent: Yes

Q-T interval: 0.36 seconds

5. AXIS

Quadrant: Right

Degrees: +120° (aVR most isoelectric)

6. HYPERTROPHY

Atrial: None

Ventricular: None

7. MYOCARDIAL INFARCTION

Q waves: Significant III, aVF

S-T displacement: No significant elevation

8. ISCHEMIA

S-T displacement: No significant depression

9. POSSIBLE DRUG EFFECTS

None noted

10. ECG ANALYSIS

The rate is 92 bpm, rhythm is regular, and the intervals are WNL. A right axis deviation is noted (net QRS deflection in lead I is negative, aVF is positive). Q waves in leads III and aVF are significant, however in lead II the Q wave is small and appears insignificant. Therefore one could not rule out an old inferior MI; however clinical correlation is again critical.

11. INTERPRETATION

Normal sinus rhythm

- Right axis deviation
- Cannot rule out old inferior MI

1. RATE

Atrial: 80 bpm

Ventricular: 80 bpm

2. RHYTHM

Atrial: Regular

Ventricular: Regular

3. WAVES

P waves present: Yes

    Appearance: Normal

    Consistent: Yes

    Relation to QRS: 1:1

Q waves present: Yes

    Leads: III

    Pathological: No

T waves present: Yes

    Morphology: Flat V_{4-6}

4. INTERVALS

P-R interval: 0.16 seconds

    Consistent: Yes

QRS: 0.08 seconds

    Appearance: Normal

    Consistent: Yes

Q-T interval: 0.38 seconds

5. AXIS

Quadrant: Left anterior hemiblock

Degrees: $-60°$ (aVF and II negative, aVR most isoelectric)

6. HYPERTROPHY

Atrial: No

Ventricular: No

7. MYOCARDIAL INFARCTION

Q waves: None significant

S-T displacement: No significant elevation

8. ISCHEMIA

S-T displacement: Flat, V_{4-6}

9. POSSIBLE DRUG EFFECTS

None noted

10. ECG ANALYSIS

The rate, rhythm, and intervals are WNL. The net QRS deflections in leads aVF and II are negative, characteristic of a left anterior hemiblock (LAHB). Nonspecific flattening of the S-T segment is noted in V_{4-6}, I, and aVL.

11. INTERPRETATION

Normal sinus rhythm

- Left anterior hemiblock (LAHB)
- Nonspecific lateral S-T changes

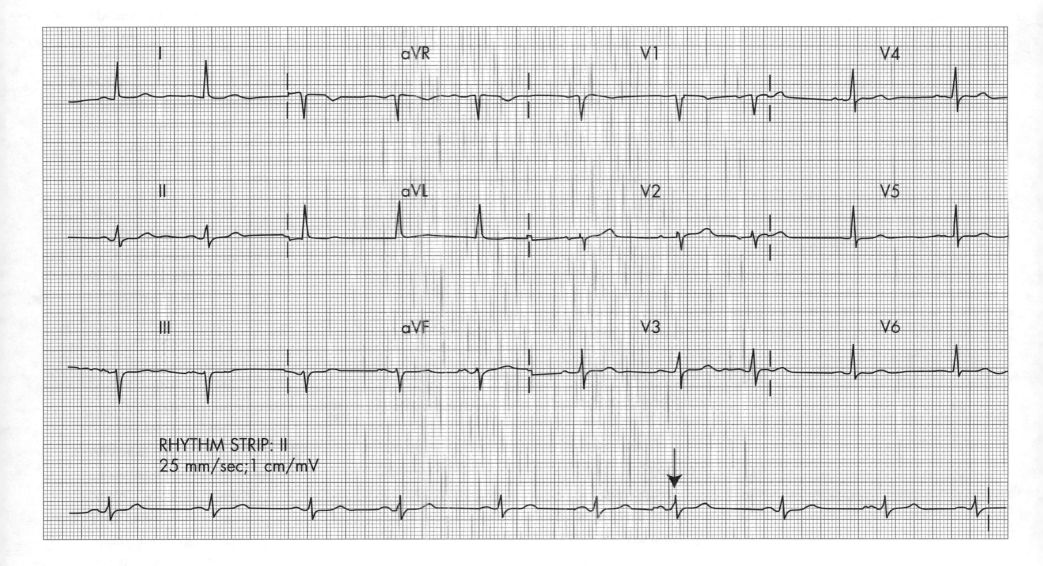

Figure 2-33
Resting 12-Lead ECG

393

1. RATE

Atrial: 55 to 80 bpm

Ventricular: 55 to 80 bpm

2. RHYTHM

Atrial: Rhythmic variation

Ventricular: Rhythmic variation

3. WAVES

P waves present: Yes

    Appearance: greater than or equal to 0.12 seconds in II

    Consistent: Yes

    Relation to QRS: 1:1

Q waves present: No

    Leads:

    Pathological:

T waves present: Yes

    Morphology: Normal

4. INTERVALS

P-R interval: 0.18 seconds

    Consistent: Yes

QRS: 0.08 seconds

    Appearance: Normal

    Consistent: Yes

Q-T interval: 0.40 seconds

5. AXIS

Quadrant: Left

Degrees: −25° (II most isoelectric, slightly positive)

6. HYPERTROPHY

Atrial: Possible

Ventricular: No

7. MYOCARDIAL INFARCTION

Q waves: None significant

S-T displacement: No significant elevation

8. ISCHEMIA

S-T displacement: No significant depression

9. POSSIBLE DRUG EFFECTS

None noted

10. ECG ANALYSIS

The rate varies from 55 to 80 bpm. Note the gradual increase and decrease in the rate that appears cyclic, probably with respiration, a trait of sinus arrhythmia. Intervals are WNL. The axis is in the left quadrant. The P waves in lead II measure 0.12 seconds and in V_1 are slightly biphasic, characteristic of left atrial enlargement. The 7th beat in the rhythm strip is early, has a P wave, and the QRS appears the same as the other beats. This beat is probably atrial in origin.

11. INTERPRETATION

Sinus arrhythmia

- Left axis deviation
- Possible LAE
- Occasional PAC

I. RATE

Atrial: 60 bpm

Ventricular: 60 bpm

2. RHYTHM

Atrial: Regular

Ventricular: Regular

3. WAVES

P waves present: Yes

   Appearance: Normal

   Consistent: Yes

   Relation to QRS: 1:1

Q waves present: No

   Leads:

   Pathological:

T waves present: Yes

   Morphology: Inverted in III and aVF, flat in II, V_{5-6}

4. INTERVALS

P-R interval: 0.18 seconds

   Consistent: Yes

QRS: 0.08 seconds

   Appearance: Normal

   Consistent: Yes

Q-T interval: 0.38 seconds

5. AXIS

Quadrant: Left

Degrees: −10° (aVF most isoelectric, slightly negative)

6. HYPERTROPHY

Atrial: None

Ventricular: None

7. MYOCARDIAL INFARCTION

Q waves: None significant

S-T displacement: No significant elevation

8. ISCHEMIA

S-T displacement: 1 mm S-T depression III and aVF

9. POSSIBLE DRUG EFFECTS

None noted

10. ECG ANALYSIS

The rate, rhythm, and intervals are all WNL. Because the net QRS deflection in lead aVF is negative, the axis lies in the left quadrant. T wave inversion and 1 mm S-T depression is noted in leads III and aVF.

II. INTERPRETATION

Normal sinus rhythm

- Left axis deviation
- Nonspecific inferior S-T and T wave changes

I. RATE

Atrial: 56 bpm

Ventricular: 56 bpm

2. RHYTHM

Atrial: Regular

Ventricular: Regular

3. WAVES

P waves present: Yes

      Appearance: Normal

      Consistent: Yes

      Relation to QRS: I:I

Q waves present: Yes

      Leads: III

      Pathological: No

T waves present: Yes

      Morphology: Normal

4. INTERVALS

P-R interval: 0.16 seconds

      Consistent: Yes

QRS: 0.06 seconds

      Appearance: Normal

      Consistent: Yes

Q-T interval: 0.40 seconds

5. AXIS

Quadrant: Left

Degrees: −5° (aVF most isoelectric, slightly negative)

6. HYPERTROPHY

Atrial: None

Ventricular: None

7. MYOCARDIAL INFARCTION

Q waves: Nonpathological

S-T displacement: No significant elevation

8. ISCHEMIA

S-T displacement: No significant depression

9. POSSIBLE DRUG EFFECTS

None noted

10. ECG ANALYSIS

The rate is less than 60 bpm. Rhythm and intervals are WNL. Slight left axis deviation is denoted by small net negative QRS deflection in lead aVF.

II. INTERPRETATION

Sinus bradycardia

    • Left axis deviation

I. RATE

Atrial: 52 bpm

Ventricular: 52 bpm

2. RHYTHM

Atrial: Regular

Ventricular: Regular

3. WAVES

P waves present: Yes

    Appearance: Normal

    Consistent: Yes

    Relation to QRS: 1:1

Q waves present: No

    Leads:

    Pathological:

T waves present: Yes

    Morphology: Flat, III, aVF

4. INTERVALS

P-R interval: 0.16 seconds

    Consistent: Yes

QRS: 0.08 seconds

    Appearance: Normal

    Consistent: Yes

Q-T interval: 0.42 seconds

5. AXIS

Quadrant: Left

Degrees: −5° (aVF most isoelectric, slightly negative)

6. HYPERTROPHY

Atrial: None

Ventricular: None

7. MYOCARDIAL INFARCTION

Q waves: None significant

S-T displacement: No significant elevation

8. ISCHEMIA

S-T displacement: Flat, III, aVF

9. POSSIBLE DRUG EFFECTS

None noted

10. ECG ANALYSIS

The rate is less than 60 bpm. Rhythm and intervals are WNL. Slight left axis deviation denoted by negative net QRS deflection in aVF. The S-T segments in II, III, and aVF are flat, which are nondiagnostic changes.

11. INTERPRETATION

Sinus bradycardia

- Slight left axis deviation
- Nonspecific inferior S-T changes

1. RATE

Atrial: 60 bpm

Ventricular: 60 bpm

2. RHYTHM

Atrial: Regular

Ventricular: Regular

3. WAVES

P waves present: Yes

    Appearance: Normal

    Consistent: Yes

    Relation to QRS: 1:1

Q waves present: No

    Leads:

    Pathological:

T waves present: Yes

    Morphology: Normal

4. INTERVALS

P-R interval: 0.16 seconds

    Consistent: Yes

QRS: 0.10 seconds

    Appearance: Normal

    Consistent: Yes

Q-T interval: 0.40 seconds

5. AXIS

Quadrant: Left anterior hemiblock

Degrees: $-40°$ (aVF and II negative and most isoelectric)

6. HYPERTROPHY

Atrial: No

Ventricular: No

7. MYOCARDIAL INFARCTION

Q waves: None significant

S-T displacement: No significant elevation

8. ISCHEMIA

S-T displacement: No significant depression

9. POSSIBLE DRUG EFFECTS

None noted

10. ECG ANALYSIS

The rate is 60 bpm, rhythm and intervals are WNL. There is a left anterior hemiblock, characterized by the net negative QRS deflections in leads aVF and II.

11. INTERPRETATION

Sinus bradycardia

    • LAHB

1. RATE

Atrial: 85 bpm

Ventricular: 85 bpm

2. RHYTHM

Atrial: Regular

Ventricular: Regular

3. WAVES

P waves present: Yes

　　Appearance: Normal

　　Consistent: Yes

　　Relation to QRS: 1:1

Q waves present: No

　　Leads:

　　Pathological:

T waves present: Yes

　　Morphology: Normal

4. INTERVALS

P-R interval: 0.12 seconds

　　Consistent: Yes

QRS: 0.08 seconds

　　Appearance: Normal

　　Consistent: Yes

Q-T interval: 0.36 seconds

5. AXIS

Quadrant: Left anterior hemiblock

Degrees: −45° (aVF and II negative, aVR and II most iscelectric)

6. HYPERTROPHY

Atrial: No

Ventricular: No

7. MYOCARDIAL INFARCTION

Q waves: None significant

S-T displacement: No significant elevation

8. ISCHEMIA

S-T displacement: No significant depression

9. POSSIBLE DRUG EFFECTS

None noted

10. ECG ANALYSIS

The rate, rhythm, and intervals are normal. There is a left anterior hemiblock characterized by net negative QRS deflections in leads aVF and II.

11. INTERPRETATION

Sinus rhythm

- LAHB

ANALYSIS 2-39

1. RATE
Atrial: 65 bpm

Ventricular: 65 bpm

2. RHYTHM
Atrial: Regular

Ventricular: Regular

3. WAVES
P waves present: Yes

    Appearance: Normal

    Consistent: Yes

    Relation to QRS: 1:1

Q waves present: Yes

    Leads: III, aVF

    Pathological: No

T waves present: Yes

    Morphology: Flat III, aVF, V_5, V_6

4. INTERVALS
P-R interval: 0.16 seconds

    Consistent: Yes

QRS: 0.08 seconds

    Appearance: Normal

    Consistent: Yes

Q-T interval: 0.40 seconds

5. AXIS
Quadrant: Normal vertical

Degrees: +90° (I most isoelectric)

6. HYPERTROPHY
Atrial: None

Ventricular: None

7. MYOCARDIAL INFARCTION
Q waves: None significant

S-T displacement: No significant elevation

8. ISCHEMIA
S-T displacement: No significant depression

9. POSSIBLE DRUG EFFECTS
None noted

10. ECG ANALYSIS
The rate, rhythm, and intervals are WNL. The axis is normal vertical because lead I is isoelectric. There are nonspecific flat S-T segments in V_{5-6} and T wave inversion in III and aVF.

11. INTERPRETATION
Normal sinus rhythm

    • Nonspecific inferior and low lateral S-T changes

1. RATE

Atrial: 103 bpm

Ventricular: 103 bpm

2. RHYTHM

Atrial: Regular

Ventricular: Regular

3. WAVES

P waves present: Yes

   Appearance: Normal

   Consistent: Yes

   Relation to QRS: 1:1

Q waves present: Yes

   Leads: III

   Pathological: No

T waves present: Yes

   Morphology: Normal

4. INTERVALS

P-R interval: 0.18 seconds

   Consistent: Yes

QRS: 0.08 seconds

   Appearance: Normal

   Consistent: Yes

Q-T interval: 0.32 seconds

5. AXIS

Quadrant: Normal

Degrees: +30° (III most isoelectric)

6. HYPERTROPHY

Atrial: No

Ventricular: No

7. MYOCARDIAL INFARCTION

Q waves: None significant

S-T displacement: No significant elevation

8. ISCHEMIA

S-T displacement: No significant depression

9. POSSIBLE DRUG EFFECTS

None noted

10. ECG ANALYSIS

The rate is 103 bpm. The rhythm, intervals, and axis are WNL. Lead III Q waves are not significant and are an isolated finding.

11. INTERPRETATION

Sinus tachycardia

ANALYSIS 2-41

1. RATE
Atrial: 128 bpm

Ventricular: 128 bpm

2. RHYTHM
Atrial: Regular

Ventricular: Regular

3. WAVES
P waves present: Yes

   Appearance: Normal

   Consistent: Yes

   Relation to QRS: 1:1

Q waves present: Yes

   Leads: III

   Pathological: No

T waves present: Yes

   Morphology: Somewhat fused to Ps

4. INTERVALS
P-R interval: 0.16 seconds

   Consistent: Yes

QRS: 0.08 seconds

   Appearance: Normal

   Consistent: Yes

Q-T interval: 0.32 seconds

5. AXIS
Quadrant: Normal

Degrees: +30° (III most isoelectric)

6. HYPERTROPHY
Atrial: None

Ventricular: None

7. MYOCARDIAL INFARCTION
Q waves: None significant

S-T displacement: No significant elevation

8. ISCHEMIA
S-T displacement: No significant depression

9. POSSIBLE DRUG EFFECTS
None noted

10. ECG ANALYSIS
The rate is 128 bpm. The rhythm, intervals, and axis are WNL. Diffuse nondiagnostic S-T and T wave abnormalities are noted.

11. INTERPRETATION
Sinus tachycardia

- Diffuse nonspecific S-T changes

1. RATE

Atrial: 100 bpm

Ventricular: 100 bpm

2. RHYTHM

Atrial: Regular

Ventricular: Regular

3. WAVES

P waves present: Yes

    Appearance: Normal

    Consistent: Yes

    Relation to QRS: 1:1

Q waves present: Yes

    Leads: III

    Pathological: No

T waves present: Yes

    Morphology: Normal

4. INTERVALS

P-R interval: 0.16 seconds

    Consistent: Yes

QRS: 0.08 seconds

    Appearance: Notched in II

    Consistent: Yes

Q-T interval: 0.32 seconds

5. AXIS

Quadrant: Normal

Degrees: +15° (aVF most isoelectric, slightly positive)

6. HYPERTROPHY

Atrial: None

Ventricular: None

7. MYOCARDIAL INFARCTION

Q waves: None significant

S-T displacement: No significant elevation

8. ISCHEMIA

S-T displacement: No significant depression

9. POSSIBLE DRUG EFFECTS

None noted

10. ECG ANALYSIS

The rate is 100 bpm. Rhythm, intervals, and axis are WNL. Wandering baseline is noted on rhythm strip and in V_6. Frontal leads show low voltage.

11. INTERPRETATION

Sinus tachycardia

ANALYSIS 2-43

1. RATE

Atrial: 108 bpm

Ventricular: 108 bpm

2. RHYTHM

Atrial: Regular

Ventricular: Regular

3. WAVES

P waves present: Yes

    Appearance: Normal

    Consistent: Yes

    Relation to QRS: 1:1

Q waves present: Yes

    Leads: III, aVF

    Pathological: No

T waves present: Yes

    Morphology: Normal

4. INTERVALS

P-R interval: 0.14 seconds

    Consistent: Yes

QRS: 0.10 seconds

    Appearance: Notched, inferior

    Consistent: Yes

Q-T interval: 0.32 seconds

5. AXIS

Quadrant: Normal

Degrees: +50° (aVL most isoelectric, slightly positive)

6. HYPERTROPHY

Atrial: None

Ventricular: None

7. MYOCARDIAL INFARCTION

Q waves: None significant

S-T displacement: No significant elevation

8. ISCHEMIA

S-T displacement: No significant depression

9. POSSIBLE DRUG EFFECTS

None noted

10. ECG ANALYSIS

The rate is 108 bpm. The rhythm, intervals, and axis are WNL. Notched QRS complexes are noted in leads II, III, and aVF, without pathological significance. Baseline artifact is also noted in limb leads.

11. INTERPRETATION

Sinus tachycardia

1. RATE

Atrial: 120 bpm

Ventricular: 120 bpm

2. RHYTHM

Atrial: Regular

Ventricular: Regular

3. WAVES

P waves present: Yes

Appearance: Normal

Consistent: Yes

Relation to QRS: 1:1

Q waves present: No

Leads:

Pathological:

T waves present: Yes

Morphology: Normal

4. INTERVALS

P-R interval: 0.16 seconds

Consistent: Yes

QRS: 0.06 seconds

Appearance: rSR' in V_2

Consistent: Yes

Q-T interval: 0.32 seconds

5. AXIS

Quadrant: Normal

Degrees: +75° (I and aVL most isoelectric)

6. HYPERTROPHY

Atrial: None

Ventricular: None

7. MYOCARDIAL INFARCTION

Q waves: None significant

S-T displacement: No significant elevation

8. ISCHEMIA

S-T displacement: No significant depression

9. POSSIBLE DRUG EFFECTS

None noted

10. ECG ANALYSIS

The rate is 120 bpm. The rhythm, intervals, and axis are WNL. Limb lead artifact is noted.

11. INTERPRETATION

Sinus tachycardia

- Limb lead artifact

1. RATE

Atrial: 130 bpm

Ventricular: 130 bpm

2. RHYTHM

Atrial: Regular

Ventricular: Regular

3. WAVES

P waves present: Yes

Appearance: Fused with T

Consistent: Yes

Relation to QRS: 1:1

Q waves present: Yes

Leads: III

Pathological: No

T waves present: Yes

Morphology: Fused with P

4. INTERVALS

P-R interval: 0.16 seconds

Consistent: Yes

QRS: 0.06 seconds

Appearance: Normal

Consistent: Yes

Q-T interval: 0.28 seconds

5. AXIS

Quadrant: Normal

Degrees: +30° (III most isoelectric)

6. HYPERTROPHY

Atrial: None

Ventricular: None

7. MYOCARDIAL INFARCTION

Q waves: None significant

S-T displacement: No significant elevation

8. ISCHEMIA

S-T displacement: Diffuse 1 mm S-T depression

9. POSSIBLE DRUG EFFECTS

None noted

10. ECG ANALYSIS

The rate is 130 bpm. Rhythm, intervals, and axis are WNL. Diffuse nondiagnostic S-T segment depression of 1 mm is noted.

11. INTERPRETATION

Sinus tachycardia

- Diffuse nondiagnostic S-T depression

1. RATE

Atrial: 50 bpm

Ventricular: 50 bpm

2. RHYTHM

Atrial: Regular

Ventricular: Regular

3. WAVES

P waves present: Yes

    Appearance: Flat

    Consistent: Yes

    Relation to QRS: 1:1

Q waves present: No

    Leads:

    Pathological:

T waves present: Yes

    Morphology: Flat, inferior

4. INTERVALS

P-R interval: 0.16 seconds

    Consistent: Yes

QRS: 0.08 seconds

    Appearance: Normal

    Consistent: Yes

Q-T interval: 0.46 seconds

5. AXIS

Quadrant: Normal

Degrees: +30° (III most isoelectric)

6. HYPERTROPHY

Atrial: None

Ventricular: None

7. MYOCARDIAL INFARCTION

Q waves: None significant

S-T displacement: No significant elevation

8. ISCHEMIA

S-T displacement: No significant depression

9. POSSIBLE DRUG EFFECTS

None noted

10. ECG ANALYSIS

The rate is 50 bpm. The rhythm, intervals, and axis are WNL. S-T flattening and T wave inversion are noted in leads III and aVF.

11. INTERPRETATION

Sinus bradycardia

- Nondiagnostic inferior T wave changes

I. RATE

Atrial: 52 bpm

Ventricular: 52 bpm

2. RHYTHM

Atrial: Regular

Ventricular: Regular

3. WAVES

P waves present: Yes

Appearance: Normal

Consistent: Yes

Relation to QRS: 1:1

Q waves present: Yes

Leads: III

Pathological: No

T waves present: Yes

Morphology: Flat V_{1-4}, slightly inverted V_{3-4}

4. INTERVALS

P-R interval: 0.16 seconds

Consistent: Yes

QRS: 0.08 seconds

Appearance: Low voltage

Consistent: Yes

Q-T interval: 0.50 seconds

5. AXIS

Quadrant: Left anterior hemiblock

Degrees: −60° (aVF and II negative, aVR most isoelectric)

6. HYPERTROPHY

Atrial: None

Ventricular: None

7. MYOCARDIAL INFARCTION

Q waves: None significant

S-T displacement: No significant elevation

8. ISCHEMIA

S-T displacement: No significant depression

9. POSSIBLE DRUG EFFECTS

None noted

10. ECG ANALYSIS

The rate is 52 bpm. The rhythm and intervals are WNL. Net QRS deflections in leads aVF and II are negative, characteristic of LAHB. There is an artifact on the rhythm strip. Poor R wave progression in V_{1-3} is characteristic of a possible old anteroseptal MI.

II. INTERPRETATION

Sinus bradycardia

- LAHB
- Cannot rule out old anteroseptal MI
- Low voltage frontal leads

1. RATE

Atrial: 54 bpm

Ventricular: 54 bpm

2. RHYTHM

Atrial: Regular

Ventricular: Regular

3. WAVES

P waves present: Yes

    Appearance: Normal

    Consistent: Yes

    Relation to QRS: 1:1

Q waves present: Yes

    Leads: II, III, aVF

    Pathological: No

T waves present: Yes

    Morphology: Normal

4. INTERVALS

P-R interval: 0.16 seconds

    Consistent: Yes

QRS: 0.08 seconds

    Appearance: Normal

    Consistent: Yes

Q-T interval: 0.40 seconds

5. AXIS

Quadrant: Normal

Degrees: +75° (aVL, I most isoelectric)

6. HYPERTROPHY

Atrial: None

Ventricular: None

7. MYOCARDIAL INFARCTION

Q waves: None significant

S-T displacement: No significant elevation

8. ISCHEMIA

S-T displacement: No significant depression

9. POSSIBLE DRUG EFFECTS

None noted

10. ECG ANALYSIS

The rate is 54 bpm. The rhythm, intervals, and axis all are WNL.

11. INTERPRETATION

Sinus bradycardia

I. RATE

Atrial: 60 to 90 bpm

Ventricular: 60 to 90 bpm

2. RHYTHM

Atrial: Variable

Ventricular: Variable

3. WAVES

P waves present: Yes

 Appearance: Normal

 Consistent: Yes

 Relation to QRS: 1:1

Q waves present: No

 Leads: II, aVF

 Pathological: No

T waves present: Yes

 Morphology: Flat, inverted III, V_{3-4}

4. INTERVALS

P-R interval: 0.18 seconds

 Consistent: Yes

QRS: 0.08 seconds

 Appearance: Normal

 Consistent: Yes

Q-T interval: 0.40 seconds

5. AXIS

Quadrant: Normal

Degrees: +45° (aVL, III most isoelectric)

6. HYPERTROPHY

Atrial: None

Ventricular: None

7. MYOCARDIAL INFARCTION

Q waves: None significant

S-T displacement: No significant elevation

8. ISCHEMIA

S-T displacement: Diffuse flattening

9. POSSIBLE DRUG EFFECTS

None noted

10. ECG ANALYSIS

The rate varies from 60 to 90 bpm. The rhythm is variable and appears cyclic, probably with respiration, a characteristic of sinus arrhythmia. Intervals and axis are WNL. Nondiagnostic diffuse S-T flattening is noted along with T wave inversion in III and V_{3-4}.

11. INTERPRETATION

Sinus arrhythmia

 • Diffuse nondiagnostic S-T and T wave changes

1. RATE
Atrial: 70 to 90 bpm

Ventricular: 70 to 90 bpm

2. RHYTHM
Atrial: Variable

Ventricular: Variable

3. WAVES
P waves present: Yes

   Appearance: Normal

   Consistent: Yes

   Relation to QRS: 1:1

Q waves present: No

   Leads:

   Pathological:

T waves present: Yes

   Morphology: Normal

4. INTERVALS
P-R interval: 0.16 seconds

   Consistent: Yes

QRS: 0.08 seconds

   Appearance: Normal

   Consistent: Yes

Q-T interval: 0.40 seconds

5. AXIS
Quadrant: Normal

Degrees: +25° (III most isoelectric, slightly negative)

6. HYPERTROPHY
Atrial: None

Ventricular: None

7. MYOCARDIAL INFARCTION
Q waves: None significant

S-T displacement: No significant elevation

8. ISCHEMIA
S-T displacement: No significant depression

9. POSSIBLE DRUG EFFECTS
None noted

10. ECG ANALYSIS
The rate varies from 70 to 90 bpm. The rhythm is variable and appears cyclic, probably with respiration, a characteristic of sinus arrhythmia. Intervals and axis are WNL.

11. INTERPRETATION
Sinus arrhythmia

1. RATE

Atrial: 50 to 90 bpm

Ventricular: 50 to 90 bpm

2. RHYTHM

Atrial: Variable

Ventricular: Variable

3. WAVES

P waves present: Yes

   Appearance: Normal

   Consistent: Yes

   Relation to QRS: 1:1

Q waves present: Yes

   Leads: II, III, aVF

   Pathological: No

T waves present: Yes

   Morphology: Normal

4. INTERVALS

P-R interval: 0.16 seconds

   Consistent: Yes

QRS: 0.08 seconds

   Appearance: Normal

   Consistent: Yes

Q-T interval: 0.38 seconds

5. AXIS

Quadrant: Normal

Degrees: +90° (I isoelectric)

6. HYPERTROPHY

Atrial: None

Ventricular: None

7. MYOCARDIAL INFARCTION

Q waves: None significant

S-T displacement: No significant elevation

8. ISCHEMIA

S-T displacement: No significant depression

9. POSSIBLE DRUG EFFECTS

None noted

10. ECG ANALYSIS

The rate varies from 50 to 90 bpm. The rhythm is variable and appears cyclic, probably with respiration, a characteristic of sinus arrhythmia. Intervals and axis are WNL.

11. INTERPRETATION

Sinus arrhythmia

1. RATE

Atrial: 50 to 75 bpm

Ventricular: 50 to 75 bpm

2. RHYTHM

Atrial: Variable

Ventricular: Variable

3. WAVES

P waves present: Yes

   Appearance: Normal

   Consistent: Yes

   Relation to QRS: 1:1

Q waves present: No

   Leads:

   Pathological:

T waves present: Yes

   Morphology: Inverted in III

4. INTERVALS

P-R interval: 0.14 seconds

   Consistent: Yes

QRS: 0.10 seconds

   Appearance: Normal

   Consistent: Yes

Q-T interval: 0.36 seconds

5. AXIS

Quadrant: Normal

Degrees: 0° (aVF isoelectric)

6. HYPERTROPHY

Atrial: None

Ventricular: None

7. MYOCARDIAL INFARCTION

Q waves: None significant

S-T displacement: No significant elevation

8. ISCHEMIA

S-T displacement: No significant depression

9. POSSIBLE DRUG EFFECTS

None noted

10. ECG ANALYSIS

The rate varies from 50 to 75 bpm. The rhythm is variable and appears cyclic, probably with respiration, a characteristic of sinus arrhythmia. Intervals and axis are WNL.

11. INTERPRETATION

Sinus arrhythmia

ANALYSIS 3-1

1. RATE

Atrial: 74 bpm

Ventricular: 74 bpm

2. RHYTHM

Atrial: Underlying rhythm, regular

Ventricular: Underlying rhythm, regular

3. WAVES

P waves present: Yes

    Appearance: Normal

    Consistent: Yes

    Relation to QRS: 1:1

Q waves present: Yes

    Leads: III, V_{1-2}

    Pathological: No

T waves present: Yes

    Morphology: Inverted III, Flat II, aVF

4. INTERVALS

P-R interval: 0.14 seconds

    Consistent: Yes

QRS: 0.08 seconds

    Appearance: Normal, except beats 3 and 4 in augmented leads

    Consistent: No

Q-T interval: 0.40 seconds

5. AXIS

Quadrant: Left anterior hemiblock

Degrees: −40° (aVF and II negative, II slightly more negative)

6. HYPERTROPHY

Atrial: None

Ventricular: None

7. MYOCARDIAL INFARCTION

Q waves: Possible

S-T displacement: No significant elevation

8. ISCHEMIA

S-T displacement: No significant depression

9. POSSIBLE DRUG EFFECTS

None noted

10. ECG ANALYSIS

The rate and intervals are within normal limits (WNL). Rhythm is interrupted by early beats in augmented leads, otherwise regular. LAHB is denoted by a positive net QRS deflection in I, negative in aVF and II. The third beat in the augmented leads appears junctional because it is the same deflection as the normal QRS and is not wide. The fourth beat appears ventricular because it is wide (greater than or equal to 0.12 seconds) and the deflection is opposite to that of the normal beat. Note the T waves in II, III, and aVF are somewhat flat, which is a nondiagnostic finding. Poor R wave progression is observed in V_{1-3}.

11. INTERPRETATION

Normal sinus rhythm

- LAHB
- Occasional PJC and PVC
- Nonspecific T wave flattening in II, III, and aVF
- Poor R wave progression in V_{1-3}, cannot rule out old anteroseptal MI

1. RATE

Atrial: 170 bpm

Ventricular: 170 bpm

2. RHYTHM

Atrial: Regular

Ventricular: Regular

3. WAVES

P waves present: Not identifiable

    Appearance: Fused with T

    Consistent:

    Relation to QRS:

Q waves present: No

    Leads:

    Pathological:

T waves present: Yes

    Morphology: Inverted, III, aVF

4. INTERVALS

P-R interval:

    Consistent:

QRS: 0.10 seconds

    Appearance: Normal

    Consistent: Yes

Q-T interval: 0.28 seconds

5. AXIS

Quadrant: Normal

Degrees: +75° (aVL, I most isoelectric)

6. HYPERTROPHY

Atrial: No

Ventricular: No

7. MYOCARDIAL INFARCTION

Q waves: None significant

S-T displacement: 2 to 3 mm S-T elevation in aVR only

8. ISCHEMIA

S-T displacement: Diffuse 1 to 2 mm S-T depression

9. POSSIBLE DRUG EFFECTS

None noted

10. ECG ANALYSIS

The rate is 170 bpm, the rhythm is regular, and the axis is WNL. There are no identifiable P waves, however because the QRS is less than 0.12 seconds; the rhythm is supraventricular. T wave inversion is noted in III and aVF, along with diffuse J point and S-T depression.

11. INTERPRETATION

Supraventricular tachycardia

- Diffuse nonspecific S-T and T wave changes

ANALYSIS 3-3

1. RATE
Atrial: 58 bpm

Ventricular: 58 bpm

2. RHYTHM
Atrial: Underlying rhythm, regular

Ventricular: Underlying rhythm, regular

3. WAVES
P waves present: Yes

    Appearance: Normal

    Consistent: Yes

    Relation to QRS: 1:1

Q waves present: Yes

    Leads: II, III, aVF

    Pathological: Possible

T waves present: Yes

    Morphology: Inverted, I and aVL

4. INTERVALS
P-R interval: 0.16 seconds

    Consistent: Yes

QRS: 0.08 seconds

    Appearance: Normal except second beat in I to III,
        and second in V_{4-6}

    Consistent: Yes

Q-T interval: 0.50 seconds

5. AXIS
Quadrant: Normal

Degrees: +40° (aVL, most isoelectric, slightly positive)

6. HYPERTROPHY
Atrial: None

Ventricular: None

7. MYOCARDIAL INFARCTION
Q waves: II, III, aVF

S-T displacement: No significant elevation

8. ISCHEMIA
S-T displacement: Flat S-T in I and aVL, slightly depressed in V_{4-6}

9. POSSIBLE DRUG EFFECTS
None noted

10. ECG ANALYSIS
The rate is 58 bpm, the rhythm is essentially regular, and the intervals and axis are WNL. The second beat in leads I to III is wide and the initial deflection is opposite to that of the normal beat, therefore, it likely originates in the ventricles. The second beat in V_{4-6} could originate in the junction (because the initial deflection is the same as the normal beat) or ventricles (because it is greater than 0.10 seconds in duration). The rhythm strip shows two PVCs from the same focci. Q waves are noted in II, III, aVF. These Q waves are slightly less than 0.04 seconds in duration and are not one-third the amplitude of the QRS, thus the significance is questionable. T wave inversion is noted in leads I and aVL, as well as nondiagnostic S-T depression in V_{4-6}.

11. INTERPRETATION
Sinus bradycardia

- Occasional PVCs
- Nondiagnostic anterolateral S-T and T wave changes
- Cannot rule out old inferior MI

1. RATE

Atrial: 45 bpm

Ventricular: 45 bpm

2. RHYTHM

Atrial:

Ventricular: Regular

3. WAVES

P waves present: Yes

    Appearance: Follow QRS

    Consistent: Yes

    Relation to QRS: Follow QRS

Q waves present: Yes

    Leads: II, III, aVF

    Pathological: No

T waves present: Yes

    Morphology: Normal

4. INTERVALS

P-R interval:

    Consistent:

QRS: 0.08 seconds

    Appearance: Normal

    Consistent: Yes

Q-T interval: 0.46 seconds

5. AXIS

Quadrant: Normal

Degrees: +70° (aVL, most isoelectric, slightly negative)

6. HYPERTROPHY

Atrial: None

Ventricular: None

7. MYOCARDIAL INFARCTION

Q waves: None significant

S-T displacement: No significant elevation

8. ISCHEMIA

S-T displacement: I mm S-T depression, I, aVL, V_{5-6}

9. POSSIBLE DRUG EFFECTS

None noted

10. ECG ANALYSIS

The rate is 45 bpm, rhythm is regular, and axis is WNL. The P waves follow the QRS complexes, thus the rhythm is not initiated in the sinus node. The QRS complex, however, is of normal duration, therefore the rhythm is junctional. The S-T segment is slightly displaced in I, aVL, and V_{1-6}. The retrograde P waves skew the configuration of the S-T segment.

11. INTERPRETATION

Junctional rhythm

    • Nonspecific anterolateral S-T changes

I. RATE

Atrial: Unable to identify

Ventricular: 70 bpm

2. RHYTHM

Atrial: Unable to identify

Ventricular: Regular

3. WAVES

P waves present: Seen occasionally throughout

Appearance: Abnormal

Consistent: No

Relation to QRS: None

Q waves present: Yes

Leads: I, aVL

Pathological: Yes

T waves present: Yes

Morphology: Deeply inverted

4. INTERVALS

P-R interval:

Consistent:

QRS: 0.16 seconds

Appearance: Wide

Consistent: Yes

Q-T interval: 0.42 seconds

5. AXIS

Quadrant: Right

Degrees: +100° (I, most isoelectric, slightly negative)

6. HYPERTROPHY

Atrial: None

Ventricular: Possible

7. MYOCARDIAL INFARCTION

Q waves: I, aVL

S-T displacement: No significant elevation

8. ISCHEMIA

S-T displacement: Diffuse S-T depression

9. POSSIBLE DRUG EFFECTS

None noted

10. ECG ANALYSIS

The rate is 70 bpm, regular, with a right axis deviation. P waves can be seen randomly throughout, however the rhythm is not initiated by those P waves. The QRS is wide indicating an intraventricular conduction delay (IVCD). The pattern does not strictly adhere to the left bundle branch block criteria (i.e., the usual LAD and wide QRS in V_{5-6} only), therefore it is less precisely termed an IVCD. Because the QRS is wide, one might think that the rhythm is ventricular, however the rate indicates an accelerated junctional rhythm with an IVCD. Diffuse S-T and T wave abnormalities should also be noted.

II. INTERPRETATION

Accelerated junctional rhythm

- RAD
- Intraventricular conduction delay (IVCD)
- Diffuse S-T and T wave abnormalities

1. RATE

Atrial: 55 bpm

Ventricular: 55 bpm

2. RHYTHM

Atrial: Slightly variable

Ventricular: Slightly variable

3. WAVES

P waves present: Yes

    Appearance: Normal

    Consistent: Yes

    Relation to QRS: 1:1

Q waves present: No

    Leads:

    Pathological:

T waves present: Yes

    Morphology: Normal

4. INTERVALS

P-R interval: 0.16 seconds

    Consistent: Yes

QRS: 0.12 seconds

    Appearance: rSR' in V_{1-2}

    Consistent: Yes

Q-T interval: 0.50 seconds

5. AXIS

Quadrant: Normal

Degrees: +90° (I most isoelectric)

6. HYPERTROPHY

Atrial: None

Ventricular: None

7. MYOCARDIAL INFARCTION

Q waves: No

S-T displacement: No

8. ISCHEMIA

S-T displacement: No

9. POSSIBLE DRUG EFFECTS

None noted

10. ECG ANALYSIS

The rate is 55 bpm, rhythm is regular, and the axis is WNL. The QRS complexes in V_{1-2} are an rSR' configuration with a duration of 0.12 seconds. These are classic characteristics of a right bundle branch block. Additionally, the Q-T interval is slightly prolonged for the rate. Information about the patient's history and medications is needed for analysis.

11. INTERPRETATION

Sinus bradycardia

- Right bundle branch block
- Q-T interval slightly long for rate

1. RATE

Atrial: 100 bpm

Ventricular: 100 bpm

2. RHYTHM

Atrial: Underlying rhythm, regular

Ventricular: Underlying rhythm, regular

3. WAVES

P waves present: Yes

Appearance: Flat in II, biphasic in V_1

Consistent: Yes

Relation to QRS: 1:1

Q waves present: No

Leads:

Pathological:

T waves present: Yes

Morphology: Flat

4. INTERVALS

P-R interval: 0.16 seconds

Consistent: Yes

QRS: 0.10 seconds

Appearance: Normal except beat 4 in augmented leads and beat 2 in V_{4-6}. Increased chest lead voltage

Consistent: No

Q-T interval: 0.40 seconds

5. AXIS

Quadrant: Normal

Degrees: +60° (aVL most isoelectric)

6. HYPERTROPHY

Atrial: Possible

Ventricular: Yes

7. MYOCARDIAL INFARCTION

Q waves: None significant

S-T displacement: 1 mm S-T elevation V_{1-2}

8. ISCHEMIA

S-T displacement: 2 mm S-T depression, II, aVF, V_{4-6}

9. POSSIBLE DRUG EFFECTS

None noted

10. ECG ANALYSIS

The rate is 100 bpm, underlying rhythm is regular, and axis and intervals are WNL. Beat 4 in augmented leads and beat 2 in V_{4-6} are early, wide, and have T waves with opposite deflection from normal Ts, therefore they are likely ventricular in origin. The sum of the S in V_1 and the R in V_5 is greater than 35 mm denoting LVH. The P waves in II are flat and 0.10 seconds in duration. In V_1 the P waves are biphasic with a prominent negative portion. Both findings are characteristics of left atrial enlargement (LAE). Diffuse nondiagnostic S-T and T wave abnormalities are also present.

11. INTERPRETATION

Sinus tachycardia

- Multiple PVCs
- LVH with strain pattern
- Possible LAE
- Diffuse nonspecific S-T and T wave changes

1. **RATE**

   Atrial: 82 to 90 bpm

   Ventricular: 82 to 90 bpm

2. **RHYTHM**

   Atrial: Regular, variable

   Ventricular: Regular, variable

3. **WAVES**

   P waves present: Yes

       Appearance: Normal

       Consistent: Yes

       Relation to QRS: 1:1

   Q waves present: No

       Leads:

       Pathological:

   T waves present: Yes

       Morphology: Normal

4. **INTERVALS**

   P-R interval: 0.18 seconds

       Consistent: Yes

   QRS: 0.08 seconds

       Appearance: Low limb lead voltage, otherwise normal except

           beat 2 in I to III

       Consistent: Yes

   Q-T interval: 0.34 seconds

5. **AXIS**

   Quadrant: Normal vertical

   Degrees: +90° (I most isoelectric)

6. **HYPERTROPHY**

   Atrial: No

   Ventricular: No

7. **MYOCARDIAL INFARCTION**

   Q waves: None significant

   S-T displacement: No significant elevation

8. **ISCHEMIA**

   S-T displacement: No significant depression

9. **POSSIBLE DRUG EFFECTS**

   None noted

10. **ECG ANALYSIS**

    The rate is 82 to 90 bpm and varies slightly, probably with respiration. The intervals and axis are WNL. The early beat in leads I to III is wide (0.10 seconds), but the T wave deflection is the same as the normal beat, therefore it is most likely junctional in origin (PJC). The second beat in V$_{1-3}$ is early and has the same morphology as the normal beat, therefore is likely atrial in origin (PAC). The QRS voltage in the limb leads is low. That combined with a vertical axis is consistent with a chronic pulmonary disease pattern.

11. **INTERPRETATION**

    Sinus arrhythmia

    • Possible chronic pulmonary pattern

    • PJC and PAC

ANALYSIS 3-9

1. RATE

Atrial: 68 bpm

Ventricular: 68 bpm

2. RHYTHM

Atrial: Regular

Ventricular: Regular

3. WAVES

P waves present: Yes

    Appearance: Normal

    Consistent: Yes

    Relation to QRS: 1:1

Q waves present: No

    Leads:

    Pathological:

T waves present: Yes

    Morphology: Flat III, aVF

4. INTERVALS

P-R interval: 0.16 seconds

    Consistent: Yes

QRS: 0.12 seconds

    Appearance: rSR' in V_{1-2}, low voltage in limb leads

    Consistent: Yes

Q-T interval: 0.40 seconds

5. AXIS

Quadrant: Normal vertical

Degrees: +90° (I most isoelectric)

6. HYPERTROPHY

Atrial: No

Ventricular: Possible

7. MYOCARDIAL INFARCTION

Q waves: None significant

S-T displacement: No significant elevation

8. ISCHEMIA

S-T displacement: No significant depression

9. POSSIBLE DRUG EFFECTS

None noted

10. ECG ANALYSIS

The rate is 68, rhythm is regular, and the intervals and axis are WNL. The rSR' in V_{1-2} is a classic indication of a right bundle branch block. Because the R in V_1 has increased voltage and large S waves are noted in V_{1-6}, there is a probability of RVH. Added to that probability is the observed low voltage in the limb leads that indicates a possible chronic pulmonary disease pattern.

11. INTERPRETATION

Sinus rhythm

- RBBB
- Probable RVH and chronic pulmonary disease pattern

1. RATE

Atrial: 92 bpm

Ventricular: 92 bpm

2. RHYTHM

Atrial: Irregular

Ventricular: Irregular

3. WAVES

P waves present: Yes

    Appearance: Flat in II, biphasic in V_1

    Consistent: Yes

    Relation to QRS: 1:1 in normal beats

Q waves present: No

    Leads:

    Pathological:

T waves present: Yes

    Morphology: Normal

4. INTERVALS

P-R interval: 0.18 seconds

    Consistent: Yes

QRS: 0.10 seconds

    Appearance: Normal

    Consistent: Yes, in normal beats

Q-T interval: 0.44 seconds

5. AXIS

Quadrant: Normal

Degrees: +60° (aVL most isoelectric)

6. HYPERTROPHY

Atrial: Possible

Ventricular: Probable

7. MYOCARDIAL INFARCTION

Q waves: None significant

S-T displacement: No significant elevation

8. ISCHEMIA

S-T displacement: S-T depression I, II, III, aVF, V_{4-6}

9. POSSIBLE DRUG EFFECTS

None noted

10. ECG ANALYSIS

The rate is 92 bpm, rhythm is irregular, and intervals and axis are WNL. There are multiple early ventricular beats. The sum of the S in V_1 and the R in V_5 is greater than 35 mm. Thus LVH is noted along with S-T abnormalities in leads V_{4-6} indicating a strain pattern. The flat P in II and biphasic P (with negative terminal portion) in V_1 may also indicate LAE.

11. INTERPRETATION

Sinus rhythm

- LVH with strain pattern
- LAE
- Multiple unifocal PVCs

1. RATE

Atrial: Unable to determine

Ventricular: 55 to 100 bpm

2. RHYTHM

Atrial: Irregular

Ventricular: Irregular

3. WAVES

P waves present: Difficult to identify

   Appearance: Fibrillation pattern

   Consistent: No

   Relation to QRS: None

Q waves present: No

   Leads:

   Pathological:

T waves present: Yes

   Morphology: Flat and inverted

4. INTERVALS

P-R interval:

   Consistent:

QRS: 0.06 seconds

   Appearance: Normal

   Consistent: Yes

Q-T interval: 0.34 seconds

5. AXIS

Quadrant: Left

Degrees: −25° (aVF negative, II most isoelectric, slightly positive)

6. HYPERTROPHY

Atrial: No

Ventricular: No

7. MYOCARDIAL INFARCTION

Q waves: None significant

S-T displacement: No significant elevation

8. ISCHEMIA

S-T displacement: Flat, diffuse depression

9. POSSIBLE DRUG EFFECTS

None noted

10. ECG ANALYSIS

The ventricular rate varies from 55 to 100 bpm. Both atrial and ventricular rhythms are irregular. Where P waves can be identified they have a fibrillation pattern. The axis is left. Nonspecific S-T and T wave abnormalities are noted throughout.

11. INTERPRETATION

Atrial fibrillation with variable ventricular response

- LAD
- Nonspecific diffuse S-T and T wave abnormalities

1. RATE

Atrial: Unable to determine

Ventricular: 75 to 150 bpm

2. RHYTHM

Atrial: Irregular

Ventricular: Irregular

3. WAVES

P waves present: Difficult to identify

Appearance: Fibrillation pattern

Consistent: No

Relation to QRS: None

Q waves present: No

Leads:

Pathological:

T waves present: Yes

Morphology: Fused with QRS

4. INTERVALS

P-R interval:

Consistent:

QRS: 0.16 seconds

Appearance: Wide, positive RS in V_6, negative QS in V_1

Consistent: Yes

Q-T interval: 0.40 seconds

5. AXIS

Quadrant: Left

Degrees: −40° (aVF and II negative, II most isoelectric slightly negative)

6. HYPERTROPHY

Atrial: No

Ventricular: No

7. MYOCARDIAL INFARCTION

Q waves: None significant

S-T displacement: S-T elevation II, III, aVF, V_{1-5}

8. ISCHEMIA

S-T displacement: S-T depression I, aVL, V_6

9. POSSIBLE DRUG EFFECTS

None noted

10. ECG ANALYSIS

The ventricular rate is 75 to 150 bpm. Atrial and ventricular rhythms are irregular. P waves can be identified in aVF. They are irregular and do not initiate the QRS. The ventricular rate is also irregular. Both findings are classic characteristics of atrial fibrillation. Left anterior hemiblock (LAHB) is denoted by the negative net QRS deflections in leads aVF and II. The broad, positive RS in V_6 with broad negative QS in V_1 are classic characteristics of left bundle branch block. Because the entire left bundle is blocked, it is more appropriate to simply note the LAHB as an LAD. The diffuse S-T abnormalities are likely secondary to the LBBB.

11. INTERPRETATION

Atrial fibrillation variable (mostly rapid) ventricular response

- LAD
- LBBB with strain pattern

1. RATE

Atrial: Unable to determine

Ventricular: 250 bpm

2. RHYTHM

Atrial: None

Ventricular: Mostly regular

3. WAVES

P waves present: Unable to identify

Appearance:

Consistent:

Relation to QRS:

Q waves present: Yes

Leads: II, III, aVF

Pathological: Yes

T waves present: Fused to QRS

Morphology:

4. INTERVALS

P-R interval:

Consistent:

QRS: 0.14 seconds

Appearance: Wide, bizarre

Consistent: Yes

Q-T interval:

5. AXIS

Quadrant: Left

Degrees: −40° (aVF and II negative, II and aVR most isoelectric)

6. HYPERTROPHY

Atrial: No

Ventricular: No

7. MYOCARDIAL INFARCTION

Q waves: II, III, aVF

S-T displacement: Elevation, II, III, aVF

8. ISCHEMIA

S-T displacement: S-T depression I, aVL, V_{2-6}

9. POSSIBLE DRUG EFFECTS

None noted

10. ECG ANALYSIS

The ventricular rate is 250 bpm, and the rhythm is regular. P waves are difficult to identify and inconsistent, thus they do not initiate the rhythm. The QRS complexes are greater than 0.12 seconds in duration, indicating an intraventricular conduction delay. The net QRS deflections in leads aVF and II are negative, denoting an LAHB. Q waves in II, III, and aVF are characteristic of an old inferior MI. The S-T segment depression is observed in leads I, aVL, V_{2-6}.

11. INTERPRETATION

Ventricular tachycardia

- LAHB
- Old inferior MI
- S-T depression secondary to IVCD and ventricular tachycardia and/or subendocardial ischemia

1. RATE

Atrial: 82 bpm

Ventricular: 82 bpm

2. RHYTHM

Atrial: Underlying rhythm, regular

Ventricular: Underlying rhythm, regular

3. WAVES

P waves present: Yes

    Appearance: Peaked in II and V_1

    Consistent: Yes

    Relation to QRS: 1:1

Q waves present: Yes

    Leads: III, aVF

    Pathological: Only in III, so not significant

T waves present: Yes

    Morphology: Inverted, II, III, aVF, V_3

4. INTERVALS

P-R interval: 0.16 seconds

    Consistent: Yes

QRS: 0.08 seconds

    Appearance: Normal except third beat of V_{4-6}

    Consistent: Yes

Q-T interval: 0.38 seconds

5. AXIS

Quadrant: Normal

Degrees: +10° (aVF most isoelectric, slightly positive)

6. HYPERTROPHY

Atrial: None

Ventricular: None

7. MYOCARDIAL INFARCTION

Q waves: None significant

S-T displacement: No significant elevation

8. ISCHEMIA

S-T displacement: Diffuse flattening

9. POSSIBLE DRUG EFFECTS

None noted

10. ECG ANALYSIS

The rate is 82 bpm with the underlying rhythm regular. Intervals and axis are WNL. Nondiagnostic S-T flattening is noted throughout. The early beats seen in the rhythm strip and in V_{4-6} are wide and have a compensatory pause, therefore are most likely ventricular in origin.

11. INTERPRETATION

Sinus rhythm

- Occasional unifocal PVC
- Diffuse nonspecific S-T flattening and T wave inversion

1. RATE

Atrial: Unable to determine

Ventricular: 170 bpm

2. RHYTHM

Atrial:

Ventricular: Regular

3. WAVES

P waves present: Buried

Appearance:

Consistent:

Relation to QRS:

Q waves present: No

Leads:

Pathological:

T waves present: Yes

Morphology:

4. INTERVALS

P-R interval:

Consistent:

QRS: 0.10 seconds

Appearance: rSR' in V_1

Consistent: Yes

Q-T interval: 0.28 seconds

5. AXIS

Quadrant: Left

Degrees: $-30°$ (aVF and II negative, II most isoelectric, slightly negative)

6. HYPERTROPHY

Atrial: No

Ventricular: Possible

7. MYOCARDIAL INFARCTION

Q waves: None significant

S-T displacement: No significant elevation

8. ISCHEMIA

S-T displacement: Flattening in V_{1-3}

9. POSSIBLE DRUG EFFECTS

None noted

10. ECG ANALYSIS

The rate is 170 bpm, and the rhythm is regular. There are no identifiable P waves. Because the QRS duration is 0.10 seconds, the rhythm is supraventricular. The mean QRS deflections in leads aVF and II are negative denoting a left anterior hemiblock. The rSR' in V_1 is characteristic of an incomplete RBBB. A combination of a LAHB and an incomplete RBBB is termed a bifascicular block, meaning the right bundle and half of the left bundle are blocked. The r and R' in V_1 have the same voltage, and persistent precordial S waves are present, therefore one must consider right ventricular hypertrophy.

11. INTERPRETATION

Supraventricular tachycardia

- Bifascicular block (ICRBBB + LAHB)
- Possible RVH

1. RATE

Atrial: greater than 300 bpm

Ventricular: 20 to 100 bpm

2. RHYTHM

Atrial: Irregular

Ventricular: Irregular

3. WAVES

P waves present: Difficult to identify, seen best in V_1

Appearance: Fibrillation pattern

Consistent: No

Relation to QRS: None

Q waves present: No

Leads:

Pathological:

T waves present: Yes

Morphology: Elevated

4. INTERVALS

P-R interval:

Consistent:

QRS: 0.12 seconds

Appearance: rSR' in V_1

Consistent: Yes

Q-T interval: 0.40 seconds

5. AXIS

Quadrant: Left anterior hemiblock

Degrees: −50° (aVF and II negative, II most isoelectric, slightly negative)

6. HYPERTROPHY

Atrial: No

Ventricular: No

7. MYOCARDIAL INFARCTION

Q waves: None significant

S-T displacement: Marked elevation, V_{2-6}: slight elevation I, aVL

8. ISCHEMIA

S-T displacement: Flattening II, III, aVF

9. POSSIBLE DRUG EFFECTS

None noted

10. ECG ANALYSIS

The ventricular rate varies from 20 to 100 bpm. The rhythm is irregular. The net QRS deflections in leads aVF and II are negative, characteristic of left anterior hemiblock. The QRS duration is 0.12 seconds, and an rSR' is observed in lead V_1. Both are classic findings of a right bundle branch block. A combination of an LAHB and an incomplete RBBB is termed a bifascicular block, meaning the right bundle and half of the left bundle are blocked. Marked S-T segment elevation is observed in V_{1-6}, symbolizing an acute anterolateral injury.

11. INTERPRETATION

Atrial fibrillation with controlled ventricular response

- Bifascicular block (LAHB + RBBB)
- Acute anterolateral MI

1. RATE

Atrial: 80 bpm

Ventricular: 80 bpm

2. RHYTHM

Atrial: Underlying rhythm, regular

Ventricular: Underlying rhythm, regular

3. WAVES

P waves present: Yes

    Appearance: Biphasic

    Consistent: Yes

    Relation to QRS: 1:1

Q waves present: Yes

    Leads: III

    Pathological: No

T waves present: Yes

    Morphology: Flat

4. INTERVALS

P-R interval: 0.16 seconds

    Consistent: Yes

QRS: 0.06 seconds

    Appearance: Normal

    Consistent: Yes, except beat 3 of leads I to III

Q-T interval: 0.36 seconds

5. AXIS

Quadrant: Left

Degrees: −10° (aVF most isoelectric, slightly negative)

6. HYPERTROPHY

Atrial: No

Ventricular: No

7. MYOCARDIAL INFARCTION

Q waves: None significant

S-T displacement: No significant elevation

8. ISCHEMIA

S-T displacement: No significant depression

9. POSSIBLE DRUG EFFECTS

None noted

10. ECG ANALYSIS

The rate is 80 bpm. The rhythm is regular, and intervals are WNL. The axis is left. The P waves in V_1 are biphasic with a larger terminal portion. In lead II the P waves are 10 seconds in duration. These findings indicate a possible LAE. Beat 3 in leads I to III is wide and has a compensatory pause, however it is the same initial deflection (in I and II) and has the same T wave deflection as the normal QRS. Because of the width it is probably ventricular in origin. Diffuse, non-diagnostic T wave flattening is also observed.

11. INTERPRETATION

Sinus rhythm

- LAD
- Occasional PVC
- Diffuse nonspecific T wave changes
- Possible LAE

1. RATE

Atrial: 75 bpm

Ventricular: 75 bpm

2. RHYTHM

Atrial: Regular

Ventricular: Regular

3. WAVES

P waves present: Yes

    Appearance: Normal

    Consistent: Yes

    Relation to QRS: 1:1

Q waves present: Yes

    Leads: III

    Pathological: No

T waves present: Yes

    Morphology: Abnormal

4. INTERVALS

P-R interval: 0.16 seconds

    Consistent: Yes

QRS: 0.16 seconds

    Appearance: Wide, RS in V_{5-6}

    Consistent: Yes

Q-T interval: 0.46 seconds

5. AXIS

Quadrant: Left

Degrees: −40° (aVF and II negative, II most isoelectric, slightly negative)

6. HYPERTROPHY

Atrial: No

Ventricular: Possible

7. MYOCARDIAL INFARCTION

Q waves: None significant

S-T displacement: S-T elevation, III, V_{1-3}

8. ISCHEMIA

S-T displacement: S-T depression, I, II, aVF, V_{4-6}

9. POSSIBLE DRUG EFFECTS

None noted

10. ECG ANALYSIS

The rate is 75 bpm, and the rhythm is regular. Left anterior hemiblock is denoted by net negative QRS deflection in leads aVF and II. The P-R interval is WNL, and the QRS is wide indicating an intraventricular conduction delay. The R-S pattern in V_{5-6} is characteristic of an LBBB. Because the left bundle is completely blocked the LAHB is more appropriately termed an LAD. The sum of the S wave in V_1 and the R wave in V_5 is greater than 35 mm, thus left ventricular hypertrophy is suspected. The first beat in the augmented leads is possibly early and has the opposite deflection of the other two beats. A pause is also noted following the ectopic beat, probably indicating it is ventricular in origin. Note: In practice it is often difficult to diagnose LVH in the presence of intraventricular conduction delays. The diffuse S-T changes are probably secondary to LVH.

11. INTERPRETATION

Sinus rhythm

- LAD
- LBBB
- Probable LVH
- S-T changes probably secondary to LVH
- PVC

I. RATE

Atrial: 80 bpm

Ventricular: 80 bpm

2. RHYTHM

Atrial: Regular

Ventricular: Regular

3. WAVES

P waves present: Yes

    Appearance: Normal

    Consistent: Yes

    Relation to QRS: 1:1

Q waves present: No

    Leads:

    Pathological:

T waves present: Yes

    Morphology: Normal

4. INTERVALS

P-R interval: 0.14 seconds

    Consistent: Yes

QRS: 0.08 seconds

    Appearance: rSR' in V_{1-2}

    Consistent: Yes

Q-T interval: 0.40 seconds

5. AXIS

Quadrant: Normal

Degrees: +75° (aVL, I most isoelectric)

6. HYPERTROPHY

Atrial: No

Ventricular: No

7. MYOCARDIAL INFARCTION

Q waves: None significant

S-T displacement: No significant elevation

8. ISCHEMIA

S-T displacement: No significant depression

9. POSSIBLE DRUG EFFECTS

None noted

10. ECG ANALYSIS

The rate, rhythm, intervals, and axis are WNL. The rSR' in V_2 is consistent with an incomplete RBBB. However, because the QRS duration is only 0.08 seconds, one might suspect that the rSR' may be due to lead placement rather than an ICRBBB.

11. INTERPRETATION

Sinus rhythm

    • ICRBBB vs. incorrect lead placement

1. RATE

Atrial: Unable to determine

Ventricular: 70 to 150 bpm

2. RHYTHM

Atrial: Irregular

Ventricular: Irregular

3. WAVES

P waves present: Difficult to identify, best seen in V_1

    Appearance: Fibrillation pattern

    Consistent: No

    Relation to QRS: None

Q waves present: No

    Leads:

    Pathological:

T waves present: Yes

    Morphology: Inverted

4. INTERVALS

P-R interval:

    Consistent:

QRS: 0.08 seconds

    Appearance: Low voltage

    Consistent: Yes

Q-T interval: 0.36 seconds

5. AXIS

Quadrant: Left anterior hemiblock

Degrees: −35° (aVL and II negative, II most isoelectric,
        slightly negative)

6. HYPERTROPHY

Atrial: No

Ventricular: No

7. MYOCARDIAL INFARCTION

Q waves: None significant

S-T displacement: No significant elevation

8. ISCHEMIA

S-T displacement: Diffuse S-T and T wave changes

9. POSSIBLE DRUG EFFECTS

None noted

10. ECG ANALYSIS

The ventricular rate varies from 70 to 150 bpm. Intervals are WNL, and the rhythm is irregular with an atrial fibrillation pattern. The mean QRS deflections in leads aVF and II are negative, which is consistent with a left anterior hemiblock. Poor R wave progression is noted in leads V_{1-3}, as well as diffuse S-T and T wave changes.

11. INTERPRETATION

Atrial fibrillation with controlled ventricular response

- Left anterior hemiblock (LAHB)
- Poor R wave progression, cannot rule out old anteroseptal MI
- Diffuse S-T and T wave abnormalities indicating possible ischemia

1. **RATE**

   Atrial: 92 bpm

   Ventricular: 92 bpm

2. **RHYTHM**

   Atrial: Underlying rhythm, regular

   Ventricular: Underlying rhythm, regular

3. **WAVES**

   P waves present: Yes

      Appearance: Normal

      Consistent: Yes

      Relation to QRS: 1:1 except beat 2 in leads I to III

   Q waves present: No

      Leads:

      Pathological:

   T waves present: Yes

      Morphology: Normal

4. **INTERVALS**

   P-R interval: 0.14 seconds

      Consistent: Yes

   QRS: 0.08 seconds

      Appearance: Normal

      Consistent: Yes

   Q-T interval: 0.36 seconds

5. **AXIS**

   Quadrant: Normal

   Degrees: +15° (III most isoelectric, slightly negative)

6. **HYPERTROPHY**

   Atrial: No

   Ventricular: No

7. **MYOCARDIAL INFARCTION**

   Q waves: None significant

   S-T displacement: No significant elevation

8. **ISCHEMIA**

   S-T displacement: No significant depression

9. **POSSIBLE DRUG EFFECTS**

   None noted

10. **ECG ANALYSIS**

    The rate, underlying rhythm, intervals, and axis are WNL. Beat 2 in leads I to III is early, not wide, and has the same deflection as the normal beat. With close observation a P wave can be detected in lead III, therefore it is probably atrial in origin.

11. **INTERPRETATION**

    Sinus rhythm
    - PAC

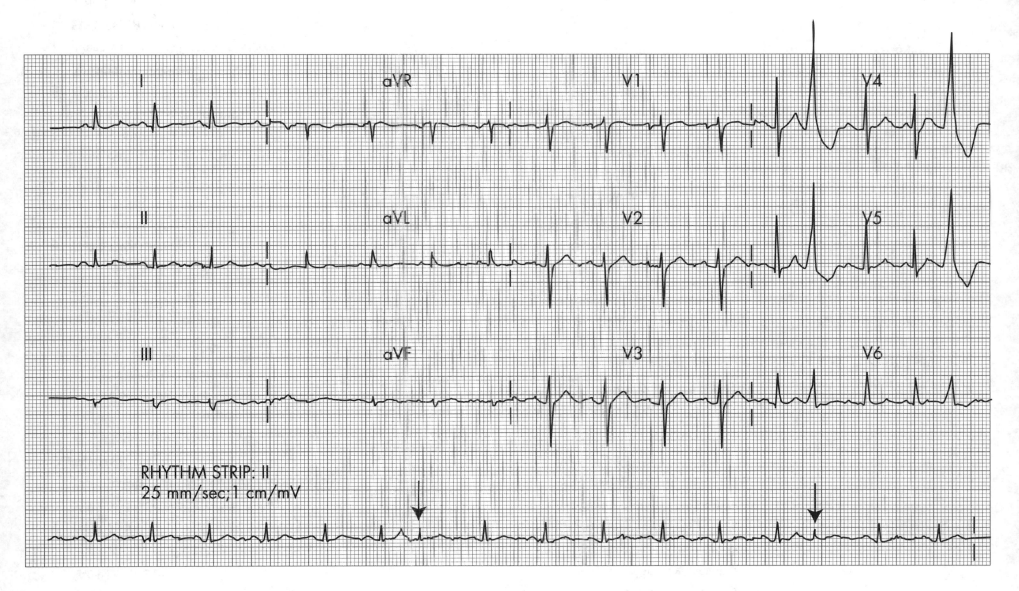

I aVR V1 V4

II aVL V2 V5

III aVF V3 V6

RHYTHM STRIP: II
25 mm/sec; 1 cm/mV

Figure 3-22
Resting 12-Lead ECG
435

1. RATE

Atrial: 102 bpm

Ventricular: 102 bpm

2. RHYTHM

Atrial: Underlying rhythm, regular

Ventricular: Underlying rhythm, regular

3. WAVES

P waves present: Yes

   Appearance: Normal

   Consistent: Yes

   Relation to QRS: 1:1

Q waves present: No

   Leads:

   Pathological:

T waves present: Yes

   Morphology: Normal

4. INTERVALS

P-R interval: 0.16 seconds

   Consistent: Yes

QRS: 0.06 seconds

   Appearance: Normal, except beats 2 and 5 in V_{4-6}

   Consistent: Yes

Q-T interval: 0.34 seconds

5. AXIS

Quadrant: Normal

Degrees: 0° (aVF most isoelectric)

6. HYPERTROPHY

Atrial: No

Ventricular: No

7. MYOCARDIAL INFARCTION

Q waves: None significant

S-T displacement: No significant elevation

8. ISCHEMIA

S-T displacement: No significant depression

9. POSSIBLE DRUG EFFECTS

None noted

10. ECG ANALYSIS

The rate is 102 bpm. The underlying rhythm is regular, and the intervals and axis are WNL. Beats 2 and 5 in V_{4-6} are wide with opposite T wave deflection from the normal beats and are probably ventricular in origin. On the rhythm strip the early beats are narrower and are likely atrial in origin.

11. INTERPRETATION

Sinus tachycardia

- Occasional PVC
- Occasional PAC

1. RATE

Atrial: Unable to determine

Ventricular: 30 to 96 bpm

2. RHYTHM

Atrial: Irregular

Ventricular: Irregular

3. WAVES

P waves present: Difficult to identify, best seen in V_1

    Appearance: Fibrillation pattern

    Consistent: No

    Relation to QRS: None

Q waves present: No

    Leads:

    Pathological:

T waves present: Yes

    Morphology: Negative, V_{4-6}

4. INTERVALS

P-R interval:

    Consistent:

QRS: 0.11 seconds

    Appearance: Normal

    Consistent: Yes

Q-T interval: 0.44 seconds

5. AXIS

Quadrant: Left anterior hemiblock

Degrees: −45° (aVF and II negative, aVR and II most isoelectric)

6. HYPERTROPHY

Atrial: No

Ventricular: No

7. MYOCARDIAL INFARCTION

Q waves: None significant

S-T displacement: No significant elevation

8. ISCHEMIA

S-T displacement: No significant depression

9. POSSIBLE DRUG EFFECTS

None noted

10. ECG ANALYSIS

The ventricular rate varies, and the rhythm is irregular. P waves can be identified and do not initiate the QRS complexes, which is a classic characteristic of atrial fibrillation. The QRS duration is slightly long (0.11 seconds) indicating an intraventricular delay. There is no clear-cut evidence as to the location of the delay. The mean QRS deflection in leads aVF and II are negative, characteristics of a left anterior hemiblock. The T waves in V_{4-6} are negative. Poor R wave progression with a significant S in V_6 may represent a pulmonary disease pattern with right ventricular enlargement. Baseline artifact should be noted.

11. INTERPRETATION

Atrial fibrillation with controlled ventricular response

- LAHB
- IVCD
- Nondiagnostic lateral T wave changes
- Possible pulmonary disease pattern with RVH

ANALYSIS 3-24

1. RATE

Atrial: 80 bpm

Ventricular: 80 bpm

2. RHYTHM

Atrial: Regular

Ventricular: Regular

3. WAVES

P waves present: Yes

    Appearance: Normal

    Consistent: Yes

    Relation to QRS: 1:1

Q waves present: Yes

    Leads: II, III, aVF

    Pathological: No

T waves present: Yes

    Morphology: Normal

4. INTERVALS

P-R interval: 0.16 seconds

    Consistent: Yes

QRS: 0.12 seconds

    Appearance: rSR' in V_1

    Consistent: Yes

Q-T interval: 0.36 seconds

5. AXIS

Quadrant: Normal

Degrees: +60° (aVL most isoelectric)

6. HYPERTROPHY

Atrial: No

Ventricular: No

7. MYOCARDIAL INFARCTION

Q waves: None significant

S-T displacement: No significant elevation

8. ISCHEMIA

S-T displacement: No significant depression

9. POSSIBLE DRUG EFFECTS

None noted

10. ECG ANALYSIS

Rate, rhythm, and axis are WNL. The QRS complex is 0.12 seconds in duration and an rSR' is noted in V_1, consistent with a right bundle branch block. The sum of S in V_1 and R in V_5 is 35 mm, indicating possible LVH. Because supporting criteria are absent (strain pattern and LAD), the probability of true LVH diminishes.

11. INTERPRETATION

Sinus rhythm

- Right bundle branch block
- Cannot rule out LVH

1. RATE

Atrial: 122 bpm

Ventricular: 122 bpm

2. RHYTHM

Atrial: Underlying rhythm, regular

Ventricular: Underlying rhythm, regular

3. WAVES

P waves present: Yes

    Appearance: Normal

    Consistent: Yes

    Relation to QRS: 1:1

Q waves present: Yes

    Leads: III, aVF

    Pathological: No

T waves present: Yes

    Morphology: Normal

4. INTERVALS

P-R interval: 0.16 seconds

    Consistent: Yes

QRS: 0.08 seconds

    Appearance: Normal, except beat 2 and 5 beat run in I to III

    Consistent: Yes

Q-T interval: 0.32 seconds

5. AXIS

Quadrant: Right

Degrees: +135° (II and aVR most isoelectric)

6. HYPERTROPHY

Atrial: No

Ventricular: No

7 MYOCARDIAL INFARCTION

Q waves: None significant

S-T displacement: No significant elevation

8. ISCHEMIA

S-T displacement: No significant depression

9. POSSIBLE DRUG EFFECTS

None noted

10. ECG ANALYSIS

The underlying rate is 122 bpm, the rhythm is regular with the exception of ectopic beats in I to III. Intervals are WNL, with a right axis deviation. The early beat (number 2) in leads I to III is wide with opposite deflection from the normal complexes, thus appearing ventricular in origin. The 5-beat run that follows appears to be of the same origin.

11. INTERPRETATION

Sinus tachycardia

- RAD
- Single PVC followed by run of ventricular tachycardia with spontaneous return to sinus tachycardia

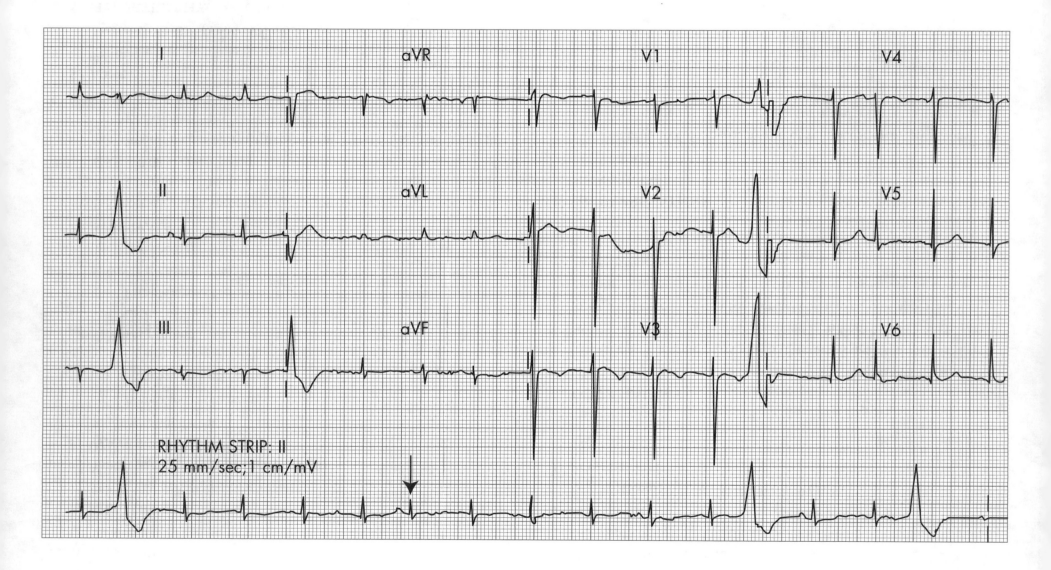

I aVR V1 V4

II aVL V2 V5

III aVF V3 V6

RHYTHM STRIP: II
25 mm/sec;1 cm/mV

Figure 3-26
Resting 12-Lead ECG
440

1. RATE

Atrial: 100 bpm

Ventricular: 100 bpm

2. RHYTHM

Atrial: Irregular

Ventricular: Irregular

3. WAVES

P waves present: Yes

Appearance: Flat

Consistent: Yes

Relation to QRS: 1:1

Q waves present: No

Leads:

Pathological:

T waves present: Yes

Morphology: Diffuse flattening

4. INTERVALS

P-R interval: 0.14 seconds

Consistent: Yes

QRS: 0.06 seconds

Appearance: Low voltage in limb leads

Consistent: No

Q-T interval: 0.40 seconds

5. AXIS

Quadrant: Normal horizontal

Degrees: 0° (aVF isoelectric)

6. HYPERTROPHY

Atrial: No

Ventricular: No

7. MYOCARDIAL INFARCTION

Q waves: None significant

S-T displacement: No significant elevation

8. ISCHEMIA

S-T displacement: No significant depression

9. POSSIBLE DRUG EFFECTS

None noted

10. ECG ANALYSIS

The rate is 100 bpm. Rhythm is irregular, and the intervals and axis are WNL. Ectopic beats vary from wide to narrow complexes. The wide complexes with opposite T wave deflection are probably ventricular in origin. The early complexes that are narrow are most likely atrial. Poor R wave progression is noted in the precordial leads. Diffuse nonspecific T wave abnormalities are also observed.

11. INTERPRETATION

Sinus tachycardia

- Occasional PVCs and PACs
- Poor R wave progression
- Diffuse nonspecific T wave abnormalities

ANALYSIS 3-27

1. RATE

Atrial: Unable to determine

Ventricular: 100 to 280 bpm

2. RHYTHM

Atrial: Irregular

Ventricular: Irregular

3. WAVES

P waves present: Difficult to identify, best seen in II, V₁

   Appearance: Fibrillation pattern

   Consistent: No

   Relation to QRS: None

Q waves present: Yes

   Leads: II, III, aVF

   Pathological: No

T waves present: Yes

   Morphology: Normal

4. INTERVALS

P-R interval:

   Consistent:

QRS: 0.08 seconds

   Appearance: Normal, low voltage in limb leads

   Consistent: Yes

Q-T interval: 0.30 seconds

5. AXIS

Quadrant: Right

Degrees: +110° (aVR most isoelectric)

6. HYPERTROPHY

Atrial: No

Ventricular: No

7. MYOCARDIAL INFARCTION

Q waves: None significant

S-T displacement: No significant elevation

8. ISCHEMIA

S-T displacement: No significant depression

9. POSSIBLE DRUG EFFECTS

None noted

10. ECG ANALYSIS

The ventricular rate is 100 to 280 bpm. The irregular rhythm and absence of regular P waves indicates atrial fibrillation. The QRS duration is WNL. A slight right axis deviation is noted in addition to borderline low limb lead voltage.

11. INTERPRETATION

Atrial fibrillation with rapid ventricular response

   • Slight right axis deviation (RAD)

1. RATE

Atrial: 50 bpm

Ventricular: 50 bpm

2. RHYTHM

Atrial: Regular

Ventricular: Regular

3. WAVES

P waves present: Yes

    Appearance: Normal

    Consistent: Yes

    Relation to QRS: 1:1

Q waves present: Yes

    Leads: II, aVF

    Pathological: No

T waves present: Yes

    Morphology: Normal

4. INTERVALS

P-R interval: 0.20 seconds

    Consistent: Yes

QRS: 0.08 seconds

    Appearance: Normal

    Consistent: Yes

Q-T interval: 0.46 seconds

5. AXIS

Quadrant: Normal

Degrees: +10° (aVF most isoelectric, slightly positive)

6. HYPERTROPHY

Atrial: No

Ventricular: No

7. MYOCARDIAL INFARCTION

Q waves: None significant

S-T displacement: No significant elevation

8. ISCHEMIA

S-T displacement: No significant depression

9. POSSIBLE DRUG EFFECTS

None noted

10. ECG ANALYSIS

Rate is 50 bpm. Rhythm is regular, and axis is WNL. The P-R interval is slightly long at 0.20 seconds, indicating a borderline first degree atrioventricular block. Other intervals are WNL. The Q waves seen in II and aVF are not significant.

11. INTERPRETATION

Sinus bradycardia

- Borderline first degree AV block

ANALYSIS 3-29

1. RATE

Atrial: 70 bpm

Ventricular: 70 bpm

2. RHYTHM

Atrial: Regular

Ventricular: Regular

3. WAVES

P waves present: Yes

Appearance: Normal

Consistent: Yes

Relation to QRS: 1:1

Q waves present: No

Leads:

Pathological:

T waves present: Yes

Morphology: Inferior inversion

4. INTERVALS

P-R interval: 0.18 seconds

Consistent: Yes

QRS: 0.16 seconds

Appearance: rSR' in V_{1-2}

Consistent: Yes

Q-T interval: 0.44 seconds

5. AXIS

Quadrant: Left anterior

Degrees: −45° (aVF and II negative, II and aVR most isoelectric)

6. HYPERTROPHY

Atrial: No

Ventricular: Possible RVH

7. MYOCARDIAL INFARCTION

Q waves: None significant

S-T displacement: No significant elevation

8. ISCHEMIA

S-T displacement: 2 to 3 mm J point depression V_{5-6}

9. POSSIBLE DRUG EFFECTS

None noted

10. ECG ANALYSIS

The rate is 70 bpm, rhythm is regular, and intervals are WNL. The rSR' in V_{2-3} is characteristic of a right bundle branch block. A left anterior hemiblock is evidenced by the negative net QRS deflections in aVF and II. A combination of an LAHB and RBBB is termed a bifascicular block, meaning the right bundle and half of the left bundle is blocked. The large R wave in V_1 indicates possible right ventricular hypertrophy. Inferior T wave inversion and S-T depression are noted throughout the chest leads.

11. INTERPRETATION

Sinus rhythm

- Bifascicular block (LAHB + RBBB)
- Possible RVH
- Diffuse S-T and T wave abnormalities indicating possible ischemia or subendocardial injury

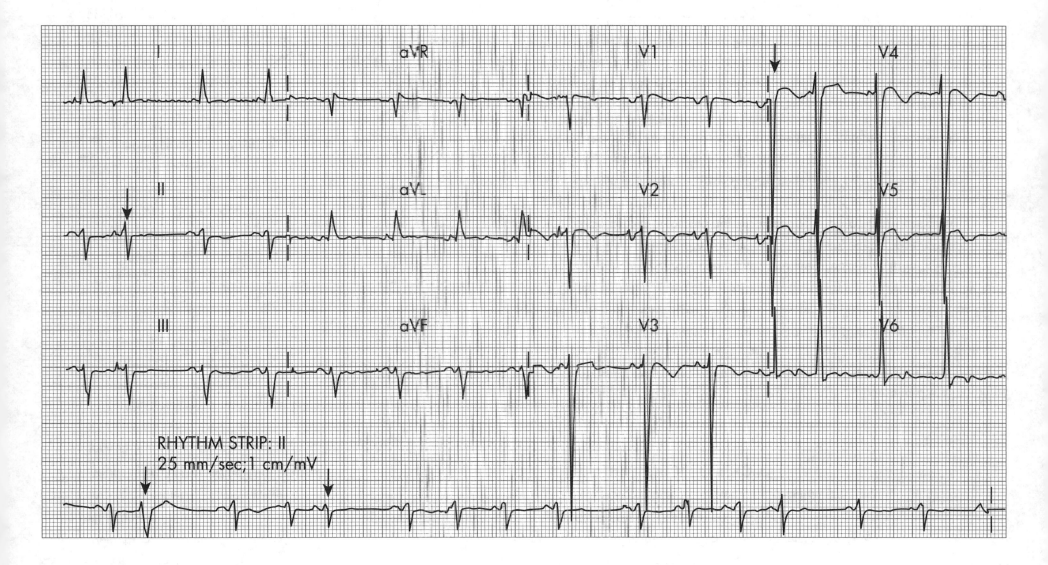

Figure 3-30
Resting 12-Lead ECG

445

1. RATE

Atrial: 90 bpm

Ventricular: 90 bpm

2. RHYTHM

Atrial: Underlying rhythm, regular

Ventricular: Underlying rhythm, regular

3. WAVES

P waves present: Yes

    Appearance: Flat in II, biphasic in V_1

    Consistent: Yes

    Relation to QRS: 1:1

Q waves present: No

    Leads:

    Pathological:

T waves present: Yes

    Morphology: Inverted V_{1-3}

4. INTERVALS

P-R interval: 0.14 seconds

    Consistent: Yes, in normal beats

QRS: 0.10 seconds

    Appearance: High voltage in V_{3-6}

    Consistent: Yes

Q-T interval: 0.40 seconds

5. AXIS

Quadrant: Left anterior hemiblock

Degrees: −40° (aVF and II negative, II most isoelectric, slightly negative)

6. HYPERTROPHY

Atrial: Possible

Ventricular: No

7. MYOCARDIAL INFARCTION

Q waves: None significant

S-T displacement: 1 to 2 mm S-T elevation V_{1-5}

8. ISCHEMIA

S-T displacement: 1 mm S-T depression, II

9. POSSIBLE DRUG EFFECTS

None noted

10. ECG ANALYSIS

The rate is 90 bpm, the underlying rhythm is regular, and the intervals are WNL. Left anterior hemiblock is evidenced by the negative net QRS deflections in aVF and II. The P waves in V_1 are negative and in II are greater than or equal to 0.12 seconds in duration, both characteristics of left atrial enlargement.

Ectopic beats (beat 2 in I to III, and beat 1 in V_{4-6}) are preceded by P waves, are narrow complexes, and are probably atrial in origin. Beat 2 on the rhythm strip is probably junctional because it is the same deflection as the normal beat and is only slightly longer in duration. As the rhythm strip continues, the P wave morphology changes indicating a possible sick sinus node or that the impulse is originating from a different focci.

Diffuse S-T and T wave abnormalities are noted indicating possible ischemia or injury.

11. INTERPRETATION

Sinus rhythm

- Multiple PACs and PJCs
- Left atrial enlargement
- LAHB
- Diffuse S-T and T wave changes suggesting possible ischemia

1. RATE

Atrial: 67 bpm

Ventricular: 67 bpm

2. RHYTHM

Atrial: Irregular

Ventricular: Irregular

3. WAVES

P waves present: Yes

   Appearance: Normal

   Consistent: Yes

   Relation to QRS: Normal beats 1:1

Q waves present: Yes

   Leads: II, III, aVF

   Pathological: Borderline

T waves present: Yes

   Morphology: Diffuse flattening

4. INTERVALS

P-R interval: 0.18 seconds

   Consistent: Yes

QRS: 0.10 seconds

   Appearance: Aberrant beats wide

   Consistent: No

Q-T interval: 0.40 seconds

5. AXIS

Quadrant: Normal

Degrees: +70° (I most isoelectric, slightly negative)

6. HYPERTROPHY

Atrial: No

Ventricular: No

7. MYOCARDIAL INFARCTION

Q waves: II, III, aVF

S-T displacement: No significant elevation

8. ISCHEMIA

S-T displacement: Flat in I, aVL, V_{2-6}

9. POSSIBLE DRUG EFFECTS

None noted

10. ECG ANALYSIS

The rate is 67 bpm. The rhythm is irregular due to ectopic beats. Intervals and axis are WNL. Ectopic beats are wide with opposite T wave deflections from normal beats. The inferior Q waves are borderline in voltage criteria for significance. However, because they occur in all three inferior leads, they are most likely pathological. S-T and T wave flattening is noted in I, aVL, and V_{2-6}.

11. INTERPRETATION

Sinus rhythm

- Frequent PVCs
- Probable old inferior MI
- Anterolateral S-T and T wave abnormalities indicating possible ischemia

1. RATE

Atrial: 100 bpm

Ventricular: 45 bpm

2. RHYTHM

Atrial: Regular

Ventricular: Regular

3. WAVES

P waves present: Yes

    Appearance: Normal

    Consistent: Yes

    Relation to QRS: Independent relation from QRS

Q waves present: Yes

    Leads: II, III, aVF

    Pathological: Possible

T waves present: Yes

    Morphology: Abnormal

4. INTERVALS

P-R interval:

    Consistent:

QRS: 0.08 seconds

    Appearance: rSR' in V_{1-2}

    Consistent: Yes

Q-T interval: 0.48 seconds

5. AXIS

Quadrant: Normal

Degrees: +70° (aVL most isoelectric, slightly negative)

6. HYPERTROPHY

Atrial: No

Ventricular: No

7. MYOCARDIAL INFARCTION

Q waves: Possibly pathological

S-T displacement: Significant elevation, V_{1-4}

8. ISCHEMIA

S-T displacement: Significant depression, V_{5-6}, I, aVL

9. POSSIBLE DRUG EFFECTS

None noted

10. ECG ANALYSIS

The atrial rate is 100, and the ventricular rate is 45 bpm. The P waves are identifiable, however, they do not initiate the QRS (i.e., the atria and ventricles are beating independently, indicating a complete third degree heart block). Because the QRS complexes are not wide, ventricular depolarization appears to be initiated in the nodal area or high in the ventricles. Marked S-T elevation is noted in V_{1-4} indicating an acute injury. S-T depression in V_{5-6}, I, and aVL, indicates possible ischemia. The Q waves in II, III, and aVF are probably evidence of an old inferior injury.

11. INTERPRETATION

AV dissociation with ventricular response of 45 bpm

- Acute anterior MI
- Probable lateral ischemia
- Cannot rule out old inferior MI

1. RATE

Atrial: 115 bpm

Ventricular: 115 bpm

2. RHYTHM

Atrial: Regular

Ventricular: Regular

3. WAVES

P waves present: Yes

   Appearance: Peaked in II, (2 mV)

   Consistent: Yes

   Relation to QRS: 1:1

Q waves present: No

   Leads:

   Pathological:

T waves present: Yes

   Morphology: Inverted II, III, aVF

4. INTERVALS

P-R interval: 0.12 seconds

   Consistent: Yes

QRS: 0.12 seconds

   Appearance: High voltage V_1, R-S in V_{5-6}

   Consistent: Yes

Q-T interval: 0.34 seconds

5. AXIS

Quadrant: Normal

Degrees: +60° (aVL most isoelectric)

6. HYPERTROPHY

Atrial: Possible

Ventricular: No

7. MYOCARDIAL INFARCTION

Q waves: None significant

S-T displacement: No significant elevation

8. ISCHEMIA

S-T displacement: Flat S-T, II, III, aVF

9. POSSIBLE DRUG EFFECTS

None noted

10. ECG ANALYSIS

The rate is 115 bpm. The rhythm is regular, and the axis is WNL. P waves in II are tall and peaked, which is evidence of possible right atrial enlargement. The QRS complexes are wide and an RS is noted in V_{5-6}, which are classic characteristics of a left bundle branch block. Flat S-Ts in V_{4-6} are probably secondary to the LBBB. Non-diagnostic T wave inversion in II, III, and aVF should be noted as well.

11. INTERPRETATION

Sinus tachycardia

- Possible RAE
- LBBB

1. RATE

Atrial: 55 bpm

Ventricular: 55 bpm

2. RHYTHM

Atrial: Regular

Ventricular: Regular

3. WAVES

P waves present: Yes

    Appearance: Normal

    Consistent: Yes

    Relation to QRS: 1:1

Q waves present: Yes

    Leads: III

    Pathological: No

T waves present: Yes

    Morphology: Flat

4. INTERVALS

P-R interval: 0.22 seconds

    Consistent: Yes

QRS: 0.08 seconds

    Appearance: Normal

    Consistent: Yes

Q-T interval: 0.44 seconds

5. AXIS

Quadrant: Normal

Degrees: +10° (aVF most isoelectric, slightly positive)

6. HYPERTROPHY

Atrial: No

Ventricular: No

7. MYOCARDIAL INFARCTION

Q waves: None significant

S-T displacement: No significant elevation

8. ISCHEMIA

S-T displacement: Diffuse nonspecific S-T changes

9. POSSIBLE DRUG EFFECTS

None noted

10. ECG ANALYSIS

The rate is 55 bpm. Rhythm is regular, and axis is WNL. The P-R interval is greater than 0.20 seconds, characteristic of a first degree AV block. Diffuse nonspecific S-T changes imply possible ischemia.

11. INTERPRETATION

Sinus bradycardia

- First degree AVB
- Diffuse nonspecific S-T and T wave changes

1. RATE

Atrial: Unable to determine

Ventricular: Variable 90 to 160 bpm

2. RHYTHM

Atrial: Irregular

Ventricular: Irregular

3. WAVES

P waves present: Difficult to identify, best seen in V_{2-3}

Appearance: Fibrillation pattern

Consistent: No

Relation to QRS: None

Q waves present: No

Leads:

Pathological:

T waves present: Yes

Morphology: No significant abnormalities

4. INTERVALS

P-R interval:

Consistent:

QRS: 0.16 seconds

Appearance: rSR' in V_{1-2}

Consistent: Yes

Q-T interval: 0.40 seconds

5. AXIS

Quadrant: Left anterior hemiblock

Degrees: −80° (Leads aVF and II negative, aVR most isoelectric, slightly positive)

6. HYPERTROPHY

Atrial: No

Ventricular: No

7. MYOCARDIAL INFARCTION

Q waves: None significant

S-T displacement: No significant elevation

8. ISCHEMIA

S-T displacement: S-T depression, V_2

9. POSSIBLE DRUG EFFECTS

None noted

10. ECG ANALYSIS

The ventricular rate varies between 90 and 160 bpm. The rhythm is irregular and P waves are difficult to identify, characteristic of atrial fibrillation. The QRS complex is wide and an rSR' is seen in V_{1-2}, consistent with a right bundle branch block. The net QRS deflections in leads aVF and II are negative, indicative of an LAHB. A combination of an RBBB and LAHB is termed a bifascicular block, meaning that the right bundle and half of the left bundle is blocked. The S-T depression noted in V_2 is probably secondary to the RBBB.

11. INTERPRETATION

Atrial fibrillation with rapid ventricular response

- Bifascicular block (LAHB + RBBB)

1. **RATE**

   Atrial: Unable to determine

   Ventricular: Variable, 80 to 160 bpm

2. **RHYTHM**

   Atrial: Irregular

   Ventricular: Irregular

3. **WAVES**

   P waves present: Difficult to identify, best seen in V_2

      Appearance: Fibrillation pattern

      Consistent: No

      Relation to QRS: None

   Q waves present: Yes

      Leads: III, aVF

      Pathological: No

   T waves present: Yes

      Morphology: Abnormal

4. **INTERVALS**

   P-R interval:

      Consistent:

   QRS: 0.12 seconds

      Appearance: rSR' in V_{1-2}

      Consistent: Yes

   Q-T interval: 0.28 seconds

5. **AXIS**

   Quadrant: Right

   Degrees: +120° (aVR most isoelectric)

6. **HYPERTROPHY**

   Atrial: No

   Ventricular: No

7. **MYOCARDIAL INFARCTION**

   Q waves: None significant

   S-T displacement: No significant elevation

8. **ISCHEMIA**

   S-T displacement: Diffuse S-T depression

9. **POSSIBLE DRUG EFFECTS**

   None noted

10. **ECG ANALYSIS**

   The ventricular rate varies from 80 to 160 bpm. The rhythm is irregular and P waves are difficult to identify, characteristic of atrial fibrillation. The axis is in the right quadrant. The rSR' in V_{1-2} denotes a right bundle branch block. An RBBB in addition to the RAD are criteria for a left posterior hemiblock (LPHB). Because the left bundle is partially blocked and the right bundle is completely blocked, the combination is more appropriately termed a bifascicular block. There are nonspecific diffuse S-T and T wave abnormalities suggesting possible ischemia.

11. **INTERPRETATION**

   Atrial fibrillation with variable ventricular response

   - RAD
   - Bifascicular block (RBBB + LPHB)
   - Diffuse S-T and T wave abnormalities suggesting possible ischemia

1. RATE

Atrial: 67 bpm

Ventricular: 67 bpm

2. RHYTHM

Atrial: Regular

Ventricular: Regular

3. WAVES

P waves present: Yes

    Appearance: Flat in limb leads

    Consistent: Yes

    Relation to QRS: 1:1

Q waves present: No

    Leads:

    Pathological:

T waves present: Yes

    Morphology: Normal

4. INTERVALS

P-R interval: 0.16 seconds

    Consistent: Yes

QRS: 0.16 seconds

    Appearance: rSR' in V_{1-2}

    Consistent: Yes

Q-T interval: 0.44 seconds

5. AXIS

Quadrant: Left

Degrees: −15° (aVF negative, aVF and II most isoelectric)

6. HYPERTROPHY

Atrial: No

Ventricular: No

7. MYOCARDIAL INFARCTION

Q waves: None significant

S-T displacement: No significant elevation

8. ISCHEMIA

S-T displacement: No significant depression

9. POSSIBLE DRUG EFFECTS

None noted

10. ECG ANALYSIS

The rate is 67 bpm. The rhythm is regular, and the axis is slightly left. The QRS complex measures 0.16 seconds in duration and there is an rSR' in V_{1-2}, which are classic characteristics of a right bundle branch block. Borderline low QRS voltage is noted in the limb leads indicating a possible chronic pulmonary disease pattern.

11. INTERPRETATION

Sinus rhythm

- LAD
- RBBB
- Possible chronic pulmonary disease pattern

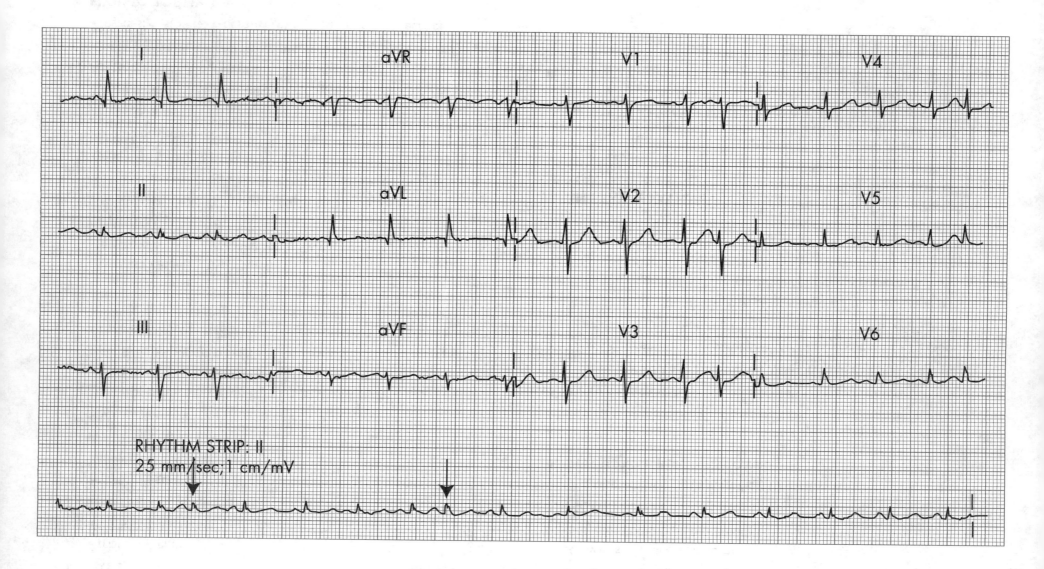

I aVR V1 V4

II aVL V2 V5

III aVF V3 V6

RHYTHM STRIP: II
25 mm/sec; 1 cm/mV

Figure 3-38
Resting 12-Lead ECG
454

1. RATE

Atrial: 98 bpm

Ventricular: 98 bpm

2. RHYTHM

Atrial: Underlying rhythm, regular

Ventricular: Underlying rhythm, regular

3. WAVES

P waves present: Yes

    Appearance: Normal

    Consistent: Yes

    Relation to QRS: 1:1

Q waves present: No

    Leads:

    Pathological:

T waves present: Yes

    Morphology: Normal

4. INTERVALS

P-R interval: 0.16 seconds

    Consistent: Yes

QRS: 0.09 seconds

    Appearance: Normal

    Consistent: Yes

Q-T interval: 0.34 seconds

5. AXIS

Quadrant: Left

Degrees: −15° (aVF negative, aVF and II most isoelectric)

6. HYPERTROPHY

Atrial: No

Ventricular: No

7. MYOCARDIAL INFARCTION

Q waves: None significant

S-T displacement: No significant elevation

8. ISCHEMIA

S-T displacement: No significant depression

9. POSSIBLE DRUG EFFECTS

None noted

10. ECG ANALYSIS

The rate is 98 bpm. The underlying rhythm is essentially regular, intervals and axis are WNL. The premature beats noted in the rhythm strip have normal appearing QRS complexes. The P waves for those beats are probably buried in the preceding T waves indicating the ectopic beat is probably atrial in origin. Beats 4 of V_{1-3} and 5 of V_{4-6}, are also early with normal QRS morphology. These early ectopic beats probably originate in the atria as well.

11. INTERPRETATION

Sinus tachycardia

- LAD
- Occasional PACs

1. RATE
Atrial: 55 bpm

Ventricular: 55 bpm

2. RHYTHM
Atrial: Regular

Ventricular: Regular

3. WAVES
P waves present: Yes

Appearance: Flat

Consistent: Yes

Relation to QRS: 1:1

Q waves present: No

Leads:

Pathological:

T waves present: Yes

Morphology: Flat

4. INTERVALS
P-R interval: 0.24 seconds

Consistent: Yes

QRS: 0.16 seconds

Appearance: R-S in V_{5-6}

Consistent: Yes

Q-T interval: 0.48 seconds

5. AXIS
Quadrant: Normal

Degrees: +45° (III and aVL most isoelectric)

6. HYPERTROPHY
Atrial: No

Ventricular: No

7. MYOCARDIAL INFARCTION
Q waves: None significant

S-T displacement: No significant elevation

8. ISCHEMIA
S-T displacement: No significant depression

9. POSSIBLE DRUG EFFECTS
None noted

10. ECG ANALYSIS
The rate is 55 bpm. Rhythm is regular. The P waves are somewhat difficult to see because they are very flat, however on closer inspection they can be seen in III and V_1. The P-R interval measures greater than 0.20 seconds, indicating a first degree AV block. The QRS complex duration is greater than 0.12 seconds, with large R-S in V_{5-6}, classic characteristics of an LBBB. Axis is normal. The S-T segment is slurred into the T wave, which is often the case with an LBBB.

11. INTERPRETATION
Sinus bradycardia

- First degree AV block
- LBBB

I. RATE

Atrial: Unable to identify

Ventricular: Variable, 75 to 100 bpm

2. RHYTHM

Atrial: Irregular

Ventricular: Irregular

3. WAVES

P waves present: Yes

    Appearance: "Sawtooth" pattern

    Consistent: No

    Relation to QRS: None consistent

Q waves present: No

    Leads:

    Pathological:

T waves present: Yes

    Morphology: Flat in V_{4-6}

4. INTERVALS

P-R interval:

    Consistent:

QRS: 0.08 seconds

    Appearance: Normal

    Consistent: Yes

Q-T interval: 0.32 seconds

5. AXIS

Quadrant: Normal

Degrees: +75° (aVL and I most isoelectric)

6. HYPERTROPHY

Atrial: No

Ventricular: No

7. MYOCARDIAL INFARCTION

Q waves: None significant

S-T displacement: No significant elevation

8. ISCHEMIA

S-T displacement: 1 mm S-T depression, II, III, aVF, V_{3-6}

9. POSSIBLE DRUG EFFECTS

None noted

10. ECG ANALYSIS

The ventricular rate varies from 75 to 100 bpm. The rhythm is irregular and the axis is WNL. The P waves are irregular and have a "sawtooth" pattern in V_{1-2}, which is a classic characteristic of atrial flutter. Poor R wave progression is observed in V_{1-3} indicating a possible old anteroseptal MI. Nondiagnostic S-T and T wave abnormalities are seen in II, III, aVF, and V_{3-6}.

11. INTERPRETATION

Atrial fibrillation/flutter with controlled ventricular response

- Cannot rule out old anteroseptal MI
- Inferior and anterolateral S-T and T wave abnormalities consistent with possible ischemia

1. RATE

Atrial: 95 bpm

Ventricular: 38 bpm

2. RHYTHM

Atrial: Regular

Ventricular: Regular

3. WAVES

P waves present: Yes

Appearance: Normal

Consistent: Yes

Relation to QRS: Independant of QRS

Q waves present: No

Leads:

Pathological:

T waves present: Yes

Morphology: Essentially normal

4. INTERVALS

P-R interval:

Consistent:

QRS: 0.10 seconds

Appearance: Normal

Consistent: Yes

Q-T interval: 0.52 seconds

5. AXIS

Quadrant: Normal

Degrees: +85° (I most isoelectric, slightly positive)

6. HYPERTROPHY

Atrial: Possible

Ventricular: No

7. MYOCARDIAL INFARCTION

Q waves: None significant

S-T displacement: 1 to 2 mm S-T elevation, V_{1-2}

8. ISCHEMIA

S-T displacement: S-T depression, II, III, V_{4-6}

9. POSSIBLE DRUG EFFECTS

None noted

10. ECG ANALYSIS

The atrial rate is 95 bpm, and the ventricular rate is 38 bpm. P waves are identified but they have no relationship with the QRS. In other words, the atria and ventricles are being conducted independently of one another and have their own rate and rhythm (complete AV dissociation or third degree heart block). No P-R interval is identified, however the QRS is WNL and the axis lies within the normal quadrant. Although the S-T segment in many leads is distorted by a P wave, S-T depression is noted in V_{5-6}, and there is slight S-T elevation noted in V_{1-2}.

11. INTERPRETATION

- Third degree block
- Inferior and anterolateral S-T and T wave abnormalities consistent with possible ischemia

1. RATE

Atrial: 90 bpm

Ventricular: 90 bpm

2. RHYTHM

Atrial: Regular

Ventricular: Regular

3. WAVES

P waves present: Yes

    Appearance: Wide in II, negative in V_1

    Consistent: Yes

    Relation to QRS: 1:1

Q waves present: No

    Leads:

    Pathological:

T waves present: Yes

    Morphology: Tall in chest leads

4. INTERVALS

P-R interval: 0.22 seconds

    Consistent: Yes

QRS: 0.16 seconds

    Appearance: Wide

    Consistent: Yes

Q-T interval: 0.36 seconds

5. AXIS

Quadrant: Left

Degrees: −75° (aVF and II negative, I and aVR most isoelectric)

6. HYPERTROPHY

Atrial: Probable

Ventricular: Probable

7. MYOCARDIAL INFARCTION

Q waves: None significant

S-T displacement: S-T elevation, V_{1-6}

8. ISCHEMIA

S-T displacement: No significant depression

9. POSSIBLE DRUG EFFECTS

None noted

10. ECG ANALYSIS

The rate is 90 bpm. Rhythm is regular. The P-R interval is greater than 0.20 seconds in duration indicating a first degree AVB. The QRS measures 0.16 seconds, a characteristic of an intraventricular conduction delay. A left anterior hemiblock is denoted by the negative net QRS deflections in aVF and II. The LAHB makes it difficult to tell if the IVCD is left or right, however, because of the deep S in V_1 the left bundle is probably involved. The P waves in lead II are 0.12 seconds in duration and in V_1 they are biphasic with a deep terminal component consistent with left atrial enlargement.

Probable evidence of left ventricular hypertrophy (LVH) exists using the Estes scoring system of 5 or more total points. Points are given for left ventricular strain [3 points], left axis deviation [2 points], left atrial enlargement [3 points], for a total of 8 points. In practice LVH is difficult to diagnose when LBBB is present. S-T elevation and tall T waves are observed in V_{1-6} probably secondary to LVH.

11. INTERPRETATION

Sinus rhythm

- Borderline first degree AVB
- LAHB
- Possible LBBB
- Probable left atrial enlargement
- Probable LVH

I. RATE

Atrial: Unable to identify, greater than or equal to 300 bpm

Ventricular: Variable, 54 to 140 bpm

2. RHYTHM

Atrial: Irregular

Ventricular: Irregular

3. WAVES

P waves present: Difficulty to identify, seen best in V_1

    Appearance: Fibrillation pattern

    Consistent: No

    Relation to QRS: None

Q waves present: No

    Leads:

    Pathological:

T waves present: Yes

    Morphology: Normal

4. INTERVALS

P-R interval:

    Consistent:

QRS: 0.08 seconds

    Appearance: Normal

    Consistent: Yes

Q-T interval: 0.36 seconds

5. AXIS

Quadrant: Normal

Degrees: +60° (aVL most isoelectric)

6. HYPERTROPHY

Atrial: No

Ventricular: No

7. MYOCARDIAL INFARCTION

Q waves: None significant

S-T displacement: No significant elevation

8. ISCHEMIA

S-T displacement: No significant depression

9. POSSIBLE DRUG EFFECTS

None noted

10. ECG ANALYSIS

The ventricular rate varies from 54 to 140 bpm. The atrial and ventricular rhythms are irregular, and the P waves in V_1 indicate a fibrillation pattern. QRS complexes and axis are WNL.

II. INTERPRETATION

Atrial fibrillation with variable ventricular response

1. RATE

Atrial: 82 bpm

Ventricular: 82 bpm

2. RHYTHM

Atrial: Underlying rhythm regular

Ventricular: Underlying rhythm regular

3. WAVES

P waves present: Yes

Appearance: Normal

Consistent: Yes

Relation to QRS: 1:1

Q waves present: Yes

Leads: III

Pathological: No

T waves present: Yes

Morphology: Inverted, I, aVL, V_{4-6}

4. INTERVALS

P-R interval: 0.20 seconds

Consistent: Yes

QRS: 0.08 seconds

Appearance: Normal

Consistent: Yes

Q-T interval: 0.36 seconds

5. AXIS

Quadrant: Normal

Degrees: +30° (III most isoelectric)

6. HYPERTROPHY

Atrial: No

Ventricular: No

7. MYOCARDIAL INFARCTION

Q waves: None significant

S-T displacement: No significant elevation

8. ISCHEMIA

S-T displacement: Diffuse S-T flattening

9. POSSIBLE DRUG EFFECTS

None noted

10. ECG ANALYSIS

The rate is 82 bpm. The rhythm is essentially regular and axis is WNL. The P-R interval measures 0.20 seconds, which is the criterion for a borderline first degree AV block. Diffuse, nondiagnostic S-T and T wave abnormalities are noted.

11. INTERPRETATION

Sinus rhythm

- Borderline first degree AV block
- Diffuse nondiagnostic S-T and T wave changes

1. RATE
Atrial: 55 bpm

Ventricular: 55 bpm

2. RHYTHM
Atrial: Regular

Ventricular: Regular

3. WAVES
P waves present: Yes

    Appearance: Normal

    Consistent: Yes

    Relation to QRS: 1:1

Q waves present: No

    Leads:

    Pathological:

T waves present: Yes

    Morphology: Normal

4. INTERVALS
P-R interval: 0.20 seconds

    Consistent: Yes

QRS: 0.10 seconds

    Appearance: rSR' in V_1

    Consistent: Yes

Q-T interval: 0.40 seconds

5. AXIS
Quadrant: Normal

Degrees: +60° (aVL most isoelectric)

6. HYPERTROPHY
Atrial: No

Ventricular: No

7. MYOCARDIAL INFARCTION
Q waves: None significant

S-T displacement: No significant elevation

8. ISCHEMIA
S-T displacement: No significant depression

9. POSSIBLE DRUG EFFECTS
None noted

10. ECG ANALYSIS
The rate is 55 bpm, rhythm is regular, and the axis is WNL. The P-R interval measures 0.20 seconds, consistent with a borderline first degree AVB. The QRS complex is slightly prolonged at 0.10 seconds. The prolonged QRS, in addition to the rSR' seen in V_1 is characteristic of an incomplete right bundle branch block.

11. INTERPRETATION
Sinus bradycardia

- Borderline first degree AV block
- Incomplete RBBB

I. RATE

Atrial: Difficult to identify

Ventricular: 210 bpm

2. RHYTHM

Atrial:

Ventricular: Yes

3. WAVES

P waves present: Difficult to identify, seen in V_1

Appearance: Fused

Consistent: No

Relation to QRS: Appear 1:1 in V_1

Q waves present: Yes

Leads: II, III, aVF

Pathological: Yes

T waves present: Yes

Morphology: Fused with QRS

4. INTERVALS

P-R interval:

Consistent:

QRS: 0.16 seconds

Appearance: R-S in V_{5-6}

Consistent: Yes

Q-T interval: Unable to identify

5. AXIS

Quadrant: Left anterior hemiblock

Degrees: −50° (aVF and II negative, II and aVR most isoelectric)

6. HYPERTROPHY

Atrial:

Ventricular: Possible

7. MYOCARDIAL INFARCTION

Q waves: II, III, aVF, V_1

S-T displacement: S-T elevation II, III, aVF

8. ISCHEMIA

S-T displacement: S-T depression I, aVL, V_{2-6}

9. POSSIBLE DRUG EFFECTS

None noted

10. ECG ANALYSIS

The ventricular rate is 210 bpm. The ventricular rhythm is regular. The QRS measures 0.16 seconds and an R-S is observed in V_{5-6}, characteristics of an LBBB. It is difficult to determine based only on the ECG tracing if this rhythm is ventricular or supraventricular because of the bundle branch block. Patient signs and symptoms would be most helpful in making a determination. Because the P waves are so clear in V_1, the rhythm is probably supraventricular. A left anterior hemiblock is evidenced by the net negative QRS deflections in aVF and II. Significant Q waves in II, III, and aVF are consistent with an old inferior MI, however the additional S-T elevation would imply a possible MI in progression. S-T depression is also noted in V_{2-6}, perhaps secondary to LBBB or reciprocal changes from an inferior MI.

II. INTERPRETATION

Supraventricular tachycardia

- LAHB
- LBBB
- Inferior MI, age indeterminate
- Diffuse S-T and T wave abnormalities, cannot rule out ischemia vs. acute injury

1. RATE

Atrial: 77 bpm

Ventricular: 77 bpm

2. RHYTHM

Atrial: Regular

Ventricular: Regular

3. WAVES

P waves present: Yes

Appearance: Biphasic V_1

Consistent: Yes

Relation to QRS: 1:1

Q waves present: No

Leads:

Pathological:

T waves present: Yes

Morphology: Inverted, I, aVL, V_{4-6}

4. INTERVALS

P-R interval: 0.18 seconds

Consistent: Yes

QRS: 0.08 seconds

Appearance: Increased voltage V_5

Consistent: Yes

Q-T interval: 0.36 seconds

5. AXIS

Quadrant: Normal

Degrees: +60° (aVL most isoelectric)

6. HYPERTROPHY

Atrial: No

Ventricular: Yes

7. MYOCARDIAL INFARCTION

Q waves: None significant

S-T displacement: No significant elevation

8. ISCHEMIA

S-T displacement: S-T depression I, II, aVF, aVL, V_{4-6}

9. POSSIBLE DRUG EFFECTS

None noted

10. ECG ANALYSIS

The rate is 77 bpm. The rhythm is regular, and the intervals and axis are within normal limits (WNL). The S wave in V_1 added to the R in V_5 equals 49 mV (greater than 35 mV indicates left ventricular hypertrophy). In addition, S-T depression is noted in leads V_{4-6}, I, II, and aVF. These findings are consistent with the LVH strain pattern indicating possible ischemia. The P wave in V_1 has a negative deflection implying left atrial enlargement. The P in lead II is less than 0.12 seconds, so supporting evidence for LAE is absent.

11. INTERPRETATION

Sinus rhythm

- LVH with strain pattern
- Cannot rule out LAE

1. RATE

Atrial: 63 bpm

Ventricular: 63 bpm

2. RHYTHM

Atrial: Regular

Ventricular: Regular

3. WAVES

P waves present: Yes

    Appearance: Normal

    Consistent: Yes

    Relation to QRS: 1:1

Q waves present: No

    Leads:

    Pathological:

T waves present: Yes

    Morphology: Abnormal

4. INTERVALS

P-R interval: 0.26 seconds

    Consistent: Yes

QRS: 0.16 seconds

    Appearance: High voltage

    Consistent: Yes

Q-T interval: 0.46 seconds

5. AXIS

Quadrant: Left

Degrees: $-10°$ (aVF, III most isoelectric)

6. HYPERTROPHY

Atrial: No

Ventricular: Yes

7. MYOCARDIAL INFARCTION

Q waves: None significant

S-T displacement: No significant elevation

8. ISCHEMIA

S-T displacement: Diffuse S-T depression

9. POSSIBLE DRUG EFFECTS

None noted

10. ECG ANALYSIS

The rate is 63 bpm, the rhythm is regular, and the axis is slightly left. The P-R interval is greater than 0.20 seconds indicating a first degree AVB. The QRS complex is greater than 0.12 seconds consistent with an intraventricular conduction delay. The prominent R-S in V_{5-6} would indicate an LBBB. The S in V_1 added to the R in V_5, equals 42 mV, and the R in aVL is greater than 12 mV. According to Estes scoring, LVH is "probable," however in practice it is difficult to diagnose LVH in the presence of an intraventricular conduction delay. The S-T segment in leads V_{4-6}, I, and aVL support a strain pattern. Left atrial enlargement is also possible because the P wave in II is greater than or equal to 0.12 seconds and the P in V_1 is biphasic.

11. INTERPRETATION

Sinus rhythm

- First degree AVB
- LAD
- LBBB
- Possible LVH with strain
- Possible LAE

ANALYSIS 4-3

1. RATE

Atrial: 98 bpm

Ventricular: 98 bpm

2. RHYTHM

Atrial: Regular

Ventricular: Regular

3. WAVES

P waves present: Yes

    Appearance: Normal

    Consistent: Yes

    Relation to QRS: 1:1

Q waves present: None significant

    Leads:

    Pathological:

T waves present: Yes

    Morphology: Inverted II, III aVF, V_{1-6}

4. INTERVALS

P-R interval: 0.18 seconds

    Consistent: Yes

QRS: 0.08 seconds

    Appearance: R greater than S in V_1

    Consistent: Yes

Q-T interval: 0.36 seconds

5. AXIS

Quadrant: Right

Degrees: +120° (aVR most isoelectric)

6. HYPERTROPHY

Atrial: No

Ventricular: Yes

7. MYOCARDIAL INFARCTION

Q waves: None significant

S-T displacement: No significant elevation

8. ISCHEMIA

S-T displacement: Diffuse S-T flattening

9. POSSIBLE DRUG EFFECTS

None noted

10. ECG ANALYSIS

The rate is 98 bpm, the rhythm is regular, and the intervals are WNL. The axis lies within the right quadrant. The R wave in V_1 has greater voltage than the S wave in the same lead, indicating RVH. Additional criteria for RVH includes the RAD and S-T and T wave abnormalities (strain pattern).

11. INTERPRETATION

Sinus rhythm

- Right axis deviation
- RVH with strain
- Diffuse nonspecific S-T and T wave changes possibly from second degree RVH

1. RATE

Atrial: 89 bpm

Ventricular: 89 bpm

2. RHYTHM

Atrial: Regular

Ventricular: Regular

3. WAVES

P waves present: Yes

    Appearance: Negative lead I

    Consistent: Yes

    Relation to QRS: 1:1

Q waves present: No

    Leads:

    Pathological:

T waves present: Yes

    Morphology: Abnormal

4. INTERVALS

P-R interval: 0.18 seconds

    Consistent: Yes

QRS: 0.10 seconds

    Appearance: High voltage, chest leads

    Consistent: Yes

Q-T interval: 0.36 seconds

5. AXIS

Quadrant: Normal

Degrees: +60° (aVL most isoelectric)

6. HYPERTROPHY

Atrial: No

Ventricular: Yes

7. MYOCARDIAL INFARCTION

Q waves: None significant

S-T displacement: 2 mm S-T elevation, V_1

8. ISCHEMIA

S-T displacement: S-T depression I, II, aVF, V_{4-6}

9. POSSIBLE DRUG EFFECTS

None noted

10. ECG ANALYSIS

The rate is 89 bpm, the rhythm is regular, and the intervals and axis are WNL. The S in V_1 plus the R in V_5 equals 47 mV, characteristic of LVH. Diffuse S-T abnormalities in I, II, aVF, V_{4-6} indicate probable LV strain pattern. The biphasic P wave in V_1 with prominent negative terminal component indicates possible left atrial enlargement.

11. INTERPRETATION

Sinus rhythm

- LVH with probable strain pattern
- Possible LAE

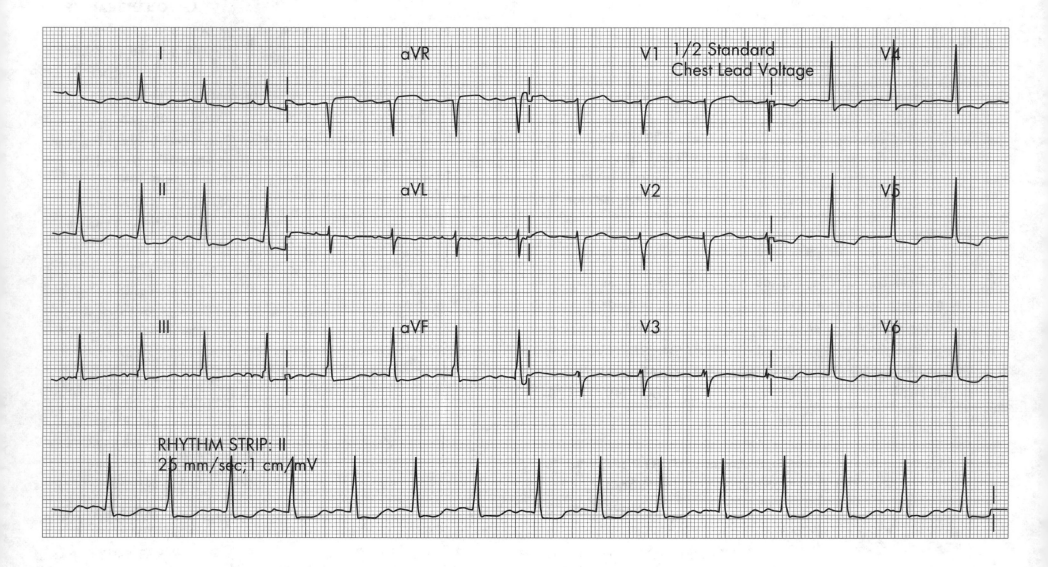

Figure 4-5
Resting 12-Lead ECG

468

1. RATE

Atrial: 92 bpm

Ventricular: 92 bpm

2. RHYTHM

Atrial: Regular

Ventricular: Regular

3. WAVES

P waves present: Yes

    Appearance: Normal

    Consistent: Yes

    Relation to QRS: 1:1

Q waves present: No

    Leads:

    Pathological:

T waves present: Yes

    Morphology: Abnormal

4. INTERVALS

P-R interval: 0.20 seconds

    Consistent: Yes

QRS: 0.08 seconds

    Appearance: High chest lead voltage

    Consistent: Yes

Q-T interval: 0.38 seconds

5. AXIS

Quadrant: Normal

Degrees: +60° (aVL most isoelectric)

6. HYPERTROPHY

Atrial: No

Ventricular: Yes

7. MYOCARDIAL INFARCTION

Q waves: None significant

S-T displacement: No significant elevation

8. ISCHEMIA

S-T displacement: S-T depression I, II, aVF, V_{4-6}

9. POSSIBLE DRUG EFFECTS

None noted

10. ECG ANALYSIS

The rate is 92 bpm, the rhythm is regular, and the axis is WNL. The P-R interval is 0.20 seconds, characteristic of a borderline first degree AVB. The other intervals are WNL. The voltage is noted to be half that of standard. With that in mind, it is evident that the S in V_1 plus the R in V_5 is greater than 35 mV, indicative of LVH. The S-T depression in I, II, aVF, and V_{4-6}, imply an LV strain pattern, however ischemia cannot be ruled out. Additionally, the poor R wave progression n V_{1-3} may indicate an old anteroseptal MI.

11. INTERPRETATION

Sinus rhythm

- Borderline first degree AVB
- LVH with strain vs. lateral ischemia
- Cannot rule out old anteroseptal MI

ANALYSIS 4-6

1. RATE
Atrial: 73 bpm

Ventricular: 73 bpm

2. RHYTHM
Atrial: Regular

Ventricular: Regular

3. WAVES
P waves present: Yes

Appearance: Negative V_1, greater than or equal to 0.12 seconds lead II

Consistent: Yes

Relation to QRS: 1:1

Q waves present: No

Leads:

Pathological:

T waves present: Yes

Morphology: Flat in limb leads

4. INTERVALS
P-R interval: 0.16 seconds

Consistent: Yes

QRS: 0.10 seconds

Appearance: High chest lead voltage

Consistent: Yes

Q-T interval: 0.44 seconds

5. AXIS
Quadrant: Left

Degrees: −10° (aVF most isoelectric, slightly negative)

6. HYPERTROPHY
Atrial: Possible

Ventricular: Yes

7. MYOCARDIAL INFARCTION
Q waves: None significant

S-T displacement: No significant elevation

8. ISCHEMIA
S-T displacement: S-T depression V_{5-6}

9. POSSIBLE DRUG EFFECTS
None noted

10. ECG ANALYSIS
The rate is 73 bpm, rhythm is regular, and intervals are WNL. The axis is left. The R waves in V_5 are greater than 35 mV, therefore LVH is evident. The S-T segment depression indicates probable LV strain pattern. The P wave in V_1 is negative and in lead II the P wave is greater than 0.12 seconds, which are characteristics of left atrial enlargement.

11. INTERPRETATION
Sinus rhythm
- LAD
- LVH with strain pattern
- Probable LAE

1. RATE

Atrial: 88 bpm

Ventricular: 88 bpm

2. RHYTHM

Atrial: Regular

Ventricular: Regular

3. WAVES

P waves present: Yes

    Appearance: Peaked in lead II (greater than or equal to 2.5 mV), biphasic V_1

    Consistent: Yes

    Relation to QRS: 1:1

Q waves present: No

    Leads:

    Pathological:

T waves present: Yes

    Morphology: Flat

4. INTERVALS

P-R interval: 0.16 seconds

    Consistent: Yes

QRS: 0.08 seconds

    Appearance: Normal

    Consistent: Yes

Q-T interval: 0.40 seconds

5. AXIS

Quadrant: Normal

Degrees: +60° (aVL most isoelectric)

6. HYPERTROPHY

Atrial: Yes

Ventricular: No

7. MYOCARDIAL INFARCTION

Q waves: None significant

S-T displacement: No significant elevation

8. ISCHEMIA

S-T displacement: Flat in I, II, III, aVF

9. POSSIBLE DRUG EFFECTS

None noted

10. ECG ANALYSIS

The rate is 88 bpm, rhythm is regular, and the intervals and axis are WNL. The P waves in lead II are tall (greater than or equal to 2.5 mV) and peaked, although in V_1, the P waves are biphasic. Both of these findings indicate right atrial enlargement. The S-T segment leads II, III, and aVF are flat. Baseline artifact is also noted.

11. INTERPRETATION

Sinus rhythm

- Right atrial enlargement (RAE)
- Nonspecific inferior S-T changes

1. RATE

Atrial: Unable to determine

Ventricular: Variable, 75 to 120 bpm

2. RHYTHM

Atrial: Irregular

Ventricular: Irregular

3. WAVES

P waves present: Difficult to identify, small P waves seen in aVF

    Appearance: Fibrillation pattern

    Consistent: No

    Relation to QRS: None

Q waves present: Yes

    Leads: III, V_2

    Pathological: II not significant, V_2 possibly significant

T waves present: Yes

    Morphology: Flat

4. INTERVALS

P-R interval:

    Consistent:

QRS: 0.08 seconds

    Appearance: Increased chest lead voltage

    Consistent: Yes

Q-T interval: 0.34 seconds

5. AXIS

Quadrant: Normal

Degrees: +30° (III most isoelectric)

6. HYPERTROPHY

Atrial: No

Ventricular: Probable

7. MYOCARDIAL INFARCTION

Q waves: V_2

S-T displacement: No significant elevation

8. ISCHEMIA

S-T displacement: Diffuse S-T flattening, S-T depression V_{4-6}

9. POSSIBLE DRUG EFFECTS

None noted

10. ECG ANALYSIS

The ventricular rate varies from 75 to 120 bpm. The rhythm is irregular and P waves are difficult to identify. Both are characteristic of atrial fibrillation. The QRS complex, Q-T interval, and axis are WNL. The S wave in V_1 measures 11 mV and the R in V_5 measures 24 mV. That total of 35 mV is borderline voltage criteria for LVH. Additionally, the R in aVL equals 7 mV (12 mV is significant for LVH). The S-T segments are flat or slightly depressed to further indicate LV strain. Poor R wave progression in V_{1-2} (significant Q in V_2) is possibly secondary to LVH or old anteroseptal MI.

11. INTERPRETATION

Atrial fibrillation with primarily controlled ventricular response

- Probable LVH with strain
- Cannot rule out old anteroseptal MI

1. **RATE**

   Atrial: 85 bpm

   Ventricular: 85 bpm

2. **RHYTHM**

   Atrial: Regular

   Ventricular: Regular

3. **WAVES**

   P waves present: Yes

       Appearance: Wide (greater than or equal to 0.12 seconds) and notched in lead II, biphasic in V_1

       Consistent: Yes

       Relation to QRS: 1:1

   Q waves present: Yes

       Leads: V_2

       Pathological: Yes

   T waves present: Yes

       Morphology: Inverted I, aVL, V_{5-6}

4. **INTERVALS**

   P-R interval: 0.18 seconds

       Consistent: Yes

   QRS: 0.08 seconds

       Appearance: Normal

       Consistent: Yes

   Q-T interval: 0.40 seconds

5. **AXIS**

   Quadrant: Normal

   Degrees: +65° (aVL most isoelectric, slightly negative)

6. **HYPERTROPHY**

   Atrial: Yes

   Ventricular: No

7. **MYOCARDIAL INFARCTION**

   Q waves: V_2

   S-T displacement: No significant elevation

8. **ISCHEMIA**

   S-T displacement: Flat S-T and T, I, aVL, V_{5-6}

9. **POSSIBLE DRUG EFFECTS**

   None noted

10. **ECG ANALYSIS**

    The rate is 85 bpm and regular, and the intervals and axis are WNL. The P waves in lead II are wide (greater than or equal to 0.12 seconds) and notched, and biphasic in V_1, both characteristics of LAE. Poor R wave progression in leads V_{1-3} indicates a possible old anteroseptal MI. The S-T segments in leads I, aVL, V_{5-6} are flat, although the T waves in the same leads are inverted, indicating a possibility of ischemia.

11. **INTERPRETATION**

    Sinus rhythm

    - Left atrial enlargement
    - Cannot rule out old anteroseptal MI
    - Nonspecific lateral S-T and T abnormalities

1. **RATE**

   Atrial: 108 bpm

   Ventricular: 108 bpm

2. **RHYTHM**

   Atrial: Regular

   Ventricular: Regular

3. **WAVES**

   P waves present: Yes

       Appearance: Tall (greater than or equal to 2.5 mV) in lead II,
   negative in lead V_1

       Consistent: Yes

       Relation to QRS: 1:1

   Q waves present: No

       Leads:

       Pathological:

   T waves present: Yes

       Morphology: Normal

4. **INTERVALS**

   P-R interval: 0.16 seconds

       Consistent: Yes

   QRS: 0.08 seconds

       Appearance: Normal

       Consistent: Yes

   Q-T interval: 0.32 seconds

5. **AXIS**

   Quadrant: Normal

   Degrees: +50° (aVL most isoelectric, slightly positive)

6. **HYPERTROPHY**

   Atrial: Yes

   Ventricular: No

7. **MYOCARDIAL INFARCTION**

   Q waves: None significant

   S-T displacement: No significant elevation

8. **ISCHEMIA**

   S-T displacement: No significant depression

9. **POSSIBLE DRUG EFFECTS**

   None noted

10. **ECG ANALYSIS**

    The rate is 108 bpm, the rhythm is regular, and the intervals and axis are WNL. The P waves in lead II are peaked and tall (greater than or equal to 2.5 mV), and in lead V_1 the P waves are primarily negative. Both of these findings are characteristic of right atrial enlargement.

11. **INTERPRETATION**

    Sinus tachycardia

    - Right atrial enlargement

1. RATE

Atrial: 100 bpm

Ventricular: 100 bpm

2. RHYTHM

Atrial: Regular

Ventricular: Regular

3. WAVES

P waves present: Yes

    Appearance: Negative in V_1, wide in II

    Consistent: Yes

    Relation to QRS: 1:1

Q waves present: No

    Leads:

    Pathological:

T waves present: Yes

    Morphology: Flat V_{5-6}

4. INTERVALS

P-R interval: 0.16 seconds

    Consistent: Yes

QRS: 0.08 seconds

    Appearance: High chest lead voltage

    Consistent: Yes

Q-T interval: 0.32 seconds

5. AXIS

Quadrant: Normal

Degrees: +20° (III most isoelectric, slightly negative)

6. HYPERTROPHY

Atrial: Yes

Ventricular: Yes

7. MYOCARDIAL INFARCTION

Q waves: None significant

S-T displacement: No significant elevation

8. ISCHEMIA

S-T displacement: 1 mm S-T depression, V_{4-6}

9. POSSIBLE DRUG EFFECTS

None noted

10. ECG ANALYSIS

The rate is 100 bpm, rhythm is regular, and the intervals and axis are WNL. The P waves in lead II are wide (greater than or equal to 0.12 seconds) and are negative in V_1 indicating LAE. The sum of the S in V_1 and the R in V_5 is greater than or equal to 35 mV, which is consistent with LVH. Additionally, the S-T segments in V_{5-6} are slightly depressed, and the T waves are flat implying possible LV strain. Poor R wave progression in V_{1-21} cannot rule out old anteroseptal MI.

11. INTERPRETATION

Sinus tachycardia

- LVH with possible strain
- LAE
- Cannot rule out old anteroseptal MI

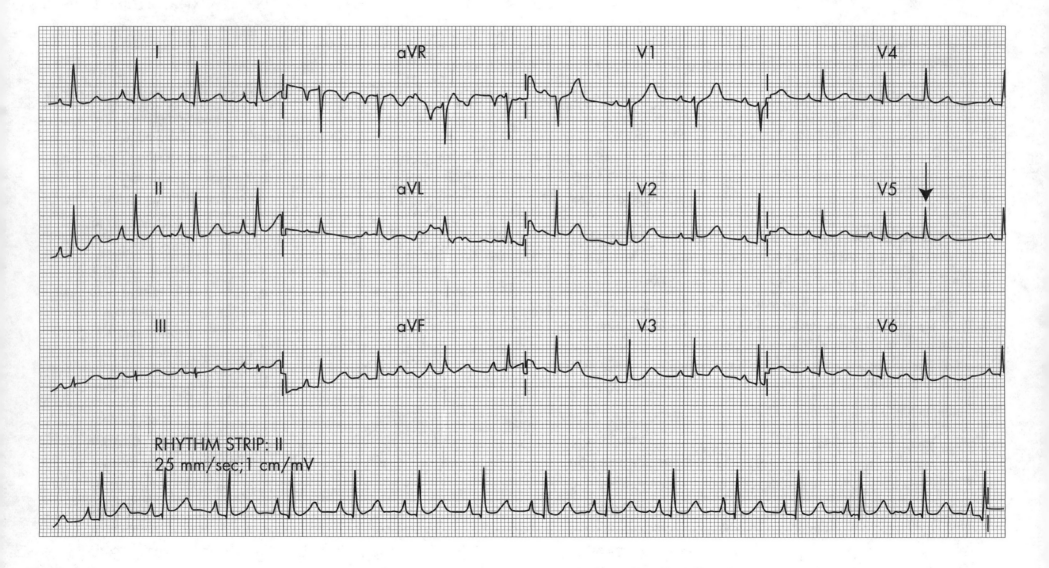

I aVR V1 V4

II aVL V2 V5

III aVF V3 V6

RHYTHM STRIP: II
25 mm/sec; 1 cm/mV

Figure 4-12
Resting 12-Lead ECG
476

1. RATE

Atrial: 92 bpm

Ventricular: 92 bpm

2. RHYTHM

Atrial: Underlying rhythm regular

Ventricular: Underlying rhythm regular

3. WAVES

P waves present: Yes

    Appearance: Tall and peaked in lead II

    Consistent: Yes

    Relation to QRS: 1:1 (exception: beat 3 V_{4-6})

Q waves present: Yes

    Leads: II

    Pathological: No

T waves present: Yes

    Morphology: Normal

4. INTERVALS

P-R interval: 0.16 seconds

    Consistent: Yes

QRS: 0.06 seconds

    Appearance: Normal

    Consistent: Yes

Q-T interval: 0.34 seconds

5. AXIS

Quadrant: Normal

Degrees: +30° (III most isoelectric)

6. HYPERTROPHY

Atrial: Yes

Ventricular: No

7. MYOCARDIAL INFARCTION

Q waves: None significant

S-T displacement: No significant elevation

8. ISCHEMIA

S-T displacement: No significant depression

9. POSSIBLE DRUG EFFECTS

None noted

10. ECG ANALYSIS

The rate is 92 bpm, the underlying rhythm is regular, and the intervals and axis are WNL. The P waves in lead II are tall (greater than or equal to 2.5 mV) and peaked indicating right atrial enlargement. However, there are no supporting criteria in V_1. Beat 3 in leads V_{4-6} is early, has a narrow complex, and is not preceded by a P wave, and therefore is probably junctional in origin. Baseline wandering is noted.

11. INTERPRETATION

Sinus rhythm

    • Possible RAE

    • PJC

1. RATE

Atrial: 122 bpm

Ventricular: 122 bpm

2. RHYTHM

Atrial: Regular

Ventricular: Regular

3. WAVES

P waves present: Yes

    Appearance: WNL

    Consistent: Yes

    Relation to QRS: 1:1

Q waves present: Yes

    Leads: II, III, aVF

    Pathological: Yes

T waves present: Yes

    Morphology: Abnormal

4. INTERVALS

P-R interval: 0.18 seconds

    Consistent: Yes

QRS: 0.08 seconds

    Appearance: R greater than S in V_1

    Consistent: Yes

Q-T interval: 0.32 seconds

5. AXIS

Quadrant: Normal

Degrees: +60° (aVL most isoelectric)

6. HYPERTROPHY

Atrial: No

Ventricular: Yes

7. MYOCARDIAL INFARCTION

Q waves: II, III, aVF

S-T displacement: No significant elevation

8. ISCHEMIA

S-T displacement: S-T depression, V_{1-4}

9. POSSIBLE DRUG EFFECTS

None noted

10. ECG ANALYSIS

The rate is 122 bpm, rhythm is regular, and the intervals and axis are WNL. Significant Q waves are observed in II, III, and aVF consistent with an old inferior MI. The R wave in V_1 exceeds the S voltage in the same lead indicating RVH or an old posterior MI. The S-T and T wave changes in leads V_{1-4} suggest ischemia, however are not diagnostic. Wandering baseline is also noted.

11. INTERPRETATION

Sinus tachycardia

- RVH vs. true posterior MI
- Old inferior MI

1. RATE

Atrial: 78 bpm

Ventricular: 78 bpm

2. RHYTHM

Atrial: Yes

Ventricular: Yes

3. WAVES

P waves present: Yes

Appearance: Wide (greater than or equal to 0. 2 seconds) in lead II, biphasic in lead V₁

Consistent: Yes

Relation to QRS: 1:1

Q waves present: No

Leads:

Pathological:

T waves present: Yes

Morphology: Normal

4. INTERVALS

P-R interval: 0.18 seconds

Consistent: Yes

QRS: 0.10 seconds

Appearance: Normal

Consistent: Yes

Q-T interval: 0.38 seconds

5. AXIS

Quadrant: Left anterior hemiblock

Degrees: −50° (leads aVF and II negative, aVR most isoelectric, slightly negative)

6. HYPERTROPHY

Atrial: Yes

Ventricular: No

7. MYOCARDIAL INFARCTION

Q waves: None significant

S-T displacement: No significant elevation

8. ISCHEMIA

S-T displacement: No significant depression

9. POSSIBLE DRUG EFFECTS

None noted

10. ECG ANALYSIS

The rate is 78 bpm, rhythm is regular, and the intervals are WNL. A left anterior hemiblock is denoted by the net negative QRS deflections in aVF and II. The P waves in lead II are wide (greater than 0.12 seconds) and biphasic in lead V₁, supporting criteria for left atrial enlargement.

11. INTERPRETATION

Sinus rhythm

- LAHB
- LAE

ANALYSIS 4-15

1. RATE

Atrial: 83 bpm

Ventricular: 83 bpm

2. RHYTHM

Atrial: Regular

Ventricular: Regular

3. WAVES

P waves present: Yes

    Appearance: Biphasic V_1

    Consistent: Yes

    Relation to QRS: 1:1

Q waves present: No

    Leads:

    Pathological:

T waves present: Yes

    Morphology: Abnormal

4. INTERVALS

P-R interval: 0.18 seconds

    Consistent: Yes

QRS: 0.10 seconds

    Appearance: High chest lead voltage

    Consistent: Yes

Q-T interval: 0.40 seconds

5. AXIS

Quadrant: Normal

Degrees: +60° (aVL most isoelectric)

6. HYPERTROPHY

Atrial: Possible

Ventricular: Yes

7. MYOCARDIAL INFARCTION

Q waves: None significant

S-T displacement: No significant elevation

8. ISCHEMIA

S-T displacement: Diffuse S-T depression

9. POSSIBLE DRUG EFFECTS

None noted

10. ECG ANALYSIS

The rate is 83 bpm, rhythm is regular, and the interval and axis are WNL. The P waves in V_1 are negative, which is a criterion for possible LAE. However, in lead II they appear normal, so supporting evidence is lacking. The sum of the S wave in lead V_1 and the R in V_5 is greater than 35 mV, indicating LVH. Diffuse S-T and T wave abnormalities imply LV strain. Some baseline artifact is noted.

11. INTERPRETATION

Sinus rhythm

- Possible LAE
- LVH with probable stain pattern

1. RATE

Atrial: 74 bpm

Ventricular: 74 bpm

2. RHYTHM

Atrial: Regular

Ventricular: Regular

3. WAVES

P waves present: Yes

    Appearance: Normal

    Consistent: Yes

    Relation to QRS: 1:1

Q waves present: Yes

    Leads: II, III, aVF, V_{1-3}

    Pathological: Yes

T waves present: Yes

    Morphology: Abnormal

4. INTERVALS

P-R interval: 0.20 seconds

    Consistent: Yes

QRS: 0.08 seconds

    Appearance: Normal

    Consistent: Yes

Q-T interval: 0.36 seconds

5. AXIS

Quadrant: Normal

Degrees: +10° (aVF most isoelectric, slightly positive)

6. HYPERTROPHY

Atrial: No

Ventricular: No

7. MYOCARDIAL INFARCTION

Q waves: II, III, aVF, V_{1-3}

S-T displacement: 4 to 5 mm S-T elevation V_{1-3}

8. ISCHEMIA

S-T displacement: No significant depression

9. POSSIBLE DRUG EFFECTS

None noted

10. ECG ANALYSIS

The rate is 74 bpm, the rhythm is regular, and the axis is within normal limits (WNL). The P-R interval measures 0.20 seconds denoting a borderline first degree AVB. Significant Q waves are noted in leads II, III and aVF indicating an old inferior MI. Significant Q waves **and** marked S-T elevation are seen in leads V_{1-3}, which are characteristic of an anteroseptal MI in progression.

11. INTERPRETATION

Sinus rhythm

- Borderline first degree AVB
- Old inferior MI
- Anteroseptal MI in progression

ANALYSIS 5-2

1. RATE
Atrial: 150 bpm

Ventricular: 150 bpm

2. RHYTHM
Atrial: Regular

Ventricular: Regular

3. WAVES
P waves present: Unable to identify

   Appearance:

   Consistent:

   Relation to QRS:

Q waves present: Yes

   Leads: II, III, aVF

   Pathological: No

T waves present: Yes

   Morphology: Abnormal

4. INTERVALS
P-R interval:

   Consistent:

QRS: 0.06 seconds

   Appearance: Normal

   Consistent: Yes

Q-T interval: 0.32 seconds

5. AXIS
Quadrant: Normal

Degrees: +80° (I most isoelectric, slightly positive)

6. HYPERTROPHY
Atrial: No

Ventricular: No

7. MYOCARDIAL INFARCTION
Q waves: None significant

S-T displacement: S-T elevation, aVR

8. ISCHEMIA
S-T displacement: Diffuse, significant S-T depression

9. POSSIBLE DRUG EFFECTS
None noted

10. ECG ANALYSIS
The ventricular rate is 150 bpm, the rhythm is regular, and the axis is WNL. No P waves are identifiable, but the QRS complexes are WNL, therefore the rhythm is initiated from above the ventricles (supraventricular tachycardia). There is diffuse, flat, S-T depression of greater than 2 mm indicating probable ischemia. Beat 6 in leads I to III, and I in leads V_{4-6} do not appear early, and are slightly wider than the normal complexes, but otherwise are very similar to the normal complexes. Thus they likely originate from the same focci as the normal complexes and are aberrantly conducted through the ventricles.

11. INTERPRETATION
Supraventricular tachycardia
- Probable diffuse ischemia
- Occasional aberrantly conducted complex

1. RATE

Atrial: 78 bpm

Ventricular: 78 bpm

2. RHYTHM

Atrial: Underlying rhythm regular

Ventricular: Underlying rhythm regular

3. WAVES

P waves present: Yes

   Appearance: Flat

   Consistent: Yes

   Relation to QRS: 1:1 except beat 3 in rhythm strip

Q waves present: Yes

   Leads: III, aVF

   Pathological: Yes

T waves present: Yes

   Morphology: Abnormal

4. INTERVALS

P-R interval: 0.22 seconds

   Consistent: Yes

QRS: 0.10 seconds

   Appearance: Abnormal

   Consistent: Yes

Q-T interval: 0.36 seconds

5. AXIS

Quadrant: Left

Degrees: −15° (aVF, II most isoelectric)

6. HYPERTROPHY

Atrial: No

Ventricular: No

7. MYOCARDIAL INFARCTION

Q waves: III, aVF

S-T displacement: Marked elevation III, aVF

8. ISCHEMIA

S-T displacement: Depression V_{2-6}, I, aVL

9. POSSIBLE DRUG EFFECTS

None noted

10. ECG ANALYSIS

The rate is 78 bpm, and the intervals and axis are WNL. The rhythm is regular with the exception of beats 3, 7, and 13 in the rhythm strip. Beat 3 appears early and the morphology of the complex is opposite of the normal, thus it is likely ventricular in origin. Following beat 6 and beat 12 in the rhythm strip, there is a noticeable sinus pause. The P-R interval measures 0.22 seconds indicating a first degree AVB. Q waves and marked S-T elevation of 4 to 5 mm are noted in III and aVF, characteristic of a recent MI in progress. The S-T depression in leads V_{2-6}, I, and aVL indicate probable lateral ischemia. Additionally, there is poor R wave progression in V_{1-3}.

11. INTERPRETATION

Sinus rhythm

- First degree AVB
- LAD
- Recent inferior MI in progression
- Probable lateral ischemia
- Cannot rule out old anteroseptal MI
- Occasional PVC
- Sinus pause × 2 of approximately 1 second

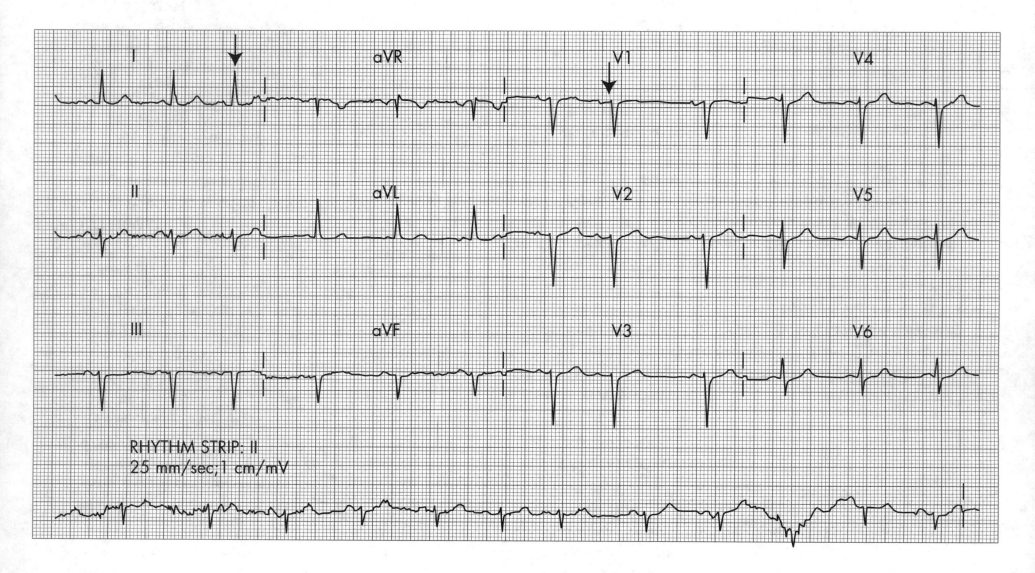

RHYTHM STRIP: II
25 mm/sec; 1 cm/mV

Figure 5-4
Resting 12-Lead ECG

484

I. RATE

Atrial: 74 bpm

Ventricular: 74 bpm

2. RHYTHM

Atrial: Underlying rhythm regular

Ventricular: Underlying rhythm regular

3. WAVES

P waves present: Yes

Appearance: Wide in II, biphasic V_1

Consistent: Yes

Relation to QRS: 1:1

Q waves present: No

Leads:

Pathological:

T waves present: Yes

Morphology: Normal

4. INTERVALS

P-R interval: 0.16 seconds

Consistent: Yes

QRS: 0.08 seconds

Appearance: Normal

Consistent: Yes

Q-T interval: 0.40 seconds

5. AXIS

Quadrant: Left anterior hemiblock

Degrees: −45° (leads aVF and II negative, II and aVR most isoelectric)

6. HYPERTROPHY

Atrial: Possible

Ventricular: No

7. MYOCARDIAL INFARCTION

Q waves: None significant

S-T displacement: No marked elevation

8. ISCHEMIA

S-T displacement: No significant depression

9. POSSIBLE DRUG EFFECTS

None noted

10. ECG ANALYSIS

The rate is 74 bpm, the rhythm is essentially regular, and the intervals are WNL. A left anterior hemiblock is denoted by a net negative QRS deflection in leads aVF and II. The P waves in lead II are greater than or equal to 0.12 seconds in duration and biphasic in V_1, characteristics of left atrial enlargement. Poor R wave progression in V_{1-3} is noted indicating a possible old anteroseptal MI. Beat 3 in leads I to III, and beat 2 in leads V_{1-3} are early, have a P wave, and have normal looking QRS complexes, and are likely atrial in origin.

II. INTERPRETATION

Sinus rhythm

- LAHB
- Cannot rule out old anteroseptal MI
- Possible LAE
- Occasional PAC

ANALYSIS 5-5

1. RATE
Atrial: 67 bpm

Ventricular: 67 bpm

2. RHYTHM
Atrial: Regular

Ventricular: Regular

3. WAVES
P waves present: Yes

    Appearance: Normal

    Consistent: Yes

    Relation to QRS: 1:1

Q waves present: Yes

    Leads: II, III, aVF

    Pathological: Yes

T waves present: Yes

    Morphology: Flat in inferior leads

4. INTERVALS
P-R interval: 0.18 seconds

    Consistent: Yes

QRS: 0.08 seconds

    Appearance: Normal

    Consistent: Yes

Q-T interval: 0.40 seconds

5. AXIS
Quadrant: Left

Degrees: −40° (leads aVF and II negative, II most isoelectric, slightly negative)

6. HYPERTROPHY
Atrial: No

Ventricular: No

7. MYOCARDIAL INFARCTION
Q waves: II, III, aVF

S-T displacement: No significant elevation

8. ISCHEMIA
S-T displacement: Flat S-T segments, III, aVF

9. POSSIBLE DRUG EFFECTS
None noted

10. ECG ANALYSIS
The rate is 67 bpm, the rhythm is regular, and the intervals are WNL. The mean QRS deflection in leads aVF and II is negative, which is characteristic of a left anterior hemiblock. Significant Q waves are noted in leads II, III, and aVF indicating an old inferior MI. The S-T segments and T waves in those leads are flat, implying some residual ischemia or that the MI is recent.

11. INTERPRETATION
Sinus rhythm

- LAHB
- Inferior MI, age indeterminate

1. RATE

Atrial: 98 bpm

Ventricular: 98 bpm

2. RHYTHM

Atrial: Regular

Ventricular: Regular

3. WAVES

P waves present: Yes

    Appearance: WNL

    Consistent: Yes

    Relation to QRS: 1:1

Q waves present: Yes

    Leads: II, III, aVF, V_{1-5}

    Pathological: Yes

T waves present: Yes

    Morphology: Flat in inferior leads

4. INTERVALS

P-R interval: 0.18 seconds

    Consistent: Yes

QRS: 0.09 seconds

    Appearance: WNL

    Consistent: Yes

Q-T interval: 0.32 seconds

5. AXIS

Quadrant: Left

Degrees: −20° (II most isoelectric, slightly positive)

6. HYPERTROPHY

Atrial: No

Ventricular: No

7. MYOCARDIAL INFARCTION

Q waves: II, III, aVF, V_{1-5}

S-T displacement: No significant elevation

8. ISCHEMIA

S-T displacement: Flat, II, III, aVF

9. POSSIBLE DRUG EFFECTS

None noted

10. ECG ANALYSIS

The rate is 98 bpm, the rhythm is regular, and the axis lies within the left quadrant. Significant Q waves are noted in leads II, III, aVF, and V_{1-5}, which is characteristic of old inferior, anterior, and anterolateral myocardial infarctions. Poor R wave progression in V_{1-2} indicates possible septal involvement. The inferior S-T segments are flat.

11. INTERPRETATION

Sinus tachycardia

- LAD
- Old inferior, anterior, anterolateral, and possible septal MI
- Nonspecific inferior S-T and T wave changes

I. RATE
Atrial: 66 bpm

Ventricular: 66 bpm

2. RHYTHM
Atrial: Regular

Ventricular: Regular

3. WAVES
P waves present: Yes

    Appearance: Normal

    Consistent: Yes

    Relation to QRS: 1:1

Q waves present: No

    Leads:

    Pathological:

T waves present: Yes

    Morphology: Tall, peaked, V_{2-4}

4. INTERVALS
P-R interval: 0.16 seconds

    Consistent: Yes

QRS: 0.08 seconds

    Appearance: WNL

    Consistent: Yes

Q-T interval: 0.44 seconds

5. AXIS
Quadrant: Normal

Degrees: +60° (aVL most isoelectric)

6. HYPERTROPHY
Atrial: No

Ventricular: No

7. MYOCARDIAL INFARCTION
Q waves: None significant

S-T displacement: Elevation, V_{1-3}

8. ISCHEMIA
S-T displacement: S-T depression V_6, II, III, aVF

9. POSSIBLE DRUG EFFECTS
None noted

10. ECG ANALYSIS
ECG #1 of 2. The rate is 66 bpm, the rhythm is regular, and the intervals and axis are WNL. Tall peaked T waves are evident in leads V_{1-4}, indicating a hyperacute anterior MI. The S-T depression seen in the low lateral and inferior leads probably indicates reciprocal changes.

II. INTERPRETATION
Sinus rhythm

    • Hyperacute anterior MI with reciprocal S-T depression

1. RATE

Atrial: 92 bpm

Ventricular: 92 bpm

2. RHYTHM

Atrial: Regular

Ventricular: Regular

3. WAVES

P waves present: Yes

Appearance: WNL

Consistent: Yes

Relation to QRS: 1:1

Q waves present: Yes

Leads: V_2

Pathological: Yes

T waves present: Yes

Morphology: Elevated, slurred with S-T segment

4. INTERVALS

P-R interval: 0.14 seconds

Consistent: Yes

QRS: 0.10 seconds

Appearance: Slurred with S-T segment

Consistent: Yes

Q-T interval: 0.32 seconds

5. AXIS

Quadrant: Left anterior hemiblock

Degrees: −75° (aVF and II negative, aVR and I most isoelectric)

6. HYPERTROPHY

Atrial: No

Ventricular: No

7. MYOCARDIAL INFARCTION

Q waves: New Q wave in V_2

S-T displacement: Marked elevation, V_{1-4}, elevation I, aVL

8. ISCHEMIA

S-T displacement: Depressed II, III, aVF, V_6

9. POSSIBLE DRUG EFFECTS

None noted

10. ECG ANALYSIS

ECG #2 of 2, taken 4 hours after #1. The rate is 92 bpm, the rhythm is regular, and the intervals are WNL. The net QRS deflection in aVF and II is negative, indicating the axis has moved more to the left than in tracing #1, and there is now an LAHB. The S-T segment has elevated more than the previous tracing, and the T waves have become less prominent. S-T depression in II, III, and aVF continues.

11. INTERPRETATION

Sinus rhythm

- LAHB
- Acute anterior MI
- Marked S-T depression, cannot rule out inferior subendocardial injury

ANALYSIS 5-9

1. RATE
Atrial: 74 bpm

Ventricular: 74 bpm

2. RHYTHM
Atrial: Regular

Ventricular: Regular

3. WAVES
P waves present: Yes

    Appearance: WNL

    Consistent: Yes

    Relation to QRS: 1:1

Q waves present: Yes

    Leads: II, III, aVF

    Pathological: Yes

T waves present: Yes

    Morphology: Inverted in II, III, aVF

4. INTERVALS
P-R interval: 0.16 seconds

    Consistent: Yes

QRS: 0.10 Seconds

    Appearance: WNL

    Consistent: Yes

Q-T interval: 0.38 seconds

5. AXIS
Quadrant: Left

Degrees: −30° (aVF negative, II most isoelectric)

6. HYPERTROPHY
Atrial: No

Ventricular: No

7. MYOCARDIAL INFARCTION
Q waves: II, III, aVF

S-T displacement: No significant elevation

8. ISCHEMIA
S-T displacement: No significant depression

9. POSSIBLE DRUG EFFECTS
None noted

10. ECG ANALYSIS
The rate is 74 bpm, the rhythm is regular, and the intervals are WNL. The axis lies within the left quadrant. Significant Q waves are noted in leads II, III, and aVF with T wave inversion remaining, indicating an inferior MI, (probably recent).

11. INTERPRETATION
Sinus rhythm

- LAD
- Inferior MI, age indeterminate

I. RATE

Atrial: 94 bpm

Ventricular: 94 bpm

2. RHYTHM

Atrial: Regular

Ventricular: Regular

3. WAVES

P waves present: Yes

    Appearance: WNL

    Consistent: Yes

    Relation to QRS: 1:1

Q waves present: Yes

    Leads: V_2

    Pathological: No

T waves present: Yes

Morphology: Inverted V_{1-2}

4. INTERVALS

P-R interval: 0.18 seconds

    Consistent: Yes

QRS: 0.12 seconds

    Appearance: RS in V_1, rSR' in V_2

    Consistent: Yes

Q-T interval: 0.40 seconds

5. AXIS

Quadrant: Left anterior hemiblock

Degrees: −60° (aVF and II negative, aVR most isoelectric)

6. HYPERTROPHY

Atrial: No

Ventricular: Possible

7. MYOCARDIAL INFARCTION

Q waves: None significant

S-T displacement: No marked elevation

8. ISCHEMIA

S-T displacement: S-T depression, V_{1-2}

9. POSSIBLE DRUG EFFECTS

None noted

10. ECG ANALYSIS

The rate is 94 bpm, and the rhythm is regular. The net QRS deflections in aVF and II are negative, indicating a left anterior hemiblock. The QRS complex is long (0.12 seconds). In leads V_{1-2} note the ventricular depolarization complexes are an R-S and rSR', respectively, indicating an RBBB. In this situation it is difficult to distinguish an RBBB from an old "true" posterior MI (ECG criteria being R greater than S in V_1). If a true RBBB exists in addition to the LAHB, a bifascicular block is also present. The R wave progression through leads V_{1-3} is poor, implying a possible old anteroseptal MI. Additionally, the R wave in aVL is greater than or equal to 12 mV, an additional criterion for LVH, although other voltage criteria do not occur.

11. INTERPRETATION

Sinus rhythm

- LAHB
- Old posterior MI vs. RBBB
- Possible bifascicular block (LAHB + RBBB)
- Possible old anteroseptal MI
- Probable LVH

1. RATE

Atrial: 98 bpm

Ventricular: 98 bpm

2. RHYTHM

Atrial: Regular

Ventricular: Regular

3. WAVES

P waves present: Yes

    Appearance: WNL

    Consistent: Yes

    Relation to QRS: 1:1

Q waves present: Yes

    Leads: V_{1-3}

    Pathological: Yes

T waves present: Yes

    Morphology: Elevated

4. INTERVALS

P-R interval: 0.16 seconds

    Consistent: Yes

QRS: 0.06 seconds

    Appearance: Low voltage

    Consistent: Yes

Q-T interval: 0.32 seconds

5. AXIS

Quadrant: Normal horizontal

Degrees: 0° (aVF isoelectric)

6. HYPERTROPHY

Atrial: No

Ventricular: No

7. MYOCARDIAL INFARCTION

Q waves: V_{1-3}

S-T displacement: 1 to 2 mm S-T elevation, V_{2-4}

8. ISCHEMIA

S-T displacement: Flat S-T, I, V_{5-6}

9. POSSIBLE DRUG EFFECTS

None noted

10. ECG ANALYSIS

The rate is 98 bpm, the rhythm is regular, and the intervals and axis are WNL. Significant Q waves are evident in leads V_{1-4} along with S-T elevation in V_{2-4}, indicating an acute anterior MI in progression. Without patient history it is difficult to determine the age of the MI. The QRS voltage is low throughout.

11. INTERPRETATION

Sinus tachycardia

- Anterior MI, possibly acute

1. RATE

Atrial: 90 bpm

Ventricular: 90 bpm

2. RHYTHM

Atrial: Regular

Ventricular: Regular

3. WAVES

P waves present: Yes

    Appearance: Greater than or equal to 0.12 seconds in II,

        negative in V_1

    Consistent: Yes

    Relation to QRS: 1:1

Q waves present: Yes

    Leads: II, III, aVF

    Pathological: Yes

T waves present: Yes

    Morphology: WNL

4. INTERVALS

P-R interval: 0.18 seconds

    Consistent: Yes

QRS: 0.08 seconds

    Appearance: WNL

    Consistent: Yes

Q-T interval: 0.32 seconds

5. AXIS

Quadrant: Left

Degrees: −30° (II most isoelectric)

6. HYPERTROPHY

Atrial: Probable

Ventricular: No

7. MYOCARDIAL INFARCTION

Q waves: II, III, aVF

S-T displacement: No significant elevation

8. ISCHEMIA

S-T displacement: 1 mm S-T depression V_5

9. POSSIBLE DRUG EFFECTS

None noted

10. ECG ANALYSIS

The rate is 90 bpm, the rhythm is regular, and the intervals and axis are WNL. The P waves in lead II are greater than or equal to 0.12 seconds in duration, and the P waves in V_1 are negative, indicating LAE. Significant Q waves are noted in leads II, III, and aVF, which is characteristic of an old inferior MI. An artifact is noted on the rhythm strip and in the limb leads.

11. INTERPRETATION

Sinus rhythm

- LAD
- LAE
- Old inferior MI

ANALYSIS 5-13

1. RATE
Atrial: 40 to 65 bpm

Ventricular: 40 to 65 bpm

2. RHYTHM
Atrial: Irregular

Ventricular: Irregular

3. WAVES
P waves present: Yes

    Appearance: WNL

    Consistent: Yes

    Relation to QRS: 1:1

Q waves present: Yes

    Leads: V_{1-4}

    Pathological: Yes

T waves present: Yes

    Morphology: Inverted V_{1-5}

4. INTERVALS
P-R interval: 0.20 seconds

    Consistent: Yes

QRS: 0.08 seconds

    Appearance: Q-S in V_{1-4}

    Consistent: Yes

Q-T interval: 0.40 seconds

5. AXIS
Quadrant: Normal

Degrees: +15° (III, aVF most isoelectric)

6. HYPERTROPHY
Atrial: Possible

Ventricular: No

7. MYOCARDIAL INFARCTION
Q waves: V_{1-4}

S-T displacement: No significant elevation

8. ISCHEMIA
S-T displacement: Diffuse S-T flattening

9. POSSIBLE DRUG EFFECTS
None noted

10. ECG ANALYSIS
The rate varies in a rhythmic fashion from 40 to 65 bpm, which is consistent with sinus arrhythmia. Intervals and axis are WNL. The P waves in lead V_1 are inverted, however in lead II they appear normal, therefore consider LAE. Significant Q waves are found in leads V_{1-4} indicating an anteroseptal MI. The T waves in those leads remain inverted, thus the infarction is probably recent. The S-T segments throughout are flat.

11. INTERPRETATION
Sinus arrhythmia

- Recent anteroseptal MI
- Diffuse nonspecific S-T abnormalities
- Possible LAE

1. RATE

Atrial: 78 bpm

Ventricular: 78 bpm

2. RHYTHM

Atrial: Regular

Ventricular: Regular

3. WAVES

P waves present: Yes

   Appearance: WNL

   Consistent: Yes

   Relation to QRS: 1:1

Q waves present: Yes

   Leads: II, III, aVF

   Pathological: Yes

T waves present: Yes

   Morphology: WNL

4. INTERVALS

P-R interval: 0.16 seconds

   Consistent: Yes

QRS: 0.08 seconds

   Appearance: WNL

   Consistent: Yes

Q-T interval: 0.38 seconds

5. AXIS

Quadrant: Left anterior hemiblock

Degrees: −40° (aVF and II negative, II most isoelectric,
   slightly negative)

6. HYPERTROPHY

Atrial: No

Ventricular: No

7. MYOCARDIAL INFARCTION

Q waves: II, III, aVF

S-T displacement: No significant elevation

8. ISCHEMIA

S-T displacement: No significant depression

9. POSSIBLE DRUG EFFECTS

None noted

10. ECG ANALYSIS

The rate is 78 bpm, the rhythm is regular, and the intervals are WNL. The mean QRS deflections in leads aVF and II are negative, indicating a left anterior hemiblock. In leads II, III, and aVF pathological Q waves are found; these are characteristic of an old inferior MI.

11. INTERPRETATION

Sinus rhythm

   • LAHB

   • Old inferior MI

1. RATE

Atrial: 140 bpm

Ventricular: 140 bpm

2. RHYTHM

Atrial: Regular

Ventricular: Regular

3. WAVES

P waves present: Fused with preceding T

Appearance: Best seen in V_1

Consistent: Appear to be

Relation to QRS: Appear 1:1

Q waves present: No

Leads:

Pathological:

T waves present: Yes

Morphology: Elevated

4. INTERVALS

P-R interval:

Consistent:

QRS: 0.08 seconds

Appearance: Fused to S-T segments in chest leads

Consistent: Yes

Q-T interval: 0.28 seconds

5. AXIS

Quadrant: Normal

Degrees: +70° (aVL most isoelectric, slightly negative)

6. HYPERTROPHY

Atrial: No

Ventricular: No

7. MYOCARDIAL INFARCTION

Q waves: No

S-T displacement: Marked elevation, V_{1-5}

8. ISCHEMIA

S-T displacement: Depression, I and aVL

9. POSSIBLE DRUG EFFECTS

None noted

10. ECG ANALYSIS

The ventricular rate is 140 bpm, the rhythm is regular, and the axis is WNL. The P waves are fused with the preceding T waves. The QRS complexes are not wide, thus the beat is most likely initiated from above the ventricles. Because the rate is less than 160 bpm, the rhythm is termed sinus tachycardia. Marked S-T elevation is noted in leads V_{1-5}, which is characteristic of an acute anterolateral MI.

A 1 mm S-T depression is also noted in I and aVL, which is possibly an ischemic response or a reciprocal change. Poor R wave progression in V_{1-5} indicates possible extended involvement. The QRS voltage is low throughout.

11. INTERPRETATION

Sinus tachycardia

- Acute anterolateral MI
- Low QRS voltage indicating possible chronic pulmonary disease

1. RATE

Atrial: Unable to identify

Ventricular: 90 bpm

2. RHYTHM

Atrial: Unable to identify

Ventricular: 90 bpm

3. WAVES

P waves present: No

Appearance:

Consistent:

Relation to QRS:

Q waves present: Yes

Leads: II, III, aVF, V_{1-6}

Pathological: Yes

T waves present: Yes

Morphology: Elevated

4. INTERVALS

P-R interval:

Consistent:

QRS: 0.14 seconds

Appearance: rSR' in V_{1-2}

Consistent: Yes

Q-T interval: 0.40 seconds

5. AXIS

Quadrant: Normal

Degrees: +30° (III most isoelectric)

6. HYPERTROPHY

Atrial: No

Ventricular: No

7. MYOCARDIAL INFARCTION

Q waves: II, III, aVF, V_{1-5}

S-T displacement: Marked elevation, V_{1-5}, I, II

8. ISCHEMIA

S-T displacement: I mm S-T depression, V_6

9. POSSIBLE DRUG EFFECTS

None noted

10. ECG ANALYSIS

The ventricular is rate 90 bpm, and the rhythm is regular. The QRS measures 0.14 seconds indicating an intraventricular delay. The rSR' in V_{1-2} is the criterion for an RBBB. No P waves can be identified, so the rhythm is initiated from the junction, although the rate is somewhat accelerated. If the rhythm was ventriculer, the QRS complexes in the limb leads would be wider and appear unusual. The axis is WNL. The Q waves in III and aVF are probably significant, characteristic of an old inferior infarction. Q waves in V_{1-5} are beginning to develop in response to the acute injury denoted by the marked S-T elevation.

11. INTERPRETATION

Accelerated junctional rhythm

- RBBB
- Cannot rule out old inferior MI
- Acute anterolateral MI with reciprocal S-T depression

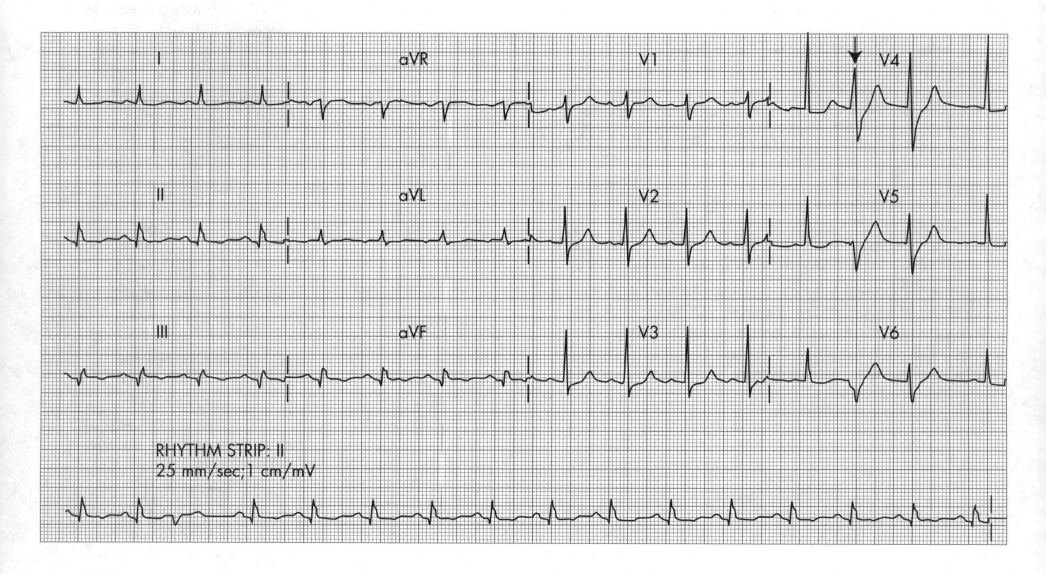

I aVR V1 V4

II aVL V2 V5

III aVF V3 V6

RHYTHM STRIP: II
25 mm/sec; 1 cm/mV

Figure 5-17
Resting 12-Lead ECG
498

1. RATE

Atrial: 94 bpm

Ventricular: 94 bpm

2. RHYTHM

Atrial: Regular

Ventricular: Regular

3. WAVES

P waves present: Yes

    Appearance: WNL

    Consistent: Yes

    Relation to QRS: 1:1

Q waves present: Yes

    Leads: II, III, aVF

    Pathological: Yes

T waves present: Yes

    Morphology: WNL

4. INTERVALS

P-R interval: 0.16 seconds

    Consistent: Yes

QRS: 0.10 seconds

    Appearance: R is greater than or equal to S in V_1

    Consistent: Yes

Q-T interval: 0.32 seconds

5. AXIS

Quadrant: Normal

Degrees: +40° (III most isoelectric, slightly positive)

6. HYPERTROPHY

Atrial: No

Ventricular:

7. MYOCARDIAL INFARCTION

Q waves: II, III, aVF

S-T displacement: No significant elevation

8. ISCHEMIA

S-T displacement: J-point depression, V_{5-6}

9. POSSIBLE DRUG EFFECTS

None noted

10. ECG ANALYSIS

The rate is 94 bpm, the rhythm is regular, and the intervals and axis are WNL. Pathological Q waves are noted in the inferior leads, which is consistent with an old inferior MI. The R wave is equal to the S in V_1, indicating either borderline RVH or a true posterior MI. In this setting (i.e., with an inferior MI) it is appropriate to think posterior MI. Beats 2 and 3 in V_{4-6} are early and are wide, thus probably ventricular in origin.

11. INTERPRETATION

Sinus rhythm

- Old inferior MI
- Possible old posterior MI vs. RVH
- Coupled multifocal PVC

ANALYSIS 5-18

1. RATE

Atrial: 94 bpm

Ventricular: 94 bpm

2. RHYTHM

Atrial: Regular

Ventricular: Regular

3. WAVES

P waves present: Yes

    Appearance: Negative in V_1

    Consistent: Yes

    Relation to QRS: 1:1

Q waves present: Yes

    Leads: V_{1-4}

    Pathological: Yes

T waves present: Yes

    Morphology: Inverted, I, aVL, $V_{1,2,4,5}$

4. INTERVALS

P-R interval: 0.16 seconds

    Consistent: Yes

QRS: 0.06 seconds

    Appearance: QS in V_{1-4}

    Consistent: Yes

Q-T interval: 0.34 seconds

5. AXIS

Quadrant: Left

Degrees: −30° (aVF negative, II most isoelectric)

6. HYPERTROPHY

Atrial: No

Ventricular: No

7. MYOCARDIAL INFARCTION

Q waves: V_{1-4}

S-T displacement: 1 to 3 mm S-T elevation, V_{2-3}

8. ISCHEMIA

S-T displacement: S-T flat, I, aVL, V_{4-6}

9. POSSIBLE DRUG EFFECTS

None noted

10. ECG ANALYSIS

The rate is 94 bpm, the rhythm is regular, and the intervals are WNL. The axis lies within the left quadrant. The P wave in V_1 is negative, however there is no supporting evidence of LAE in lead II. Marked Q waves in leads V_{1-4} with S-T elevation indicate an acute anterior MI, probably recent. Possible ischemia is also indicated by S-T depression and T wave inversion in V_{4-6}, I, and aVL.

11. INTERPRETATION

Sinus rhythm

- LAD
- Anterior MI, probably recent
- Nonspecific lateral S-T and T wave abnormalities, possible ischemia

I. RATE

Atrial: 68 bpm

Ventricular: 68 bpm

2. RHYTHM

Atrial: Regular

Ventricular: Regular

3. WAVES

P waves present: Yes

    Appearance: Negative V_1

    Consistent: Yes

    Relation to QRS: 1:1

Q waves present: Yes

    Leads: III, aVF

    Pathological: Yes

T waves present: Yes

    Morphology: Flat, inverted, I, aVL, V_{2-6}

4. INTERVALS

P-R interval: 0.20 seconds

    Consistent: Yes

QRS: 0.08 seconds

    Appearance: WNL

    Consistent: Yes

Q-T interval: 0.34 seconds

5. AXIS

Quadrant: Normal

Degrees: 0° (aVF most isoelectric)

6. HYPERTROPHY

Atrial: No

Ventricular: No

7. MYOCARDIAL INFARCTION

Q waves: III, aVF

S-T displacement: No significant elevation

8. ISCHEMIA

S-T displacement: 1 mm S-T depression, V_{3-6}

9. POSSIBLE DRUG EFFECTS

None noted

10. ECG ANALYSIS

The rate is 68 bpm, the rhythm is regular, and the axis is WNL. The P-R interval is 0.20 seconds indicating a borderline first degree AVB. The P wave in V_1 is negative, however there is no supporting evidence of LAE in lead II. The Q waves in leads III and aVF are significant, but there is no Q in lead II, making the diagnosis of old inferior MI more difficult. The S-T depression and T wave inversion in V_{3-6}, I, and aVL are nonspecific.

11. INTERPRETATION:

Sinus rhythm

- Borderline first degree AVB
- Possible old inferior MI
- Nonspecific anterolateral S-T and T wave abnormalities

1. RATE

Atrial: 122 bpm

Ventricular: 122 bpm

2. RHYTHM

Atrial: Regular

Ventricular: Regular

3. WAVES

P waves present: Yes

Appearance: Tall, peaked in II

Consistent: Yes

Relation to QRS: 1:1

Q waves present: Yes

Leads: II, III, aVF

Pathological: Yes

T waves present: Yes

Morphology: Flat

4. INTERVALS

P-R interval: 0.12 seconds

Consistent: Yes

QRS: 0.08 seconds

Appearance: WNL

Consistent: Yes

Q-T interval: 0.32 seconds

5. AXIS

Quadrant: Indeterminate

Degrees: Each limb lead appears isoelectric

6. HYPERTROPHY

Atrial: Right

Ventricular: No

7. MYOCARDIAL INFARCTION

Q waves: II, III, aVF

S-T displacement: No significant elevation

8. ISCHEMIA

S-T displacement: Diffuse flattening

9. POSSIBLE DRUG EFFECTS

None noted

10. ECG ANALYSIS

The rate is 122 bpm, with a regular rhythm, and the intervals are WNL. The axis is indeterminate because each of the limb leads is isoelectric. The P waves in II are tall and peaked, indicating right atrial enlargement. The significant Q waves in II, III, and aVF are consistent with a possible old inferior MI. There is diffuse nondiagnostic S-T flattening and low limb lead voltage.

11. INTERPRETATION:

Sinus tachycardia

- RAE
- Probable old inferior MI
- Nondiagnostic S-T and T wave changes

1. RATE

Atrial: 122 bpm

Ventricular: 122 bpm

2. RHYTHM

Atrial: Regular

Ventricular: Regular

3. WAVES

P waves present: Yes

    Appearance: WNL

    Consistent: Yes

    Relation to QRS: 1:1

Q waves present: Yes

    Leads: II, III, aVF

    Pathological: Yes

T waves present: Yes

    Morphology: Abnormal

4. INTERVALS

P-R interval: 0.18 seconds

    Consistent: Yes

QRS: 0.08 seconds

    Appearance: R greater than S in V_1

    Consistent: Yes

Q-T interval: 0.32 seconds

5. AXIS

Quadrant: Normal

Degrees: +60° (aVL most isoelectric, slightly positive)

6. HYPERTROPHY

Atrial: No

Ventricular: Possible

7. MYOCARDIAL INFARCTION

Q waves: II, III, aVF

S-T displacement: 1 mm S-T elevation III, aVF

8. ISCHEMIA

S-T displacement: 1-2 mm S-T depression, V_{1-4}

9. POSSIBLE DRUG EFFECTS

None noted

10. ECG ANALYSIS

The rate is 122 bpm, the rhythm is regular, and the intervals and axis are WNL. Significant Q waves are found in II, III, and aVF, which is consistent with an old inferior MI. The R in V_1 is greater than the S indicating either an old posterior MI or RVH. Because of the inferior infarction, it is reasonable to lean toward a posterior MI. The S-T and T wave changes in leads V_{1-4}, although not diagnostic, suggest ischemia. Also the baseline artifact is noted.

11. INTERPRETATION

Sinus tachycardia

- Old inferior MI
- Possible old posterior MI vs. RVH
- Nonspecific anteroseptal S-T and T wave changes

ANALYSIS 5-22

1. RATE

Atrial: 84 bpm

Ventricular: 84 bpm

2. RHYTHM

Atrial: Regular

Ventricular: Regular

3. WAVES

P waves present: Yes

    Appearance: WNL

    Consistent: Yes

    Relation to QRS: 1:1

Q waves present: Yes

    Leads: II, III, aVF

    Pathological: Yes

T waves present: Yes

    Morphology: Deeply inverted V_{3-5}

4. INTERVALS

P-R interval: 0.18 seconds

    Consistent: Yes

QRS: 0.08 seconds

    Appearance: Low voltage

    Consistent: Yes

Q-T interval: 0.40 seconds

5. AXIS

Quadrant: Left anterior hemiblock

Degrees: −45° (aVf and II negative, II and aVR most isoelectric)

6. HYPERTROPHY

Atrial: No

Ventricular: No

7. MYOCARDIAL INFARCTION

Q waves: II, III, aVF

S-T displacement: Deep symmetrical T waves V_{3-4}

8. ISCHEMIA

S-T displacement: Deep symmetrical T waves V_{3-4}

9. POSSIBLE DRUG EFFECTS

None noted

10. ECG ANALYSIS

The rate is 84 bpm, the rhythm is regular, and the intervals are WNL. The net QRS deflections in leads aVF and II are negative, denoting an LAHB. The significant Q waves in leads II, III, and aVF indicate an old inferior MI. Deep T wave inversion in V_{3-4} is characteristic of anterior, subendocardial injury. The S-T and T waves in the lateral leads are nondiagnostic, but flat, implying ischemia. Additionally, low limb lead voltage is noted.

11. INTERPRETATION

Sinus rhythm

- LAHB
- Old inferior MI
- Acute anterior subendocardial infarction
- Low limb lead voltage

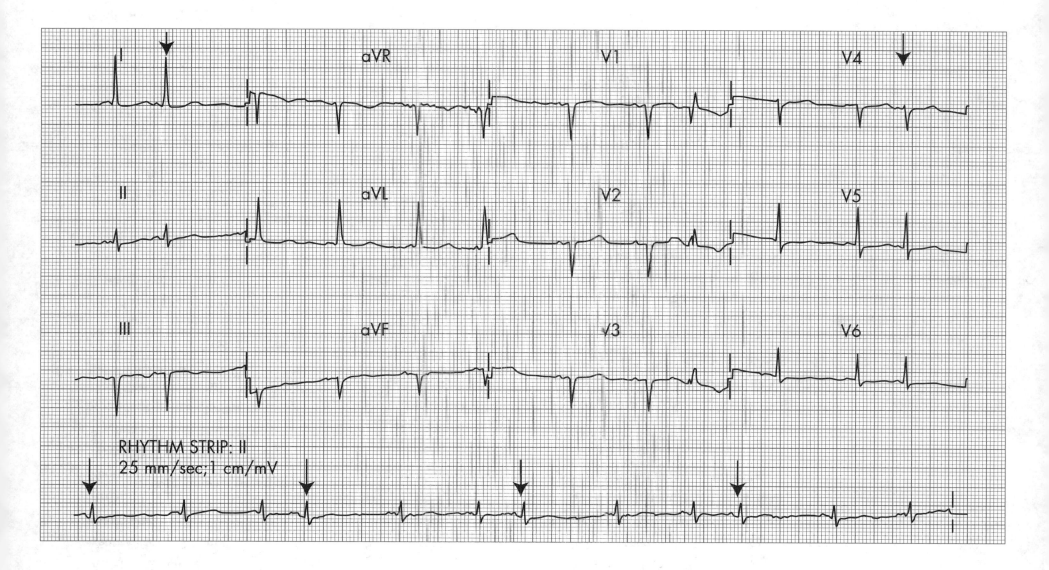

RHYTHM STRIP: II
25 mm/sec;1 cm/mV

Figure 5-23
Resting 12-Lead ECG

505

I. RATE

Atrial: 72 bpm

Ventricular: 72 bpm

2. RHYTHM

Atrial: Irregular

Ventricular: Irregular

3. WAVES

P waves present: Yes

    Appearance: WNL

    Consistent: Yes

    Relation to QRS: 1:1

Q waves present: Yes

    Leads: II, V_{2-3}

    Pathological: Yes

T waves present: Yes

    Morphology: Flat

4. INTERVALS

P-R interval: 0.14 seconds

    Consistent: No

QRS: 0.08 seconds

    Appearance: QS in V_{2-3}, III

    Consistent: Yes

Q-T interval: 0.44 seconds

5. AXIS

Quadrant: Left

Degrees: −25° (II most isoelectric, slightly positive)

6. HYPERTROPHY

Atrial: No

Ventricular: No

7. MYOCARDIAL INFARCTION

Q waves: III, aVF, V_{1-3}

S-T displacement: No significant elevation

8. ISCHEMIA

S-T displacement: Diffuse flattening

9. POSSIBLE DRUG EFFECTS

None noted

10. ECG ANALYSIS

The rate is 72 bpm, and the rhythm is irregular with trigeminal ectopic beats; the intervals are WNL and LAD. The Q waves in III and V_{2-3} indicate old inferior and anteroseptal infarctions respectively. The ectopic beats indicated by the arrows are preceded by a P wave, are not wide, and appear much the same as the normal beats. These are characteristic of atrial ectopies. Nonspecific diffuse S-T and T wave changes are also noted.

11. INTERPRETATION

Sinus rhythm

- LAD
- Trigeminal PACs
- Possible old inferior MI
- Old anteroseptal MI
- Diffuse nonspecific S-T and T wave changes

1. RATE

Atrial: 76 bpm

Ventricular: 76 bpm

2. RHYTHM

Atrial: Regular

Ventricular: Regular

3. WAVES

P waves present: Yes

    Appearance: WNL

    Consistent: Yes

    Relation to QRS: 1:1

Q waves present: Yes

    Leads: V_{1-3}

    Pathological: Yes

T waves present: Yes

    Morphology: Inverted, V_{1-3}

4. INTERVALS

P-R interval: 0.12 seconds

    Consistent: Yes

QRS: 0.08 seconds

    Appearance: QS in V_{1-3}

    Consistent: Yes

Q-T interval: 0.36 seconds

5. AXIS

Quadrant: Normal

Degrees: +60° (aVL most isoelectric)

6. HYPERTROPHY

Atrial: No

Ventricular: No

7. MYOCARDIAL INFARCTION

Q waves: V_{1-3}

S-T displacement: Marked elevation V_{1-3}

8. ISCHEMIA

S-T displacement: 1 mm S-T depression II, V_{5-6}

9. POSSIBLE DRUG EFFECTS

None noted

10. ECG ANALYSIS

The rate is 76 bpm, the rhythm is regular, and the axis is WNL. The P-R interval is slightly short symbolizing accelerated AV conduction. The significant Q waves and S-T elevation in leads V_{1-3} are consistent with an acute anteroseptal MI. Because the S-T segment is returning to baseline, the MI appears to be evolving. Nonspecific, 1 mm S-T depression is noted in II and V_{5-6}.

11. INTERPRETATION

Sinus rhythm

- Accelerated AV conduction
- Acute/evolving anteroseptal MI
- Nonspecific lateral S-T changes

ANALYSIS 5-25

I. RATE

Atrial: 66 bpm

Ventricular: 66 bpm

2. RHYTHM

Atrial: Regular

Ventricular: Regular

3. WAVES

P waves present: Yes

   Appearance: WNL

   Consistent: Yes

   Relation to QRS: 1:1

Q waves present: Yes

   Leads: V_{1-2}

   Pathological: V_2

T waves present: Yes

   Morphology: WNL

4. INTERVALS

P-R interval: 0.14 seconds

   Consistent: Yes

QRS: 0.08 seconds

   Appearance: QS in V_2

   Consistent: Yes

Q-T interval: 0.40 seconds

5. AXIS

Quadrant: Left

Degrees: −5° (aVF most isoelectric, slightly negative)

6. HYPERTROPHY

Atrial: No

Ventricular: No

7. MYOCARDIAL INFARCTION

Q waves: V_2

S-T displacement: No significant elevation

8. ISCHEMIA

S-T displacement: 1 mm S-T depression, V_{4-6}

9. POSSIBLE DRUG EFFECTS

None noted

10. ECG ANALYSIS

The rate is 66 bpm, the rhythm is regular, and the intervals and axis are slightly left. The poor R wave progression in leads V_{1-3} possibly indicates an old anteroseptal MI. The S-T depression seen in V_{4-6} is only 1 mm and therefore not considered diagnostic for ischemia.

11. INTERPRETATION

Sinus rhythm

- LAD
- Possible old anteroseptal MI
- Nondiagnostic anterolateral S-T depression

1. RATE

Atrial: Greater than 250 bpm

Ventricular: 75 to 150 bpm

2. RHYTHM

Atrial: Irregular

Ventricular: Irregular

3. WAVES

P waves present: Difficult to identify, present in II, V_1

Appearance: Fibrillation pattern

Consistent: No

Relation to QRS: None

Q waves present: Yes

Leads: III, V_{1-3}

Pathological: Yes

T waves present: Yes

Morphology: Abnormal

4. INTERVALS

P-R interval:

Consistent:

QRS: 0.08 seconds

Appearance: QS in V_{1-3}, III

Consistent: Yes, with the exception of ectopic beats

Q-T interval: 0.36 seconds

5. AXIS

Quadrant: Left

Degrees: −30° (II is most isoelectric)

6. HYPERTROPHY

Atrial: No

Ventricular: No

7. MYOCARDIAL INFARCTION

Q waves: V_{1-3}, III, aVF

S-T displacement: No significant elevation

8. ISCHEMIA

S-T displacement: Diffuse flattening

9. POSSIBLE DRUG EFFECTS

None noted

10. ECG ANALYSIS

The ventricular rate varies from 75 to 150 bpm. The rhythm is irregular and no P waves are identifiable, which are characteristic of atrial fibrillation. The axis is left. The Q waves in III and V_{1-3} indicate possible old inferior and anteroseptal infarctions respectively. The ectopic beats are wider than the normal QRS complexes. Because of the atrial fibrillation, these complexes may be ventricular in origin or simply aberrantly conducted through the ventricles.

11. INTERPRETATION

Atrial fibrillation with primarily uncontrolled ventricular response

- LAD
- Cannot rule out old inferior MI
- Cannot rule out old anteroseptal MI
- Occasional aberrantly conducted ectopic beats

1. RATE

Atrial: Greater than 300 bpm

Ventricular: 50 to 95 bpm

2. RHYTHM

Atrial: Irregular

Ventricular: Irregular

3. WAVES

P waves present: Difficult to identify

Appearance: Fibrillation pattern

Consistent: No

Relation to QRS: None

Q waves present: Yes

Leads: II, III, aVF, V_{1-5}

Pathological: Yes

T waves present: Yes

Morphology: Inverted V_6, I, aVL

4. INTERVALS

P-R interval:

Consistent:

QRS: 0.11 seconds

Appearance: Q-S, II, III, aVF, V_{1-5}

Consistent: Yes

Q-T interval: 0.40 seconds

5. AXIS

Quadrant: Left

Degrees: −80° (aVF and II negative, I most isoelectric, slightly positive)

6. HYPERTROPHY

Atrial: No

Ventricular: No

7. MYOCARDIAL INFARCTION

Q waves: II, III, aVF, V_{1-5}

S-T displacement: 1 to 2 mm elevation, V_{3-4}

8. ISCHEMIA

S-T displacement: 1 to 2 mm S-T depression V_5, I and aVL

9. POSSIBLE DRUG EFFECTS

None noted

10. ECG ANALYSIS

The ventricular rate varies from 50 to 95 bpm, the rhythm is irregular, and the P waves are difficult to identify. There is an underlying rhythm and atrial fibrillation. The QRS complexes measure 0.11 seconds, which is characteristic of an intraventricular conduction delay. The R-S in V_6 indicates the delay is in the left bundle. The net QRS in leads aVF and II are negative, which is characteristic of an LAHB. Large Q waves in leads II, III, aVF, and V_{1-5} are properties of old inferior and anterior MIs respectively. The S-T segments in leads V_6, I, and aVL are depressed and down-sloping, therefore possible lateral ischemia is suspected.

11. INTERPRETATION

Atrial fibrillation with slow ventricular response

- LAHB
- Old inferior MI
- Extensive old anterior MI
- IVCD, probably LBBB
- Nondiagnostic lateral S-T changes

1. RATE

Atrial: 89 bpm

Ventricular: 89 bpm

2. RHYTHM

Atrial: Regular

Ventricular: Regular

3. WAVES

P waves present: Yes

    Appearance: WNL

    Consistent: Yes

    Relation to QRS: 1:1

Q waves present: Yes

    Leads: II, III, aVF

    Pathological: Yes, possible

T waves present: Yes

    Morphology: Flat

4. INTERVALS

P-R interval: 0.16 seconds

    Consistent: Yes

QRS: 0.08 seconds

    Appearance: WNL

    Consistent: Yes

Q-T interval: 0.36 seconds

5. AXIS

Quadrant: Normal

Degrees: +60° (aVL most isoelectric)

6. HYPERTROPHY

Atrial: No

Ventricular: No

7. MYOCARDIAL INFARCTION

Q waves: II, III, aVF

S-T displacement: No significant elevation

8. ISCHEMIA

S-T displacement: Diffuse S-T depression

9. POSSIBLE DRUG EFFECTS

None noted

10. ECG ANALYSIS

The rate is 89 bpm, the rhythm is regular, and the intervals and axis are WNL. The Q waves in II, III, and aVF are borderline significant, (i.e., they are only 1 mm in width and less than one third the height of the QRS). Nonspecific S-T and T wave abnormalities occur in I, aVL, and V_{2-6}.

11. INTERPRETATION:

Sinus rhythm

- Cannot rule out old inferior MI
- Diffuse nonspecific anterolateral S-T and T wave abnormalities

ANALYSIS 5-29

1. RATE
Atrial: Greater than 300 bpm

Ventricular: 110 to 150 bpm

2. RHYTHM
Atrial: Irregular

Ventricular: Irregular

3. WAVES
P waves present: Difficult to identify, best seen V_1

    Appearance: Fibrillation pattern

    Consistent: No

    Relation to QRS: None

Q waves present: Yes

    Leads: V_{1-3}

    Pathological: Yes

T waves present: Yes

    Morphology: Flat in V_{4-6}, I, and aVL

4. INTERVALS
P-R interval:

    Consistent:

QRS: 0.06 seconds

    Appearance: QS in V_{1-3}

    Consistent: Yes

Q-T interval: 0.24 seconds

5. AXIS
Quadrant: Left

Degrees: −20° (II most isoelectric, slightly positive)

6. HYPERTROPHY
Atrial: No

Ventricular: No

7. MYOCARDIAL INFARCTION
Q waves: V_{1-3}

S-T displacement: 1 to 2 mm S-T elevation V_{1-3}

8. ISCHEMIA
S-T displacement: Flat, V_{4-6}, I, aVL

9. POSSIBLE DRUG EFFECTS
None noted

10. ECG ANALYSIS
The ventricular rate varies from 110 to 150 bpm. The rhythm is irregular, and there is not a P wave for each QRS, which are classic characteristics of atrial fibrillation. The mean QRS deflection in lead aVF is negative, thus the axis is left. The large Q waves in V_{1-3} indicate with 1 to 2 mm S-T elevation an anteroseptal MI, age indeterminate. Poor R wave progression is also noted. Nonspecific S-T and T wave abnormalities are also seen in leads V_{4-6}, I, and aVL.

11. INTERPRETATION
Atrial fibrillation with rapid ventricular response

- LAD
- Anteroseptal MI, age indeterminate
- Nonspecific lateral S-T and T wave abnormalities

1. RATE

Atrial: 97 bpm

Ventricular: 97 bpm

2. RHYTHM

Atrial: Regular

Ventricular: Regular

3. WAVES

P waves present: Yes

  Appearance: Negative in V_1

  Consistent: Yes

  Relation to QRS: 1:1

Q waves present: Yes

  Leads: II, III, aVF

  Pathological: Yes

T waves present: Yes

  Morphology: Elevated V_{2-3}, inverted III and aVF

4. INTERVALS

P-R interval: 0.14 seconds

  Consistent: Yes

QRS: 0.08 seconds

  Appearance: Q-S in II and aVF

  Consistent: Yes

Q-T interval: 0.36 seconds

5. AXIS

Quadrant: Left

Degrees: −10° (aVF slightly negative, II most isoelectric, slightly postiive)

6. HYPERTROPHY

Atrial: Possible

Ventricular: No

7. MYOCARDIAL INFARCTION

Q waves: II, III, aVF

S-T displacement: No significant elevation

8. ISCHEMIA

S-T displacement: No significant depression

9. POSSIBLE DRUG EFFECTS

None noted

10. ECG ANALYSIS

The rate is 97 bpm, the rhythm is regular, and the intervals are WNL. The P waves in V_1 are negative, but lead II lends no supporting evidence for atrial hypertrophy. The axis is slightly left. Significant Q waves in leads II, III, and aVF indicate an old inferior MI. The T waves in those leads are inverted, characteristic of an MI that is resolving. Nonspecific S-T and T wave changes occur in V_{4-6}, I, II, III, aVL, and aVF.

11. INTERPRETATION

Sinus rhythm

- LAD
- Inferior MI, age indeterminate
- Diffuse nonspecific S-T and T wave changes

1. RATE

Atrial: 78 bpm

Ventricular: 78 bpm

2. RHYTHM

Atrial: Regular

Ventricular: Regular

3. WAVES

P waves present: Yes

    Appearance: WNL

    Consistent: Yes

    Relation to QRS: 1:1

Q waves present: Yes

    Leads: II, III, aVF, V_{1-5}

    Pathological: Yes

T waves present: Yes

    Morphology: Elevated V_{1-5}

4. INTERVALS

P-R interval: 0.14 seconds

    Consistent: Yes

QRS: 0.08 seconds

    Appearance: Q-S II, V_{1-5}

    Consistent: Yes

Q-T interval: 0.40 seconds

5. AXIS

Quadrant: Left

Degrees: −15° (II and aVF most isoelectric)

6. HYPERTROPHY

Atrial: No

Ventricular: No

7. MYOCARDIAL INFARCTION

Q waves: II, III, aVF, V_{1-5}

S-T displacement: S-T elevation V_{1-5}

8. ISCHEMIA

S-T displacement: Acute changes

9. POSSIBLE DRUG EFFECTS

None noted

10. ECG ANALYSIS

ECG #1 of 2. The rate is 78 bpm, the rhythm is regular, and the intervals are WNL. The axis is slightly left. Significant Q waves in leads II, III, and aVF indicate an old inferior MI. Significant Q waves in leads V_{1-5} **with** S-T elevation indicate an extensive anterior MI (probably recent).

11. INTERPRETATION

Sinus rhythm

- LAD
- Old inferior MI
- Extensive anterior MI, probably recent

I. RATE

Atrial: 90 bpm

Ventricular: 90 bpm

2. RHYTHM

Atrial: Regular

Ventricular: Regular

3. WAVES

P waves present: Yes

    Appearance: WNL

    Consistent: Yes

    Relation to QRS: 1:1

Q waves present: Yes

    Leads: II, III, aVF, V_{1-5}

    Pathological: Yes

T waves present: Yes

    Morphology: Elevated

4. INTERVALS

P-R interval: 0.14 seconds

    Consistent: Yes

QRS: 0.08 seconds

    Appearance: Q-S in II, III, aVF, V_{1-5}

    Consistent: Yes

Q-T interval: 0.36 seconds

5. AXIS

Quadrant: Left

Degrees: −70° (aVF and II negative, aVR most isoelectric,
slightly positive)

6. HYPERTROPHY

Atrial: No

Ventricular: No

7. MYOCARDIAL INFARCTION

Q waves: II, III, aVF, V_{1-5}

S-T displacement: Elevation V_{1-5}

8. ISCHEMIA

S-T displacement: Acute changes

9. POSSIBLE DRUG EFFECTS

None noted

10. ECG ANALYSIS

ECG #2 of 2. The rate is 90 bpm, the rhythm is regular, and the intervals are WNL. From the preceding ECG taken 1 day earlier, LAHB has developed. The S-T segments in V_{1-2} have begun to return to the baseline, however they remain somewhat elevated and prominent in V_{3-5}.

11. INTERPRETATION

Sinus rhythm

- Recent LAHB
- Old inferior MI
- Evolving extensive anterior MI

1. RATE

Atrial: 52 bpm

Ventricular: 52 bpm

2. RHYTHM

Atrial: Regular

Ventricular: Regular

3. WAVES

P waves present: Yes

    Appearance: WNL

    Consistent: Yes

    Relation to QRS: 1:1

Q waves present: Yes

    Leads: III, V_1

    Pathological: Yes

T waves present: Yes

    Morphology: Elevated I, II, III, aVF, V_{5-6}

4. INTERVALS

P-R interval: 0.20 seconds

    Consistent: Yes

QRS: 0.11 seconds

    Appearance: Fused with S-T

    Consistent: Yes

Q-T interval: 0.40 seconds

5. AXIS

Quadrant: Normal

Degrees: +30° (III most isoelectric)

6. HYPERTROPHY

Atrial: No

Ventricular: No

7. MYOCARDIAL INFARCTION

Q waves: Developing in III, V_1

S-T displacement: Marked elevation, I, II, III, aVF, V_{5-6}

8. ISCHEMIA

S-T displacement: Acute changes

9. POSSIBLE DRUG EFFECTS

None noted

10. ECG ANALYSIS

ECG #1 of 3. The rate is 52 bpm, the rhythm is regular, and the axis is WNL. The P-R interval of 0.20 seconds is consistent with a borderline first degree AVB. The QRS duration is 0.11 seconds, which is characteristic of an intraventricular conduction delay. The R-S in V_{5-6} indicates an incomplete left bundle branch block. Marked S-T elevation in leads I, II, III, aVF, V_{5-6}, symbolize acute inferior and lateral infarctions. Poor R wave progression in V_{1-3} may indicate an old anteroseptal MI. Artifact is also noted in II, III, and aVF.

11. INTERPRETATION

Sinus bradycardia

- Borderline first degree AVB
- Acute inferolateral MI
- Cannot rule out old anteroseptal MI
- Incomplete LBBB

1. RATE

Atrial: 56 bpm

Ventricular: 56 bpm

2. RHYTHM

Atrial: Regular

Ventricular: Regular

3. WAVES

P waves present: Yes

    Appearance: WNL

    Consistent: Yes

    Relation to QRS: 1:1

Q waves present: Yes

    Leads: III, V_1

    Pathological: Yes

T waves present: Yes

    Morphology: Elevated I, II, III, aVF, V_{5-6}, inverted V_1

4. INTERVALS

P-R interval: 0.20 seconds

    Consistent: Yes

QRS: 0.11 seconds

    Appearance: Fused with S-T

    Consistent: Yes

Q-T interval: 0.38 seconds

5. AXIS

Quadrant: Normal

Degrees: +30° (III most isoelectric)

6. HYPERTROPHY

Atrial: No

Ventricular: No

7. MYOCARDIAL INFARCTION

Q waves: Developing, III and V_1

S-T displacement: Acute S-T elevation, II, III, aVF, V_{5-6}

8. ISCHEMIA

S-T displacement: Acute changes

9. POSSIBLE DRUG EFFECTS

None noted

10. ECG ANALYSIS

ECG #2 of 3. There are few changes 10 minutes following the first ECG. There are continued acute inferior and lateral infarctions.

11. INTERPRETATION

Sinus rhythm

- Borderline first degree AVB
- Acute inferolateral MI, in progression
- Cannot rule out old anteroseptal MI
- Incomplete LBBB

1. RATE

Atrial: 62 bpm

Ventricular: 62 bpm

2. RHYTHM

Atrial: Regular

Ventricular: Regular

3. WAVES

P waves present: Yes

    Appearance: WNL

    Consistent: Yes

    Relation to QRS: 1:1

Q waves present: Yes

    Leads: III, V_1

    Pathological: Yes

T waves present: Yes

    Morphology: Slightly elevated

4. INTERVALS

P-R interval: 0.20 seconds

    Consistent: Yes

QRS: 0.11 seconds

    Appearance: Q-S in III and V_1

    Consistent: Yes

Q-T interval: 0.38 seconds

5. AXIS

Quadrant: Normal

Degrees: +15° (III and aVF most isoelectric)

6. HYPERTROPHY

Atrial: No

Ventricular: No

7. MYOCARDIAL INFARCTION

Q waves: Developing acute inferior Q waves

S-T displacement: Less acute elevation I, II, III, aVF, V_{2-5}

8. ISCHEMIA

S-T displacement: Acute changes

9. POSSIBLE DRUG EFFECTS

None noted

10. ECG ANALYSIS

ECG #3 of 3. Taken 70 minutes following ECG #2. Inferolateral MI is resolving, and the Q wave is becoming more defined in aVF. The S-T segment is less elevated.

11. INTERPRETATION:

Sinus rhythm

- Borderline first degree AVB
- Acute inferolateral MI, in progression
- Cannot rule out old anteroseptal MI
- Incomplete LBBB

1. RATE
Atrial: 90 bpm
Ventricular: 90 bpm

2. RHYTHM
Atrial: Irregular
Ventricular: Regular

3. WAVES
P waves present: Best seen on rhythm strip
    Appearance: Tall and peaked
    Consistent: Yes
    Relation to QRS: 1:1
Q waves present: Unable to determine
    Leads:
    Pathological:
T waves present: Yes
    Morphology: Inverted in lead II (rhythm strip)

4. INTERVALS
P-R interval: 0.16 seconds
    Consistent: Yes
QRS: 0.12 seconds
    Appearance: Ventricular pacemaker
    Consistent: Yes
Q-T interval: 0.40 seconds

5. AXIS
Quadrant: Unable to determine
Degrees:

6. HYPERTROPHY
Atrial: Possible
Ventricular: Unable to determine

7. MYOCARDIAL INFARCTION
Q waves: Unable to determine
S-T displacement: Unable to determine

8. PACEMAKER TYPE
Spikes present: Yes
Relationship to P wave: No P wave
AV delay: None
Relationship to QRS: 1:1

9. PACEMAKER RATE
Atrial:
Ventricular: 90 bpm

10. PACEMAKER SENSING
Unexpected pauses: No

11. PACEMAKER CAPTURE
Spikes without depolarization: No

12. POSSIBLE DRUG EFFECTS
None noted

13. ECG ANALYSIS
The rate is 90 bpm, and the ventricular rhythm is regular. All complexes on the 12-lead tracing are paced at a rate of 90 bpm. The **VVI** pacemaker is sensing and pacing the ventricle. The mode of response to an intrinsic complex inhibits pacing. The first nine beats of the rhythm strip appear to be sinus (i.e., the complexes are initiated by a P wave). The P waves of those first nine beats are tall and peaked, which is characteristic of a possible right atrial enlargement. The QRS complexes are wide, indicating an intraventricular conduction delay. The six complexes that follow are initiated by the pacemaker and have a different configuration. The axis is indeterminate due to the pacemaker function. Further analysis cannot be performed due to the dominant pacemaker rhythm.

14. INTERPRETATION
Underlying rhythm:
- Sinus rhythm
    - IVCD
    - Probable RAE

Mechanical pacemaker:
- **VVI**
    - 100% sensing and capture

I. RATE
Atrial: 70 bpm
Ventricular: 70 to 75 bpm

2. RHYTHM
Atrial: Regular
Ventricular: Regular

3. WAVES
P waves present: On rhythm strip only
    Appearance: Normal
    Consistent: Yes
    Relation to QRS: 1:1
Q waves present: Yes
    Leads: II (rhythm strip)
    Pathological: Yes, however only one lead available
T waves present: Yes
    Morphology: Inverted, lead II (rhythm strip)

4. INTERVALS
P-R interval: 0.12 seconds
    Consistent: Yes
QRS: 0.08 seconds
    Appearance: Q wave
    Consistent: Yes
Q-T interval: 0.40 seconds

5. AXIS
Quadrant: Unable to determine
Degrees:

6. HYPERTROPHY
Atrial: Unable to determine
Ventricular: Unable to determine

7. MYOCARDIAL INFARCTION
Q waves: Unable to determine
S-T displacement: Unable to determine

8. PACEMAKER TYPE
Spikes present: Yes
Relationship to P wave: None
AV delay: None
Relationship to QRS: 1:1

9. PACEMAKER RATE
Atrial: None
Ventricular: 70 bpm

10. PACEMAKER SENSING
Unexpected pauses: None

11. PACEMAKER CAPTURE
Spikes without depolarization: None

12. POSSIBLE DRUG EFFECTS
None noted

13. ECG ANALYSIS
The rate is 70 to 75 bpm, and the ventricular rhythm is regular. All complexes on the 12-lead tracing, with the exception of the last beat in leads V$_{4-6}$, are paced at a rate of 70 bpm. The **VVI** pacemaker is sensing and pacing the ventricles, and the mode of response inhibits pacing. The first six beats of the rhythm strip are sinus (i.e., they appear to be initiated by a P wave). The QRS complexes of those first six beats have significant Q waves. Because the 12-lead is nearly 100% paced, it is impossible to determine the significance of those Q waves. Otherwise the tracing is unremarkable.

14. INTERPRETATION
Underlying rhythm:
    • Sinus rhythm
Mechanical pacemaker:
    • **VVI**
    • 100% sensing and capture

1. RATE
Atrial: Unable to determine
Ventricular: 70 to 100 bpm

2. RHYTHM
Atrial: Irregular
Ventricular: Irregular

3. WAVES
P waves present: Difficult to identify, best seen on rhythm strip
    Appearance: Fibrillation pattern
    Consistent: No
    Relation to QRS: None
Q waves present: Yes
    Leads: V_{1-3}
    Pathological: Yes
T waves present: Yes
    Morphology: Inverted in II, peaked in V_{2-3}

4. INTERVALS
P-R interval:
    Consistent: No
QRS: 0.06 seconds (intrinsic complex)
    Appearance: Q-S in V_{1-3}
    Consistent: Yes
Q-T interval: 0.34 seconds

5. AXIS
Quadrant: Unable to determine
Degrees:

6. HYPERTROPHY
Atrial: Unable to determine
Ventricular: Unable to determine

7. MYOCARDIAL INFARCTION
Q waves: V_{1-3}
S-T displacement: 2 to 4 mm S-T depression V_{4-6}

8. PACEMAKER TYPE
Spikes present: Yes
Relationship to P wave: None
AV delay: None
Relationship to QRS: 1:1

9. PACEMAKER RATE
Atrial:
Ventricular: 70 bpm

10. PACEMAKER SENSING
Unexpected pauses: No

11. PACEMAKER CAPTURE
Spikes without depolarization: No

12. POSSIBLE DRUG EFFECTS
None noted

13. ECG ANALYSIS
The rate varies from 70 to 100 bpm. The underlying atrial and ventricular rhythms are irregular and the P waves do not have a 1:1 relationship with the QRS, which are characteristics of atrial fibrillation. The S-T segments in leads II (rhythm strip), aVF, and V_{4-6} are depressed, indicating possible ischemia. The Q waves are noted (non-paced beats) in leads V_{1-3} symbolizing an old anteroseptal MI. The VVI pacemaker is sensing and pacing the ventricles, and the mode of response inhibits pacing. The pacemaker rate is 75 bpm.

14. INTERPRETATION
Underlying rhythm:
- Atrial fibrillation with controlled ventricular response
- Old anteroseptal MI
- Probable inferolateral ischemia

Mechanical pacemaker:
- **VVI**
- 100% sensing and capture

ANALYSIS 6-4

1. RATE
Atrial: 65 bpm
Ventricular: 65 bpm

2. RHYTHM
Atrial: Regular
Ventricular: Regular

3. WAVES
P waves present: Yes
    Appearance: Follow pacemaker spike
    Consistent: Yes
    Relation to QRS: 1:1
Q waves present: Yes
    Leads: II, III, aVF
    Pathological: No
T waves present: Yes
    Morphology: Normal

4. INTERVALS
P-R interval:
    Consistent:
QRS: 0.10 seconds
    Appearance: Within normal limits (WNL)
    Consistent: Yes
Q-T interval: 0.40 seconds

5. AXIS
Quadrant: Normal
Degrees: +75° (I and aVL most isoelectric)

6. HYPERTROPHY
Atrial: No
Ventricular: Yes

7. MYOCARDIAL INFARCTION
Q waves: None significant
S-T displacement: No significant elevation

8. PACEMAKER TYPE
Spikes present: Yes
Relationship to P wave: Immediately prior to P
AV delay: 0.18 seconds
Relationship to QRS: 1:1

9. PACEMAKER RATE
Atrial: 65 bpm
Ventricular: 65 bpm

10. PACEMAKER SENSING
Unexpected pauses: No

11. PACEMAKER CAPTURE
Spikes without depolarization: No

12. POSSIBLE DRUG EFFECTS
None noted

13. ECG ANALYSIS
The rate is 65 bpm, the rhythm is regular, and all complexes are paced. The **AAI** pacemaker is sensing and pacing the atria. The mode of response to a P wave inhibits pacing. The sum S wave is V_1 and the R wave in V_5 is greater than or equal to 35 mm, which are voltage criteria for left ventricular hypertrophy. The S-T segment in II, III, and aVF is flat.

14. INTERPRETATION
Underlying rhythm:
    • Unable to determine
Mechanical pacemaker:
    • **AAI**
    • 100% sensing and capture
    • LVH
    • Nonspecific inferior S-T changes

1. RATE
Atrial: Unable to determine
Ventricular: 65 bpm

2. RHYTHM
Atrial: Unable to determine
Ventricular: 65 bpm

3. WAVES
P waves present: No
   Appearance:
   Consistent:
   Relation to QRS:
Q waves present: Unable to determine
   Leads:
   Pathological:
T waves present: Yes
   Morphology: Paced

4. INTERVALS
P-R interval:
   Consistent:
QRS: 0.16 seconds
   Appearance: Ventricular pacemaker
   Consistent: Yes
Q-T interval: 0.52 seconds

5. AXIS
Quadrant: Unable to determine
Degrees:

6. HYPERTROPHY
Atrial: Unable to determine
Ventricular: Unable to determine

7. MYOCARDIAL INFARCTION
Q waves: Unable to determine
S-T displacement: Unable to determine

8. PACEMAKER TYPE
Spikes present: Yes
Relationship to P wave: None
AV delay: None
Relationship to QRS: 1:1

9. PACEMAKER RATE
Atrial: None
Ventricular: 65 bpm

10. PACEMAKER SENSING
Unexpected pauses: No

11. PACEMAKER CAPTURE
Spikes without depolarization: No

12. POSSIBLE DRUG EFFECTS
None noted

13. ECG ANALYSIS
The ventricular rate is 65 bpm, the rhythm is regular, and all complexes are paced. The **VVI** pacemaker is sensing and pacing the ventricles. The mode of response to a spontaneous QRS inhibits pacing. Further analysis cannot be performed due to the dominant pacemaker rhythm.

14. INTERPRETATION
Underlying rhythm:
   • Unable to determine
Mechanical pacemaker:
   • **VVI**
   • 100% sensing and capture

1. RATE
Atrial: Unable to detemine
Ventricular: Varies from 70 to 120 bpm

2. RHYTHM
Atrial: Irregular
Ventricular: Irregular

3. WAVES
P waves present: Difficult to identify, best seen in V$_1$
   Appearance: Fibrillation pattern
   Consistent: No
   Relation to QRS: None
Q waves present: No
   Leads:
   Pathological:
T waves present: Yes
   Morphology: Flat

4. INTERVALS
P-R interval:
   Consistent:
QRS: 0.12 seconds
   Appearance: Wide
   Consistent: Yes
Q-T interval: 0.36 seconds

5. AXIS
Quadrant: Left anterior hemiblock
Degrees: −60° (aVF and II negative, aVR most isoelectric)

6. HYPERTROPHY
Atrial: No
Ventricular: No

7. MYOCARDIAL INFARCTION
Q waves: None significant
S-T displacement: No significant elevation

8. PACEMAKER TYPE
Spikes present: Yes
Relationship to P wave: None

AV delay: None
Relationship to QRS: 1:1, paced beats

9. PACEMAKER RATE
Atrial:
Ventricular: 70 bpm

10. PACEMAKER SENSING
Unexpected pauses: No

11. PACEMAKER CAPTURE
Spikes without depolarization: No

12. POSSIBLE DRUG EFFECTS
None noted

13. ECG ANALYSIS
The ventricular rate varies from 70 to 120 bpm. The rhythm is irregular and the P waves are difficult to identify and have no relationship to the QRS complexes. The underlying rhythm is atrial fibrillation with a controlled ventricular response. The nonpaced QRS complexes in leads aVF and II are negative, characteristic of a left anterior hemiblock. The QRS complexes are 0.12 seconds in duration, indicating an intraventricular conduction delay. Beat 3 in the augmented leads is wide and has opposite T wave deflection of the normal beats. It is probably ventricular in origin, but may simply be aberrantly conducted through the ventricles. It is very difficult to be accurate because of the IVCD. The paced complexes are noted throughout when the rate drops below 70 bpm. The **VVI** pacemaker is sensing and pacing the ventricles. The mode of response is inhibiting to a sensed QRS.

14. INTERPRETATION
Underlying rhythm:
- Atrial fibrillation with controlled ventricular response
  - LAHB
  - Occasional ventricular aberrancy
  - IVCD

Mechanical pacemaker:
- **VVI**
- 25% paced
- 100% sensing and capture

1. RATE
Atrial: Unable to determine
Ventricular: 72 bpm

2. RHYTHM
Atrial: Unable to determine
Ventricular: Regular

3. WAVES
P waves present: No
    Appearance:
    Consistent:
    Relation to QRS:
Q waves present: Unable to determine
    Leads:
    Pathological:
T waves present: Yes
    Morphology: Unable to analyze

4. INTERVALS
P-R interval:
    Consistent:
QRS: 0.16 seconds
    Appearance: Paced
    Consistent: Yes
Q-T interval: 0.48 seconds

5. AXIS
Quadrant: Unable to determine
Degrees:

6. HYPERTROPHY
Atrial: Unable to determine
Ventricular: Unable to determine

7. MYOCARDIAL INFARCTION
Q waves: Unable to determine
S-T displacement: Unable to determine

8. PACEMAKER TYPE
Spikes present: Yes
Relationship to P wave: No P waves identified
AV delay: 0.16 seconds
Relationship to QRS: 2:1

9. PACEMAKER RATE
Atrial: 72 bpm
Ventricular: 72 bpm

10. PACEMAKER SENSING
Unexpected pauses: No

11. PACEMAKER CAPTURE
Spikes without depolarization: No

12. POSSIBLE DRUG EFFECTS
None noted

13. ECG ANALYSIS
The rate is 72 bpm, the rhythm is regular, and all complexes are paced. The **DDD** pacemaker is in the AV sequential mode, pacing both the atria and ventricle and sensing the ventricle. The mode of response to a normal complex inhibits pacing. Further analysis cannot be performed due to dominant pacemaker rhythm.

14. INTERPRETATION
Underlying rhythm:
- Unable to determine

Mechanical pacemaker:
- **DDD**
  - **DVI** (AV sequential mode)
  - 100% sensing and capture

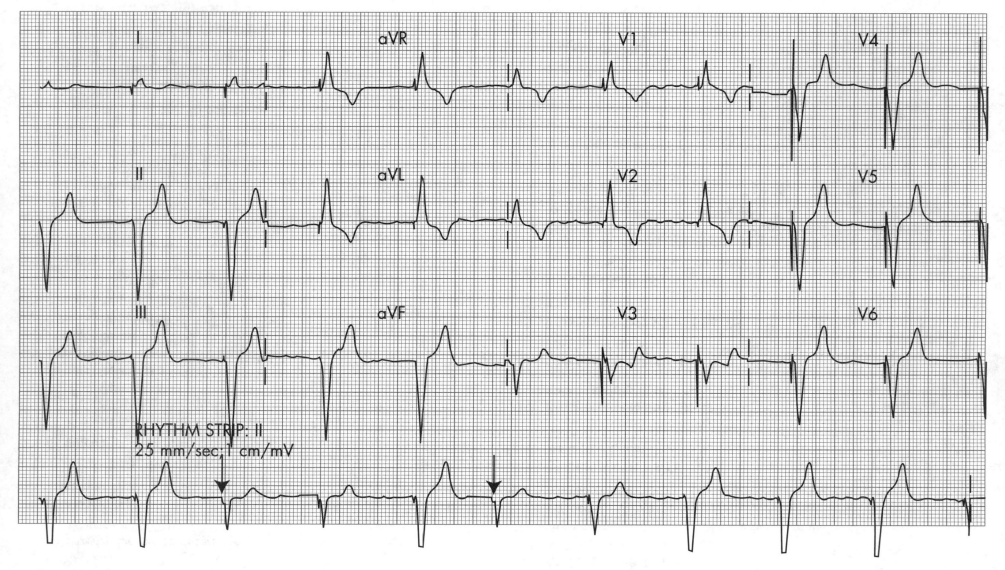

RHYTHM STRIP: II
25 mm/sec; 1 cm/mV

Figure 6-8
Resting 12-Lead ECG

1. RATE
Atrial: Unable to determine
Ventricular: 60 bpm

2. RHYTHM
Atrial: Unable to determine
Ventricular: Regular

3. WAVES
P waves present: No
   Appearance:
   Consistent:
   Relation to QRS:
Q waves present: Unable to determine
   Leads:
   Pathological:
T waves present: Yes
   Morphology: Unable to determine

4. INTERVALS
P-R interval:
   Consistent:
QRS: 0.16 seconds
   Appearance: Paced
   Consistent: Yes
Q-T interval: 0.44 seconds

5. AXIS
Quadrant: Unable to determine
Degrees:

6. HYPERTROPHY
Atrial: Unable to determine
Ventricular: Unable to determine

7. MYOCARDIAL INFARCTION
Q waves: Unable to determine
S-T displacement: Unable to determine

8. PACEMAKER TYPE
Spikes present: Yes
Relationship to P wave: None
AV delay: None
Relationship to QRS: 1:1

9. PACEMAKER RATE
Atrial:
Ventricular: 60 bpm

10. PACEMAKER SENSING
Unexpected pauses: No

11. PACEMAKER CAPTURE
Spikes without depolarization: No

12. POSSIBLE DRUG EFFECTS
None noted

13. ECG ANALYSIS
The ventricular rate is 60 bpm, the rhythm is regular, and all complexes are paced. The **VVI** pacemaker senses and paces the ventricle. The mode of response to a normal QRS inhibits pacing. Further analysis cannot be performed due to the dominant pacemaker rhythm.

14. INTERPRETATION
Underlying rhythm:
   • Unable to determine
Mechanical pacemaker:
   • **VVI**
   • 100% sensing and capture

ANALYSIS 6-9

I. RATE
Atrial: 70 to 75 bpm
Ventricular: 70 to 75 bpm

2. RHYTHM
Atrial: Irregular
Ventricular: Irregular

3. WAVES
P waves present: Yes
   Appearance: Intrinsic complexes, WNL
   Consistent: No
   Relation to QRS: Variable
Q waves present: Unable to determine
   Leads:
   Pathological:
T waves present: Yes
   Morphology: Intrinsic complexes, tall V_{2-5}

4. INTERVALS
P-R interval: 0.14 seconds (intrinsic complexes)
   Consistent: Yes
QRS: 0.08 seconds (intrinsic complexes)
   Appearance: WNL
   Consistent: Yes
Q-T interval: 0.36 seconds

5. AXIS
Quadrant: Unable to determine
Degrees:

6. HYPERTROPHY
Atrial: Unable to determine
Ventricular: No

7. MYOCARDIAL INFARCTION
Q waves: None significant
S-T displacement: S-T depression (J-point) V_{2-5}

8. PACEMAKER TYPE
Spikes present: Yes
Relationship to P wave: None
AV delay: None
Relationship to QRS: 1:1 (paced complexes)

9. PACEMAKER RATE
Atrial:
Ventricular: 70 bpm

10. PACEMAKER SENSING
Unexpected pauses: No

11. PACEMAKER CAPTURE
Spikes without depolarization: No

12. POSSIBLE DRUG EFFECTS
None noted

13. ECG ANALYSIS
The rate varies from 70 to 75 bpm. The rhythm is irregular. The underlying rhythm, seen in V_{1-6}, is sinus. All variables are WNL. The limb leads are primarily paced complexes with a ventricular ectopic beat noted in leads I to III. The rhythm strip is mixed with sinus complexes, ventricular ectopic complexes, and VVI paced complexes. The **VVI** pacemaker is sensing and pacing the ventricle. The mode of response to a sinus or ventricular complex inhibits pacing. The S-T segments (J points in particular) in leads V_{2-5} are 1 to 2 mm depressed, a nondiagnostic finding. Further analysis cannot be performed due to dominant pacemaker rhythm.

14. INTERPRETATION
Underlying rhythm:
- Sinus rhythm
  - Multiple PVCs

Mechanical pacemaker:
- **VVI**
- 25% pacing
- 100% sensing and capture

1. RATE

Atrial: Paced, 72 bpm
Ventricular: Paced, 72 bpm

2. RHYTHM

Atrial: Regular
Ventricular: Regular

3. WAVES

P waves present: No
 Appearance:
 Consistent:
 Relation to QRS:
Q waves present: Unable to determine
 Leads:
 Pathological:
T waves present: Yes
 Morphology: Morphology distorted by pacemaker

4. INTERVALS

P-R interval:
 Consistent:
QRS: 0.20 seconds
 Appearance: Paced
 Consistent: Yes
Q-T interval: 0.40 seconds

5. AXIS

Quadrant: Unable to determine
Degrees:

6. HYPERTROPHY

Atrial: Unable to determine
Ventricular: Unable to determine

7. MYOCARDIAL INFARCTION

Q waves:
S-T displacement:

8. PACEMAKER TYPE

Spikes present: Yes
Relationship to P wave: None
AV delay: 0.16 seconds
Relationship to QRS: 2:1

9. PACEMAKER RATE

Atrial: 72 bpm
Ventricular: 72 bpm

10. PACEMAKER SENSING

Unexpected pauses: No

11. PACEMAKER CAPTURE

Spikes without depolarization: None

12. POSSIBLE DRUG EFFECTS

None noted

13. ECG ANALYSIS

The rate is 72 bpm, the rhythm is regular, and all complexes are paced. The **DDD** pacemaker is in the AV sequential mode (**DVI**). Both the atrium and the ventricle are paced with an AV delay of 0.16 seconds. The ventricle is sensed and the mode of response to an intrinsic complex inhibits pacing. Further analysis cannot be performed due to dominant pacemaker rhythm.

14. INTERPRETATION

Underlying rhythm:
 • Unable to determine
Mechanical pacemaker:
 • **DDD**
  • **DVI** (AV sequential mode)
  • 100% sensing and capture

1. RATE
Atrial: Unable to determine
Ventricular: 62 bpm

2. RHYTHM
Atrial: Irregular
Ventricular: Regular

3. WAVES
P waves present: Yes
    Appearance: Abnormal
    Consistent: No
    Relation to QRS: None
Q waves present: Unable to determine
    Leads:
    Pathological:
T waves present: Yes
    Morphology: Unable to determine

4. INTERVALS
P-R interval:
    Consistent:
QRS: 0.20 seconds
    Appearance: Paced
    Consistent: Yes
Q-T interval: 0.52 seconds

5. AXIS
Quadrant: Unable to determine
Degrees:

6. HYPERTROPHY
Atrial: Unable to determine
Ventricular: Unable to determine

7. MYOCARDIAL INFARCTION
Q waves:
S-T displacement:

8. PACEMAKER TYPE
Spikes present: Yes
Relationship to P wave: None
AV delay: None
Relationship to QRS: 1:1

9. PACEMAKER RATE
Atrial: Unable to determine
Ventricular: 62 bpm

10. PACEMAKER SENSING
Unexpected pauses: No

11. PACEMAKER CAPTURE
Spikes without depolarization: No

12. POSSIBLE DRUG EFFECTS
None noted

13. ECG ANALYSIS
The ventricular rate is 62 bpm, the rhythm is regular, and all complexes are paced. P waves are noted throughout the tracing. They do not initiate a QRS complex, indicating that the underlying rhythm is probably complete heart block. The **VVI** pacemaker is sensing and pacing the ventricle. The mode of response to an intrinsic complex inhibits pacing. Further analysis cannot be performed due to dominant pacemaker rhythm.

14. INTERPRETATION
Underlying rhythm:
    • Probable complete heart block
Mechanical pacemaker:
    • **VVI**
    • 100% sensing and capture

1. RATE

Atrial: 68 bpm

Ventricular: 68 bpm

2. RHYTHM

Atrial: Regular

Ventricular: Regular

3. WAVES

P waves present: Yes

    Appearance: Normal

    Consistent: Yes

    Relation to QRS: 1:1

Q waves present: No

    Leads:

    Pathological:

T waves present: Yes

    Morphology: Inverted, V_{5-6}, I, aVL

4. INTERVALS

P-R interval: 0.22 seconds

    Consistent: Yes

QRS: 0.12 seconds

    Appearance: Wide

    Consistent: Yes

Q-T interval: 0.32 seconds

5. AXIS

Quadrant: Left anterior hemiblock

Degrees: −60° (aVF and II negative, aVR most isoelectric)

6. HYPERTROPHY

Atrial: No

Ventricular: No

7. MYOCARDIAL INFARCTION

Q waves: None significant

S-T displacement: 1 to 2 mm S-T elevation V_{1-3}

8. ISCHEMIA

S-T displacement: 1 mm S-T depression V_{5-6}, I, and aVL

9. POSSIBLE DRUG EFFECTS

None noted

10. ECG ANALYSIS

The rate is 68 bpm, and the rhythm is regular. The P-R interval measures 0.22 seconds, which is characteristic of a first degree AVB. The QRS complex measures 0.12 seconds indicative of a nonspecific intraventricular conduction delay. The Q-T interval measures 0.32 seconds, which is short for a rate of 60 bpm. This finding may indicate hypocalcemia. A left anterior hemiblock (LAHB) is denoted by the net negative QRS deflections in leads aVF and II. Poor R wave progression with slight S-T elevation in leads V_{1-3} may indicate an anterior MI. Nonspecific S-T and T wave abnormalities are noted in leads V_{5-6}, I, and aVL.

11. INTERPRETATION

Sinus rhythm

- First degree AVB
- LAHB
- Nonspecific IVCD
- Possible hypocalcemia
- Possible anterior MI, age indeterminate
- Nonspecific lateral S-T and T wave abnormalities

ANALYSIS 6-13

1. RATE

Atrial: 64 to 74 bpm

Ventricular: 64 to 74 bpm

2. RHYTHM

Atrial: Slightly variable

Ventricular: Slightly variable

3. WAVES

P waves present: Yes

    Appearance: Normal

    Consistent: Yes

    Relation to QRS: 1:1

Q waves present: No

    Leads:

    Pathological:

T waves present: Yes

    Morphology: Flat, inverted in III, V_{5-6}

4. INTERVALS

P-R interval: 0.16 seconds

    Consistent: Yes

QRS: 0.08 seconds

    Appearance: Normal

    Consistent: Yes

Q-T interval: 0.44 seconds

5. AXIS

Quadrant: Normal

Degrees: +10° (aVF most isolectric, slightly positive)

6. HYPERTROPHY

Atrial: No

Ventricular: No

7. MYOCARDIAL INFARCTION

Q waves: None significant

S-T displacement: No significant elevation

8. ISCHEMIA

S-T displacement: No significant depression

9. POSSIBLE DRUG EFFECTS

The patient is on long term lasix therapy. Prolonged Q-T interval and flat T waves may be a consequence of hypokalemia.

10. ECG ANALYSIS

The rate is 64 to 74 bpm, the rhythm varies slightly, probably in sequence with breathing. The axis is WNL. The intervals are WNL, with the exception of Q-T noted above. No U waves are noted. Diffuse nonspecific T wave abnormalities are noted.

11. INTERPRETATION

Sinus arrhythmia

- Prolonged Q-T interval and flat T waves
    - Possible hypokalemia secondary to long term lasix therapy
- Diffuse nonspecific T wave abnormalities

1. RATE

Atrial: 72 bpm

Ventricular: 72 bpm

2. RHYTHM

Atrial: Underlying rhythm regular

Ventricular: Underlying rhythm regular

3. WAVES

P waves present: Yes

   Appearance: Normal

   Consistent: Yes

   Relation to QRS: 1:1

Q waves present: No

   Leads:

   Pathological:

T waves present: Yes

   Morphology: Flat II, inverted III

4. INTERVALS

P-R interval: 0.16 seconds

   Consistent: Yes

QRS: 0.08 seconds

   Appearance: WNL

   Consistent: Yes

Q-T interval: 0.48 seconds

5. AXIS

Quadrant: Left

Degrees: $-10°$ (aVF most isoelectric, slightly negative)

6. HYPERTROPHY

Atrial: No

Ventricular: No

7. MYOCARDIAL INFARCTION

Q waves: None significant

S-T displacement: No significant elevation

8. ISCHEMIA

S-T displacement: No significant depression

9. POSSIBLE DRUG EFFECTS

None noted

10. ECG ANALYSIS

The rate is 72 bpm, the underlying rhythm is regular, and the axis is slightly left. The P-R intervals and QRS complexes are WNL. The Q-T intervals are prolonged and U waves are noted in the chest leads. These findings are characteristic of possible antiarrhythmic or phenothiazine medication use, which is impossible to isolate without patient history. Another possibility is an electrolyte disturbance, particularly hypokalemia.

Beat 2 in the augmented leads is slightly early and is wide, therefore probably ventricular in origin.

11. INTERPRETATION

Sinus rhythm

- LAD
- Prolonged Q-T interval, undetermined origin
- U waves V_{2-6}
- Rare PVC

ANALYSIS 6-15

1. RATE

Atrial: Unable to determine

Ventricular: Variable, 50 to 75 bpm

2. RHYTHM

Atrial: Irregular

Ventricular: Irregular

3. WAVES

P waves present: Difficult to identify, best seen in V_1

    Appearance: Fibrillation pattern

    Consistent: No

    Relation to QRS: None

Q waves present: No

    Leads:

    Pathological:

T waves present: Yes

    Morphology: Flat, limb leads

4. INTERVALS

P-R interval:

    Consistent:

QRS: 0.10 seconds

    Appearance: WNL

    Consistent: Yes

Q-T interval: 0.48 to 0.60 seconds

5. AXIS

Quadrant: Left anterior hemiblock

Degrees: −90° (aVF and II negative, I most isoelectric)

6. HYPERTROPHY

Atrial: No

Ventricular: Possible

7. MYOCARDIAL INFARCTION

Q waves: None significant

S-T displacement: No significant elevation

8. ISCHEMIA

S-T displacement: No significant depression

9. POSSIBLE DRUG EFFECTS

None noted

10. ECG ANALYSIS

The ventricular rate varies from 50 to 75 bpm. The rhythm is irregular and the P waves have a distinct fibrillation pattern. A left anterior hemiblock is denoted by the negative net QRS deflections in aVF and II. The Q-T interval is prolonged and varies with the rate from 0.48 to 0.60 seconds. Although difficult to see clearly, U waves are noted in $V_{2-3-5-6}$. The significance of the prolonged Q-T interval and U waves is indeterminate without patient history. The R wave voltage in V_6 is 30 mV indicating LVH.

11. INTERPRETATION

Atrial fibrillation with controlled ventricular response

- LAHB
- Prolonged Q-T interval, undetermined origin
- LVH

1. RATE

Atrial: 83 bpm

Ventricular: 83 bpm

2. RHYTHM

Atrial: Regular

Ventricular: Regular

3. WAVES

P waves present: Yes

Appearance: Flat

Consistent: Yes

Relation to QRS: 1:1

Q waves present: Yes

Leads: II, III, aVF

Pathological: Yes

T waves present: Yes

Morphology: Elevated

4. INTERVALS

P-R interval: 0.24 seconds

Consistent: Yes

QRS: 0.16 seconds

Appearance: $rSR'V_1$

Consistent: Yes

Q-T interval: 0.48 seconds

5. AXIS

Quadrant: Left anterior hemiblock

Degrees: −60° (aVF and II negative, aVR most isoelectric)

6. HYPERTROPHY

Atrial: Possible

Ventricular: No

7. MYOCARDIAL INFARCTION

Q waves: II, III, aVF

S-T displacement: Significant elevation II, III, aVF, V_{4-5}

8. ISCHEMIA

S-T displacement: Significant depression I, aVL, V_2

9. POSSIBLE DRUG EFFECTS

Patient on Quinidex and digoxin

10. ECG ANALYSIS

The rate is 83 bpm, and the rhythm is regular. The prolonged P-R interval is indicative of a first degree AVB. A left anterior hemiblock is denoted by the net negative QRS deflections in aVF and II. The wide QRS and rSR' in V_1 are characteristic of a complete RBBB. Because both bundle branches are affected, the block is more appropriately termed a bifascicular block. Significant Q waves and S-T segment elevation in leads II, III, and aVF indicate an acute inferior MI. The prolonged Q-T interval may be an effect of the Quinidex medication, however this cannot be confirmed without serum quinidine levels. The "scooped" appearance of the S-T segment in lead V_2 could be an effect of the medication digoxin. Digoxin could also be the underlying cause of the first degree AVB.

11. INTERPRETATION

Sinus rhythm

- First degree AVB
- Bifascicular block (LAHB + RBBB)
- Acute inferior MI
- Possible quinidine toxicity
- Possible digoxin effect

ANALYSIS 6-17

1. RATE

Atrial: 72 bpm

Ventricular: 72 bpm

2. RHYTHM

Atrial: Underlying rhythm regular

Ventricular: Underlying rhythm regular

3. WAVES

P waves present: Yes

    Appearance: Flat

    Consistent: Yes

    Relation to QRS: 1:1

Q waves present: No

    Leads:

    Pathological:

T waves present: Yes

    Morphology: Flat

4. INTERVALS

P-R interval: 0.26 seconds

    Consistent: Yes

QRS: 0.08 seconds

    Appearance: WNL

    Consistent: Yes

Q-T interval: 0.40 seconds

5. AXIS

Quadrant: Normal

Degrees: +30° (III most isoelectric)

6. HYPERTROPHY

Atrial: No

Ventricular: No

7. MYOCARDIAL INFARCTION

Q waves: None significant

S-T displacement: No significant elevation

8. ISCHEMIA

S-T displacement: Significant depression, V_{2-5}

9. POSSIBLE DRUG EFFECTS

Patient taking Lanoxin (digitalis preparation)

10. ECG ANALYSIS

The rate is 72 bpm, the rhythm is regular, and the axis is WNL. The P-R interval is prolonged indicating a first degree AVB, possibly caused by the Lanoxin. Beat 3 in leads V_{1-3} is early, slightly wider than the normal beat and thus is probably ventricular in origin. The S-T segment depression in leads V_{2-6}, is down sloping, which may indicate anterolateral ischemia or subendocardial injury. The "scooped" appearance of the S-T segments in leads I and II are characteristic of a digitalis effect.

11. INTERPRETATION

Sinus rhythm

- First degree AVB
- Probable acute anterolateral subendocardial injury
- Occasional PVC
- Digitalis effect

1. RATE

Atrial: 28 to 45 bpm

Ventricular: 28 to 45 bpm

2. RHYTHM

Atrial: Essentially regular

Ventricular: Essentially regular

3. WAVES

P waves present: Yes

Appearance: WNL

Consistent: Yes

Relation to QRS: 1:1

Q waves present: No

Leads:

Pathological:

T waves present: Yes

Morphology: Flat

4. INTERVALS

P-R interval: 0.18 seconds

Consistent: Yes

QRS: 0.08 seconds

Appearance: WNL

Consistent: Yes

Q-T interval: 0.44 seconds

5. AXIS

Quadrant: Normal

Degrees: +30° (III most isoelectric)

6. HYPERTROPHY

Atrial: No

Ventricular: No

7. MYOCARDIAL INFARCTION

Q waves: None significant

S-T displacement: No significant elevation

8. ISCHEMIA

S-T displacement: No significant depression

9. POSSIBLE DRUG EFFECTS

Patient on Lanoxin (digitalis preparation)

10. ECG ANALYSIS

The rate is 28 to 45 bpm and probably varies with respiration. Intervals and axis are WNL. The rhythm is essentially regular, but in the rhythm strip a slight irregularity is noted that probably coincides with breathing. The S-T segments throughout are slightly depressed and have a "scooped" appearance characteristic of a digitalis effect. No other abnormalities are noted.

11. INTERPRETATION

Sinus arrhythmia (slow)

• Possible digitalis effect

Part VIII
Continuing Education

How to obtain continuing education credit

Registered nurses may receive 16 contact hours by completing the ECG analysis in Parts 2 through 6 and successfully answering the posttest questions in Part 8.

Taking the test

1. Read each test question and record your answer on the answer sheet provided. **Do not duplicate this answer sheet, a photocopy will be rejected by the scanner.**
2. Follow the instructions on the answer sheet exactly. Use only a **No. 2 pencil,** and do not make any stray marks on the answer sheet. It is important that you PRINT your name, address, and Social Security number correctly; failure to do so will result in rejection of your answer sheet by the computer.

Payment:

Check or money order in the amount of $55.00
Payable to: Mosby

Mail to:

Mosby
Division of Continuing Education
11830 Westline Industrial Drive
St. Louis, MO 63146-3318

Continuing education

Mosby, Division of Continuing Education and Training (DCET) is accredited as a provider of continuing education in nursing by the American Nurses Credentialing Center Commission on Accreditation. This approval is reciprocal in all states and for all specialty organizations who recognize the ANCC approval process.

Mosby, DCET contact hours are applicable for recertification/relicensure requirements for all professional associations and in all states requiring mandatory continuing education that recognize the ANCC approval process.

Receiving your results

Your posttest will be graded, and you will be advised of your results by postcard within 90 days of receipt of your completed answer sheet. A score of 70% or higher is required.

PLEASE KEEP THE POSTCARD; IT IS YOUR CERTIFICATE OF CONTACT HOURS EARNED.

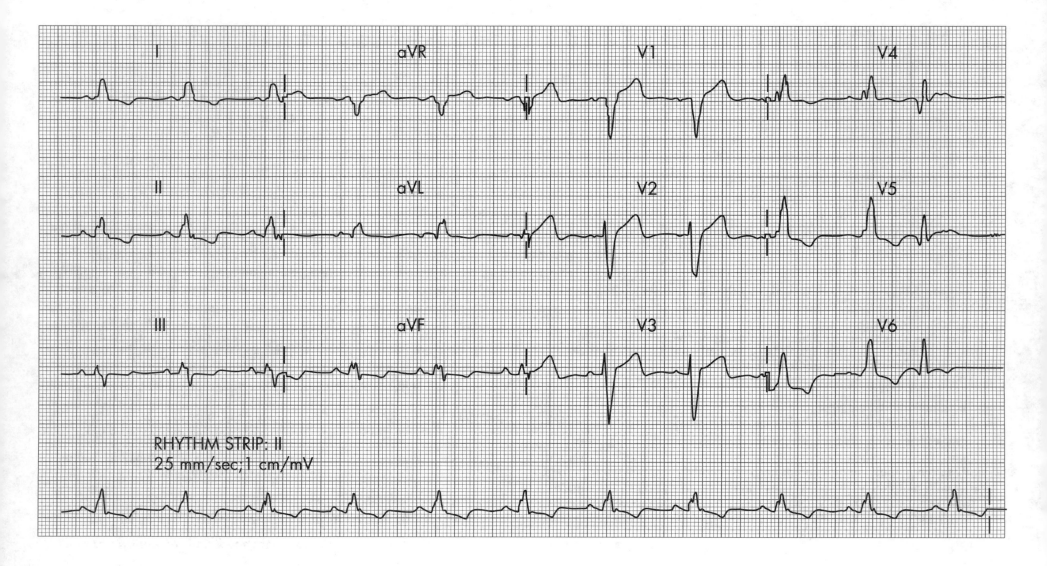

RHYTHM STRIP: II
25 mm/sec; 1 cm/mV

Figure 8-1
Resting 12-Lead ECG

1. The underlying rhythm in this ECG is which of the following?

   a. Sinus

   b. Sinus bradycardia

   c. Junctional

   d. Ventricular

2. The duration of the QRS complex is which of the following?

   a. 0.08 seconds

   b. 0.10 seconds

   c. 0.12 seconds

   d. 0.16 seconds

3. The wide QRS and the R-S in V_{5-6} are characteristics of which of the following?

   a. Incomplete LBBB

   b. Complete LBBB

   c. Incomplete RBBB

   d. Complete RBBB

4. Beat 3 in leads V_{4-6} probably originates in which of the following?

   a. Atria

   b. Junction

   c. Ventricles

   d. None of the above

5. The S-T segment abnormalities are which of the following?

   a. Diagnostic changes of an acute MI

   b. Nondiagnostic and probably secondary to the LBBB

   c. Nonspecific without patient history

   d. B and C

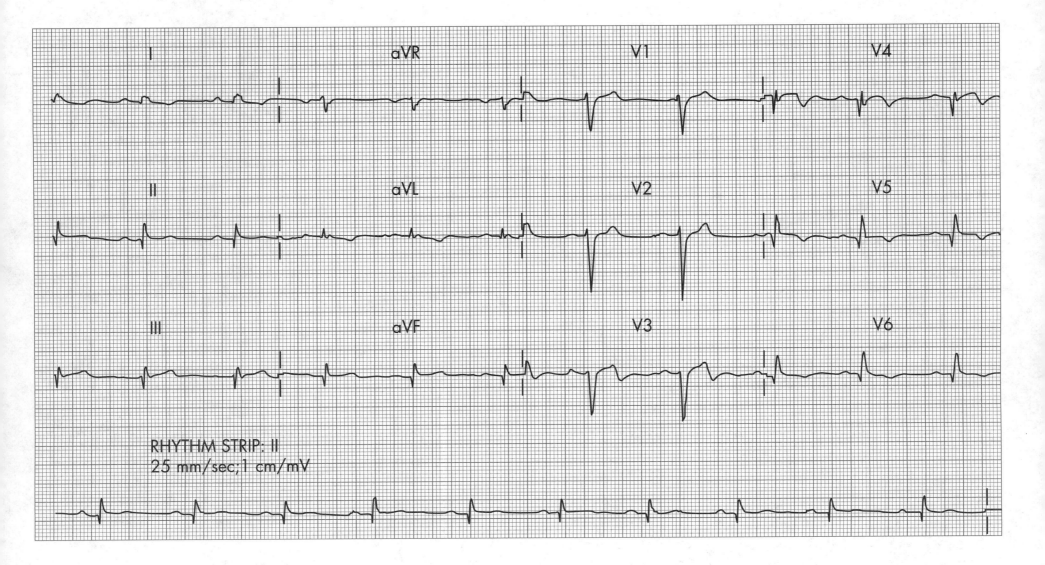

I aVR V1 V4

II aVL V2 V5

III aVF V3 V6

RHYTHM STRIP: II
25 mm/sec;1 cm/mV

Figure 8-2
Resting 12-Lead ECG

1. The underlying rhythm in this ECG is which of the following?

    a.   Sinus

    b.   Sinus with a first degree AVB

    c.   Junctional

    d.   Accelerated junctional

2. The axis is which of the following?

    a.   Normal quadrant

    b.   Right quadrant

    c.   Left quadrant

    d.   Left quadrant, greater than −30°

3. The Q waves in leads II, III, and aVF indicate which of the following?

    a.   Acute inferior MI

    b.   Old inferior MI

    c.   Old anteroseptal MI

    d.   True posterior MI

4. The Q waves and T wave inversion is leads V_{4-6} indicate which of the following?

    a.   Acute inferior MI

    b.   Old inferior MI

    c.   Old posterior MI

    d.   Anterolateral MI, age indeterminate

5. The poor R wave progression in V_{1-3} may indicate which of the following?

    a.   Acute inferior MI

    b.   Old anterolateral MI

    c.   Possible old anterior MI

    d.   True posterior MI

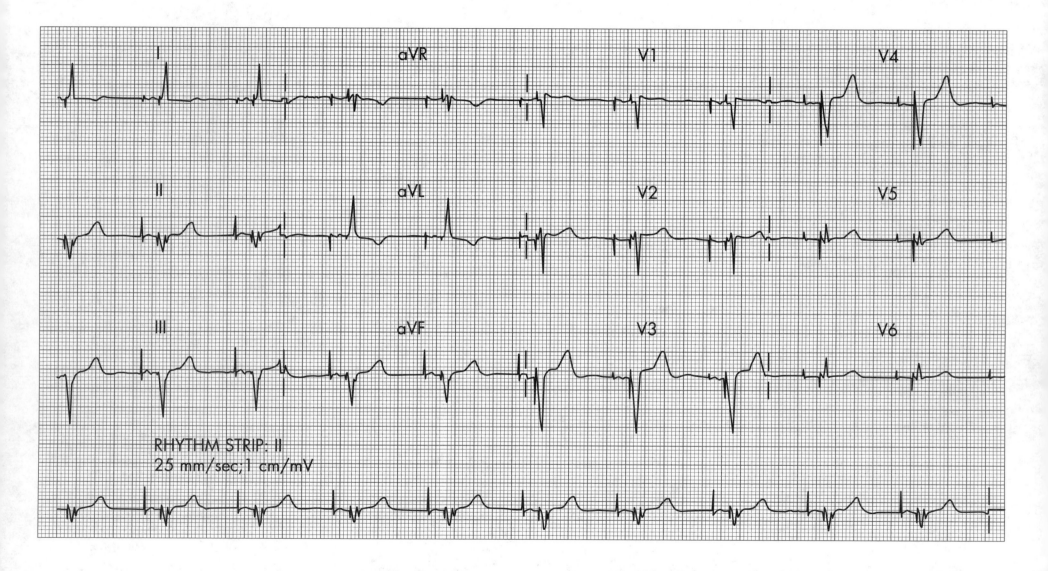

I   aVR   V1   V4

II   aVL   V2   V5

III   aVF   V3   V6

RHYTHM STRIP: II
25 mm/sec;1 cm/mV

Figure 8-3
Resting 12-Lead ECG

1. The P-R interval is how long?

    a. 0.10 seconds

    b. 0.12 seconds

    c. 0.14 seconds

    d. None of the above

2. The underlying rhythm is probably which of the following?

    a. Atrial fibrillation

    b. Complete heart block (3° HB)

    c. Asystole

    d. Unable to determine

3. The pacemaker rate is set at which of the following?

    a. 60 bpm

    b. 65 bpm

    c. 70 bpm

    d. None of the above

4. The pacemaker in this tracing is which of the following?

    a. Single chamber pacemaker

    b. Dual chamber pacemaker

5. The type of pacemaker in this tracing is which of the following?

    a. DDD, VVI

    b. DDD, AAI

    c. DDD, DVI (atrial-ventricular sequential mode)

    d. DDD, VAT

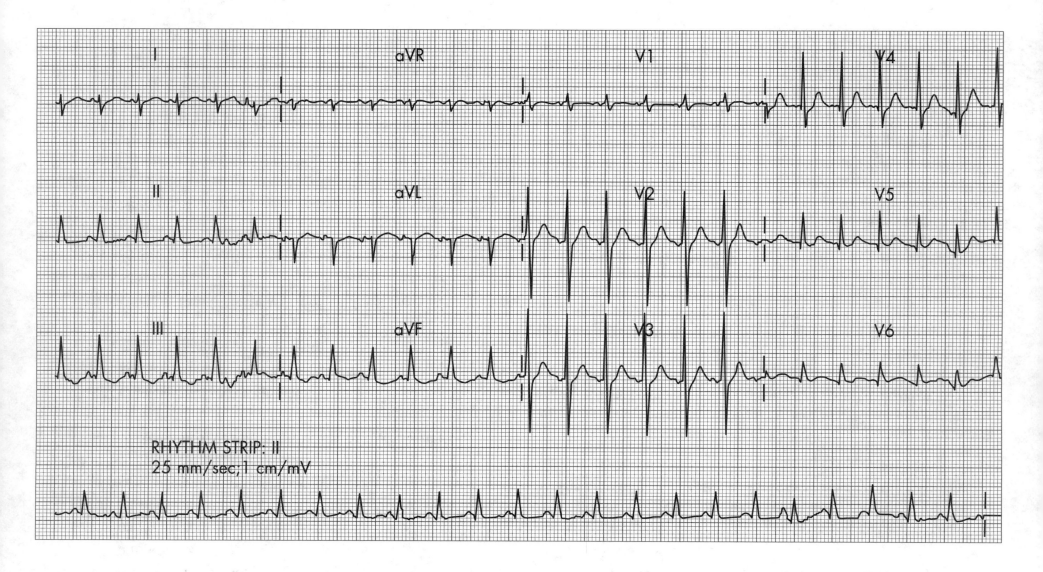

Figure 8-4
Resting 12-Lead ECG

1. The ventricular rate is which of the following?

     a.　100 bpm

     b.　120 bpm

     c.　145 bpm

     d.　160 bpm

2. The axis is which of the following?

     a.　Normal quadrant

     b.　Right quadrant

     c.　Left quadrant

     d.　Left quadrant, greater than −30°

3. The R greater than S in V_1 probably indicates which of the following?

     a.　LVH

     b.　RBBB

     c.　RVH

     d.　RAE

4. The Q waves in leads II, III, and aVF indicate which of the following?

     a.　Old inferior MI

     b.　Acute inferior MI

     c.　Anterior MI

     d.　Nondiagnostic Q waves

5. The best interpretation for this ECG is which of the following?

     a.　PAT with LAD and RVH

     b.　SVT with LAD and RBBB

     c.　Sinus tachycardia with RAD and RVH

     d.　Sinus tachycardia with RAD and RBBB

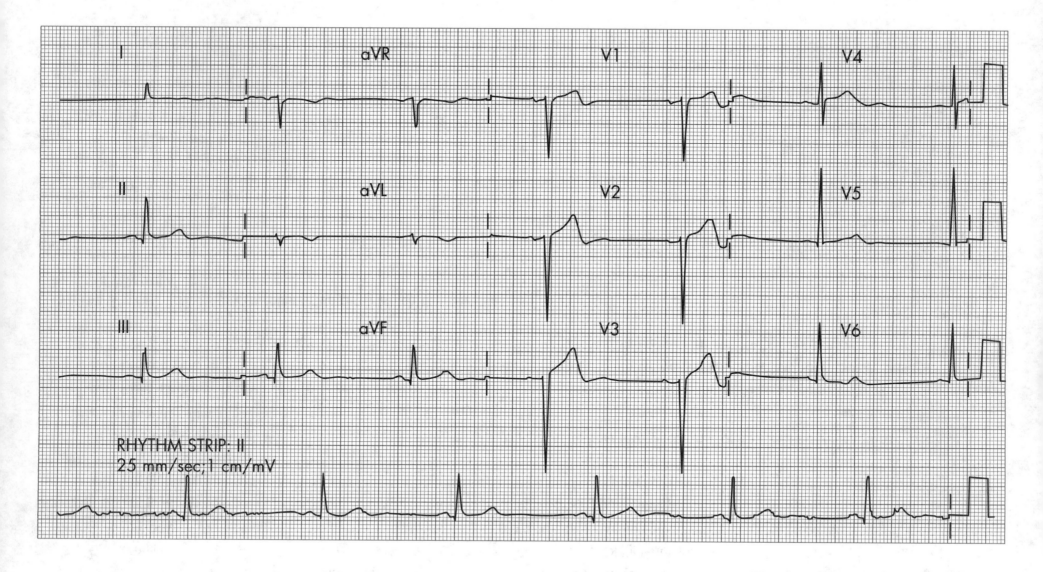

I aVR V1 V4

II aVL V2 V5

III aVF V3 V6

RHYTHM STRIP: II
25 mm/sec; 1 cm/mV

Figure 8-5
Resting 12-Lead ECG

550

1. The rate is which of the following?

   a. 40 bpm

   b. 50 bpm

   c. 60 bpm

   d. 70 bpm

2. The axis is which of the following?

   a. Normal quadrant

   b. Right quadrant

   c. Left quadrant

   d. Left quadrant, greater than −30°

3. The S wave in V_1 plus the R wave in V_5 are voltage criteria for which of the following?

   a. RVH

   b. RAE

   c. LVH

   d. LAE

4. The poor R wave progression and S-T elevation in V_{1-3} probably indicate which of the following?

   a. Recent anterior MI

   b. Recent inferior MI

   c. Recent inferolateral MI

   d. Recent lateral MI

5. The best interpretation for this ECG is which of the following?

   a. Sinus rhythm with LVH and recent anterior MI

   b. Sinus bradycardia with LVH and recent anterior MI

   c. Sinus bradycardia with LVH and old anterolateral MI

   d. Sinus rhythm with LVH and old anterolateral MI

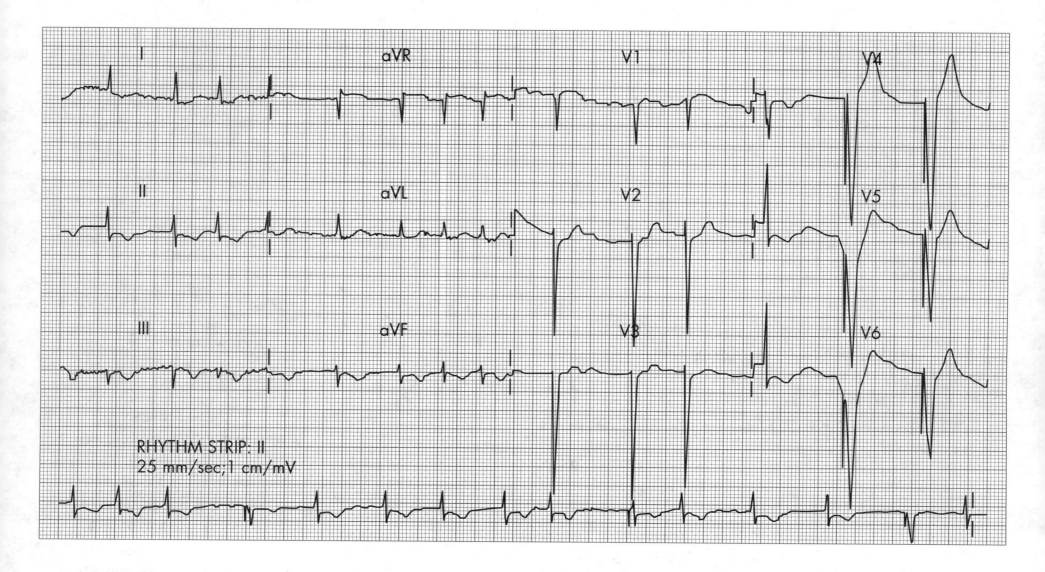

Figure 8-6
Resting 12-Lead ECG

552

1. The atrial rate is which of the following?

    a.   100 bpm

    b.   200 bpm

    c.   250 bpm

    d.   Unable to determine

2. The ventricular rhythm is which of the following?

    a.   Regular

    b.   Irregular

    c.   Mostly regular

    d.   Mostly paced

3. The axis is which of the following?

    a.   Normal quadrant

    b.   Right quadrant

    c.   Left quadrant

    d.   Left quadrant, greater than −30°

4. The underlying rhythm is which of the following?

    a.   Atrial fibrillation

    b.   Supraventricular tachycardia

    c.   Accelerated junctional rhythm

    d.   Idioventricular rhythm

5. The best interpretation for this ECG is which of the following?

    a.   Atrial fibrillation with controlled ventricular response

    b.   Atrial fibrillation with uncontrolled ventricular response

    c.   Atrial fibrillation with dual chamber (DDD) pacemaker

    d.   Atrial fibrillation with ventricular demand (VVI) pacemaker

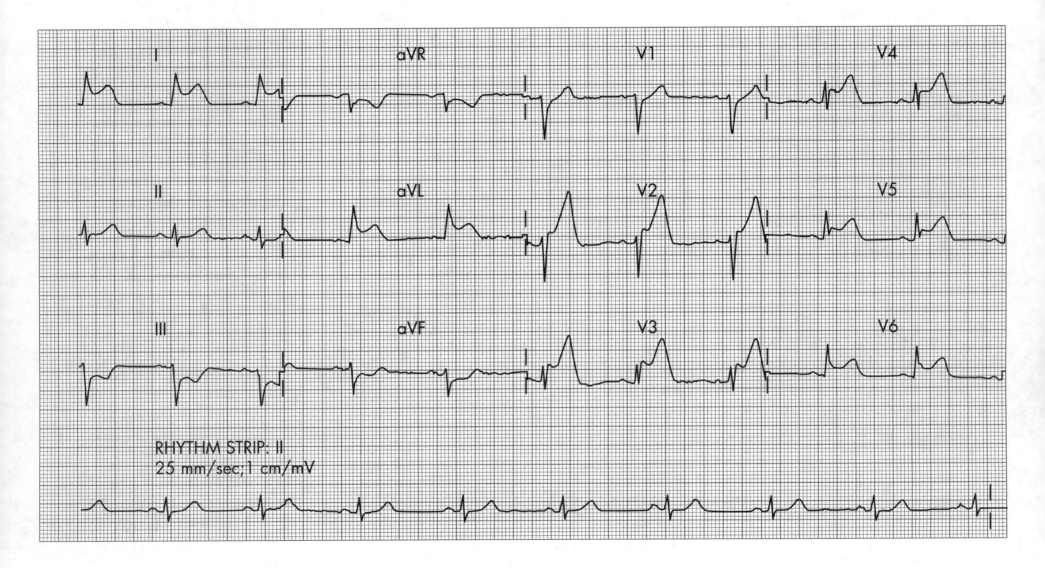

Figure 8-7
Resting 12-Lead ECG

1. The ventricular rate is which of the following?

    a.   58 bpm

    b.   70 bpm

    c.   85 bpm

    d.   90 bpm

2. The axis is which of the following?

    a.   Normal quadrant

    b.   Right quadrant

    c.   Left quadrant

    d.   Left quadrant, greater than −30°

3. The underlying rhythm is which of the following?

    a.   Sinus

    b.   Junctional

    c.   Accelerated junctional

    d.   Ventricular

4. The S-T elevation in leads V_{2-6}, I, and aVL indicate which of the following?

    a.   Old inferior MI

    b.   Old anteroseptal MI

    c.   Acute anterolateral MI

    d.   Acute posterior MI

5. The best interpretation for this ECG is which of the following?

    a.   Sinus rhythm, left axis deviation, acute anterolateral MI

    b.   Sinus rhythm, acute anterolateral MI

    c.   Sinus rhythm, left axis deviation, old inferior MI

    d.   Sinus rhythm, old inferior MI

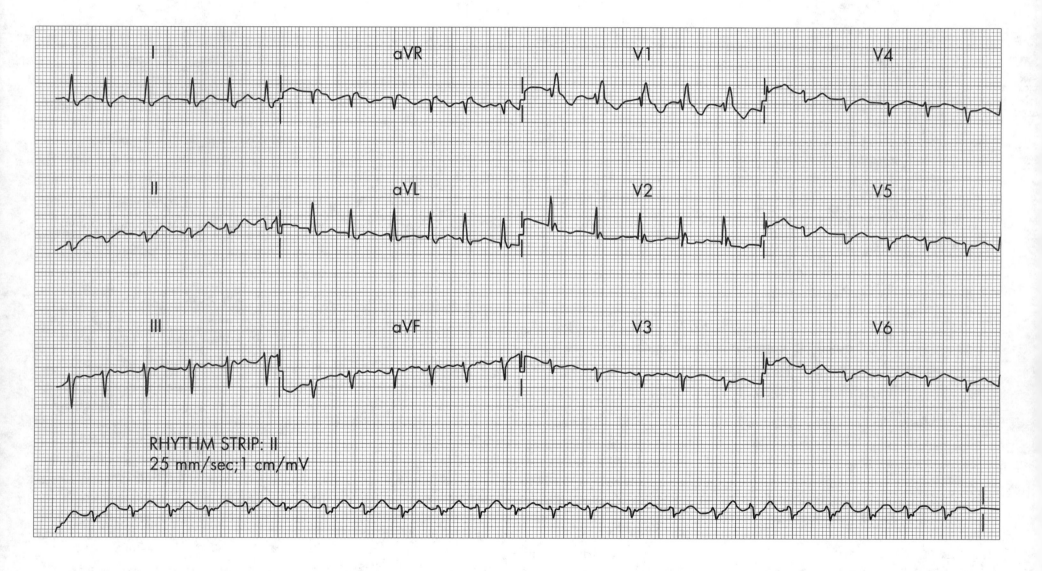

I aVR V1 V4

II aVL V2 V5

III aVF V3 V6

RHYTHM STRIP: II
25 mm/sec; 1 cm/mV

Figure 8-8
Resting 12-Lead ECG

1. The atrial rate is which of the following?

   a. 100 bpm

   b. 150 bpm

   c. 200 bpm

   d. Unable to determine

2. The ventricular rate is approximately which of the following?

   a. 100 bpm

   b. 140 bpm

   c. 180 bpm

   d. 200 bpm

3. The axis is which of the following?

   a. Normal quadrant

   b. Right quadrant

   c. Left quadrant

   d. Left quadrant, greater than −30°

4. The rSR' in V_1 indicates which of the following?

   a. LVH

   b. RVH

   c. LBBB

   d. RBBB

5. The best interpretation for this ECG is which of the following?

   a. Sinus tachycardia, left axis deviation, LBBB

   b. Atrial fibrillation, left axis deviation, RBBB

   c. Atrial fibrillation, bifascicular block, possible old anterolateral MI

   d. Sinus tachycardia, bifascicular block, possible old anterolateral MI

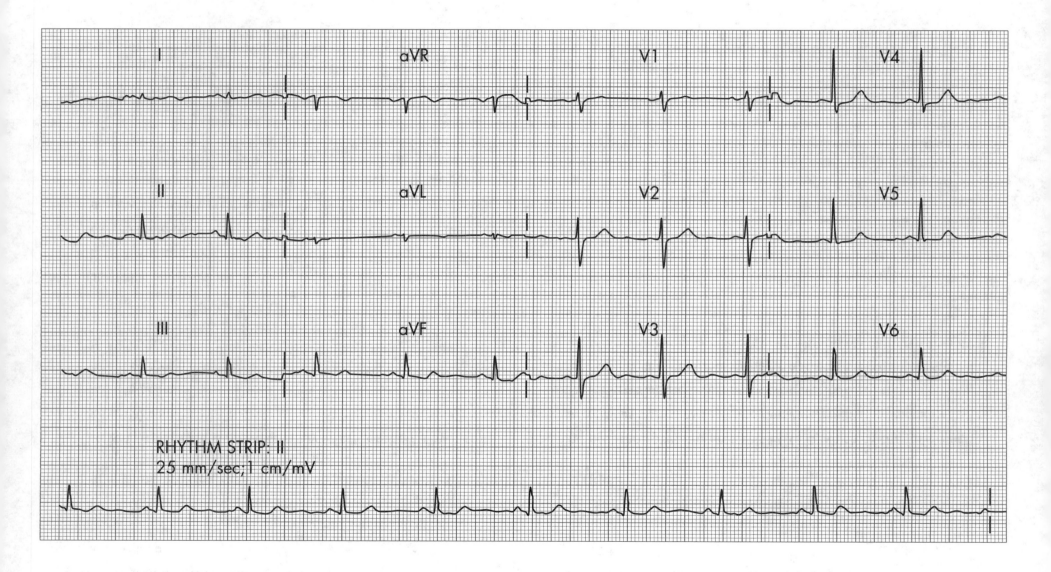

I aVR V1 V4

II aVL V2 V5

III aVF V3 V6

RHYTHM STRIP: II
25 mm/sec; 1 cm/mV

Figure 8-9
Resting 12-Lead ECG

1. The atrial rate is which of the following?

    a.   63 bpm

    b.   80 bpm

    c.   90 bpm

    d.   95 bpm

2. The rhythm is which of the following?

    a.   Ventricular

    b.   Accelerated junctional

    c.   Junctional

    d.   Sinus

3. The axis is which of the following?

    a.   Normal quadrant

    b.   Right quadrant

    c.   Left quadrant

    d.   Left quadrant, greater than −30°

4. The S-T depression in leads II, III, and aVF is which of the following?

    a.   Diagnostic of inferior subendocardial injury

    b.   Nondiagnostic without patient history

    c.   Of no consequence and should not be noted

    d.   Diagnostic of inferior acute injury

5. The best interpretation for this ECG is which of the following?

    a.   Sinus bracycardia with first degree AVB

    b.   Sinus rhythm with first degree AVB

    c.   Sinus rhythm with nondiagnostic inferior S-T changes

    d.   Sinus rhythm with inferior subendocardial injury

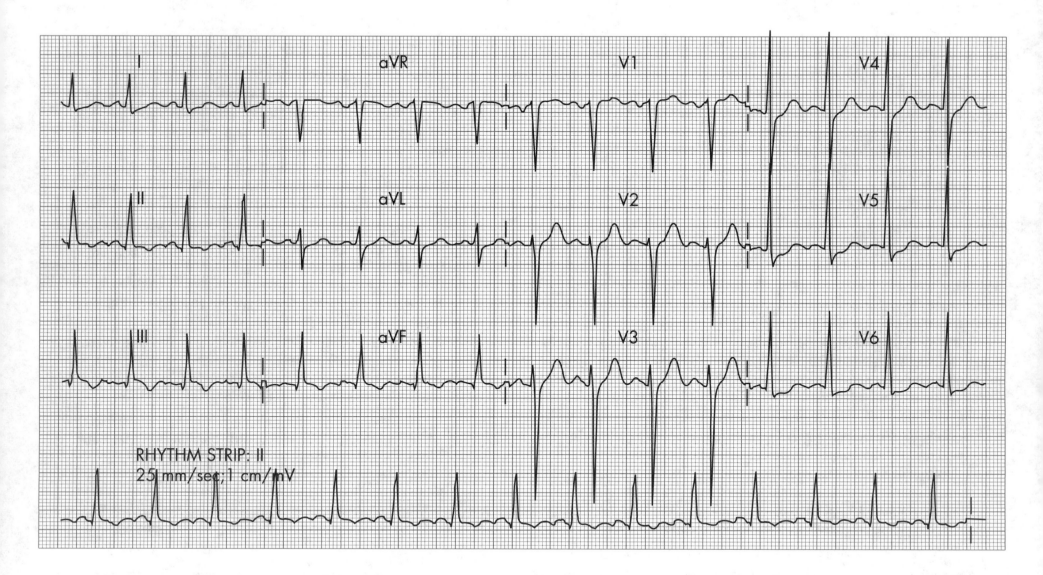

I aVR V1 V4

II aVL V2 V5

III aVF V3 V6

RHYTHM STRIP: II
25 mm/sec; 1 cm/mV

Figure 8-10
Resting 12-Lead ECG

1. The ventricular rate is which of the following?

   a. 85 bpm

   b. 98 bpm

   c. 115 bpm

   d. 118 bpm

2. The axis is which of the following?

   a. Normal quadrant

   b. Right quadrant

   c. Left quadrant

   d. Left quadrant, greater than −30°

3. The P wave in lead II measures 0.12 seconds, and in V_1 the P wave is biphasic with a primarily negative component. These findings would indicate which of the following?

   a. LVH

   b. RVH

   c. RAE

   d. LAE

4. Left ventricular hypertrophy is evidenced in this tracing by which of the following?

   a. R greater than S in V_1

   b. S greater than R in V_1

   c. R wave voltage in aVL greater than 12 mV

   d. R wave in V_1 plus S in V_5 greater than or equal to 35 mV

5. The best interpretation for this ECG is which of the following?

   a. Sinus tachycardia with LBBB, nonspecific inferior S-T changes

   b. Sinus tachycardia with LVH, nonspecific inferior S-T changes

   c. Sinus rhythm, LVH with strain pattern, nonspecific inferior S-T changes

   d. Sinus tachycardia, LVH with strain pattern, nonspecific inferior S-T changes

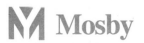 **Mosby**

DO NOT DUPLICATE THIS ANSWER SHEET

PURE PRACTICE FOR 12-LEAD ECGs
DIVISION OF CONTINUING EDUCATION & TRAINING
HOME STUDY ANSWER SHEET

| TEST ID |
| 29705A |

IMPORTANT:
Please read and follow all instructions carefully. We suggest you keep a photocopy of your answer sheet in case it is lost in the mail. In order to receive continuing education credit, a grade of 70% or greater must be achieved.

MARKING INSTRUCTIONS

- COMPLETE ALL REQUESTED INFORMATION. Your test results will be sent to your name and address EXACTLY as coded on this sheet. Coding errors could result in you never receiving your grade or certificate.
- Mark only one oval for each question.
- Use a No. 2 or softer pencil.
- Make all marks black and glossy.
- Erase cleanly any mark you wish to change.
- See the correct and incorrect examples to the right.
- Only fold along dotted fold lines.

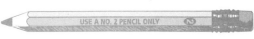

USE A NO. 2 PENCIL ONLY

CORRECT MARK   INCORRECT MARKS

EXAM 1
A B C D E
1 (T)(F)○○○
2 (T)(F)○○○
3 (T)(F)○○○
4 (T)(F)○○○
5 (T)(F)○○○

EXAM 3
A B C D E
1 (T)(F)○○○
2 (T)(F)○○○
3 (T)(F)○○○
4 (T)(F)○○○
5 (T)(F)○○○

EXAM 5
A B C D E
1 (T)(F)○○○
2 (T)(F)○○○
3 (T)(F)○○○
4 (T)(F)○○○
5 (T)(F)○○○

EXAM 7
A B C D E
1 (T)(F)○○○
2 (T)(F)○○○
3 (T)(F)○○○
4 (T)(F)○○○
5 (T)(F)○○○

EXAM 9
A B C D E
1 (T)(F)○○○
2 (T)(F)○○○
3 (T)(F)○○○
4 (T)(F)○○○
5 (T)(F)○○○

EXAM 2
A B C D E
1 (T)(F)○○○
2 (T)(F)○○○
3 (T)(F)○○○
4 (T)(F)○○○
5 (T)(F)○○○

EXAM 4
A B C D E
1 (T)(F)○○○
2 (T)(F)○○○
3 (T)(F)○○○
4 (T)(F)○○○
5 (T)(F)○○○

EXAM 6
A B C D E
1 (T)(F)○○○
2 (T)(F)○○○
3 (T)(F)○○○
4 (T)(F)○○○
5 (T)(F)○○○

EXAM 8
A B C D E
1 (T)(F)○○○
2 (T)(F)○○○
3 (T)(F)○○○
4 (T)(F)○○○
5 (T)(F)○○○

EXAM 10
A B C D E
1 (T)(F)○○○
2 (T)(F)○○○
3 (T)(F)○○○
4 (T)(F)○○○
5 (T)(F)○○○

PROGRAM EVALUATION

Rate the following where
1= strongly disagree to 5 = strongly agree

	Strongly Disagree				Strongly Agree
1. The material was presented clearly.	①	②	③	④	⑤
2. The material met stated objectives.	①	②	③	④	⑤
3. The content was appropriate.	①	②	③	④	⑤
4. The level of difficulty of the test was appropriate.	①	②	③	④	⑤

5. Time needed to complete this program:
○ Less than 1 hour   ○ 1 - 2 hours   ○ 2 - 3 hours   ○ more than 3 hours

---

Payment to Mosby by check or money order must be included for your test to be processed.
Results will be mailed to you within 90 days of receipt of your answer sheet.

Return form in business sized envelope to:

Mosby
Division of Continuing Education & Training
Home Study Program
11830 Westline Industrial Drive
St. Louis, MO 63146

MARKING INSTRUCTIONS

— **COMPLETE ALL REQUESTED INFORMATION.** Your test results will be sent to your name and address EXACTLY as coded on this sheet. Coding errors could result in you never receiving your grade or certificate.

LAST NAME

FIRST NAME   MI

SOCIAL SECURITY

ZIP CODE

STREET NUMBER AND NAME

CITY   STATE

Daytime Phone # _____

_____

_____

Printed in U.S.A.   Mark Reflex® by NCS MM207470-1   321   ED11